Surgical Management of Childhood Glaucoma

Alana L. Grajewski • Elena Bitrian
Maria Papadopoulos
Sharon F. Freedman
Editors

Surgical Management of Childhood Glaucoma

Clinical Considerations and Techniques

Springer

Editors
Alana L. Grajewski, MD
Samuel & Ethel Balkan International Pediatric Glaucoma Center
Bascom Palmer Eye Institute
University of Miami Miller School of Medicine
Miami, FL
USA

Maria Papadopoulos, MBBS, FRCOphth
Glaucoma Service
Moorfields Eye Hospital
London
United Kingdom

Elena Bitrian, MD
Department of Ophthalmology
Mayo Clinic
Rochester, MN
USA

Sharon F. Freedman, MD
Department of Ophthalmology
Duke University Medical Center
Durham, NC
USA

ISBN 978-3-030-09609-0 ISBN 978-3-319-54003-0 (eBook)
https://doi.org/10.1007/978-3-319-54003-0

Softcover re-print of the Hardcover 1st edition 2018

This Springer imprint is published by the registered company Springer Nature Switzerland AG
The registered company address is: Gewerbestrasse 11, 6330 Cham, Switzerland

Preface

Childhood glaucoma is a vision threatening but relatively uncommon disease, which often requires surgery. These characteristics make childhood glaucoma challenging for the surgeon, who must master all the different modalities of treatment, acquire new surgical techniques, and furthermore transfer these skills to trainees.

For a child and their parents to receive a diagnosis of glaucoma is a stressful event and a learning process for the child's entire family and support circle. These young patients and their families are usually surprised by the diagnosis, understandably perceiving glaucoma to be a "disease of the elderly." This element of surprise, coupled with anxiety, also adds to the emotional burden of the situation.

Perhaps also unique to glaucoma management in the pediatric age group is that often the clinical scenario is not complete without subjecting the child to an examination under anesthesia (EUA). Then given the desire to minimize anesthetic sessions in affected children, the surgeon must be prepared to gather and interpret clinical data for rapid clinical decision-making immediately after the EUA, including choosing the appropriate surgical intervention, if necessary. Furthermore, preparing the family for all possible options, including the risks, benefits, and expected postoperative management of the possible surgical interventions, is necessary and presents an additional challenge to the pediatric glaucoma surgeon.

Most pediatric glaucoma surgery is based on the principle of restoring or bypassing the obstruction to aqueous flow. From the tried and tested, the old and new, each of these surgical options has its own set of advantages and disadvantages. It is our hope that this text will be a helpful guide to the evaluation and surgical management of those who are our smallest of patients, but who deserve our greatest efforts.

Miami, FL, USA — Alana L. Grajewski
Rochester, MN, USA — Elena Bitrian
London, UK — Maria Papadopoulos
Durham, NC, USA — Sharon F. Freedman

Contents

Contributors

Oscar Albis-Donado, MD Department of Glaucoma, Instituto Mexicano de Oftalmolgía IAP, Querétaro, Mexico

Shveta Bali, MBBS, MD Department of Ophthalmology, The Ottawa Hospital, University of Ottawa, Ottawa, ON, Canada

Michael R. Banitt, MD, MHA Department of Ophthalmology, University of Washington, Seattle, WA, USA

Allen D. Beck, MD Department of Ophthalmology, Emory University, Atlanta, GA, USA

Elena Bitrian, MD Department of Ophthalmology, Mayo Clinic, Rochester, MN, USA

James D. Brandt, MD Department of Ophthalmology and Vision Science, University of California, Davis, Sacramento, CA, USA

Ta Chen Peter Chang, MD Bascom Palemr Eye Institute, University of Miami Miller School of Medicine, Miami, FL, USA

Teresa C. Chen, MD Department of Ophthalmology, Massachusetts Eye and Ear Infirmary, Harvard Medical School, Boston, MA, USA

Tanuj Dada, MBBS, MD Glaucoma Services, Department of Ophthalmology, Dr. Rajendra Prasad Centre for Ophthalmic Sciences, All India Institute of Medical Sciences, New Delhi, India

Beth Edmunds, MBChB, FRCOphth, MD Casey Eye Institute, Oregon Health and Science University, Portland, OR, USA

Mahmoud A. Fayed, MD Glaucoma Service, Massachusetts Eye and Ear Infirmary, Harvard Medical School, Boston, MA, USA

Cecilia Fenerty, MD, FRCOphth Manchester Royal Eye Hospital, University of Manchester, Manchester, UK

Sharon F. Freedman, MD Department of Ophthalmology, Duke University Medical Center, Durham, NC, USA

Alexander Foster, MD Department of Ophthalmology, University of Washington, Seattle, WA, USA

Alana L. Grajewski, MD Samuel & Ethel Balkan International Pediatric Glaucoma Center, Bascom Palmer Eye Institute, University of Miami Miller School of Medicine, Miami, FL, USA

Franz Grehn, MD, PhD Department of Ophthalmology, University Hospitals Würzburg, Würzburg, Germany

Naama Hammel, MD Departrment of Ophthalmology and Vision Science, University of California, Davis, Sacramento, CA, USA

Elizabeth Hodapp, MD Bascom Palmer Eye Institute, Department of Ophthalmology, University of Miami Miller School of Medicine, Miami, FL, USA

Esther Hoffmann, MD Department of Ophthalmology, Childhood Glaucoma Center, University Medical Center Mainz, Mainz, Germany

Karen M. Joos, MD, PhD Vanderbilt Eye Institute, Vanderbilt Univeristy Medical Center, Nashville, TN, USA

Dorothea Kadarian-Baumgard, MD Division of Pediatric Anesthesia, Department of Anesthesiology, Holtz Children's Hospital at Jackson Memorial Hospital, University of Miami Miller School of Medicine, Miami, FL, USA

Tanya Karaconji, MD, FRANZCO Manchester Royal Eye Hospital, University of Manchester, Manchester, UK

Peng Tee Khaw, PhD, FRCP, FRCS, FRCOphth, CBiol National Institute for Health Research Biomedical Research Centre, Moorfields Eye Hospital and University College London Institute of Ophthalmology, London, UK

Anne Ko, MD Department of Ophthalmology, University of Washington, Seattle, WA, USA

Anil K. Mandal, MD, FAMS Department of Glaucoma and Pediatric Ophthalmology, L. V. Prasad Eye Institute, Hyderabad, Telangana, India

Maria Papadopoulos, MBBS, FRCOphth Glaucoma Service, Moorfields Eye Hospital, London, United Kingdom

Sirisha Senthil, MS, FRCS Department of Glaucoma and Pediatric Ophthalmology, L. V. Prasad Eye Institute, Hyderabad, Telangana, India

Alecia L. S. Stein, MD, MSc Division of Pediatric Anesthesiology, Department of Anesthesiology, Perioperative Medicine and Pain Management, University of Miami Health Centers, FL, USA

Jackson Memorial Hospital, University of Miami Miller School of Medicine, FL, USA

Jacqueline L. Tutiven, MD Pediatric Anesthesia Fellowship, University of Miami Department of Anesthesiology, University of Miami Miller School of Medicine, Miami, FL, USA

David S. Walton, MD Department of Ophthalmology, Massachusetts Eye and Ear Infirmary, Boston, MA, USA

List of videos

Video 4.1 Nasal goniotomy technique, shown using locking forceps at the superior and inferior limbus, and a Barkan goniotomy lens modified with the addition of a handle, sitting on a cushion of viscoelastic applied to the cornea. A 25-gauge needle is used to enter the anterior chamber and to make a cleft to either side, while the assistant stabilizes the globe and rotates it to expose additional angle. Note that the needle entry is closed with a single buried10-0 polyglactin suture. (Courtesy of Sharon F. Freedman, MD)

Video 4.2 Nasal goniotomy technique without traction suture or assistant using modified Swan Jacob lens. The anterior chamber is maintained with viscoelastic and a 25-gauge needle. (Courtesy of Alana L. Grajewski, MD)

Video 4.3 Nasal goniotomy without an assistant using a standard Swan Jacob lens and a 25-gauge needle on viscoelastic. (Courtesy of and narrated by Elizabeth Hodapp, MD)

Video 5.1 Conventional trabeculotomy with metal trabeculotome. (Courtesy of Professor Nader Bayoumi, Alexandria University, Egypt)

Video 5.2 Circumferential trabeculotomy, ab externo, with illuminated microcatheter. (Courtesy of Beth Edmunds, MBChB, FRCOphth, MD)

Video 5.3 Circumferential trabeculotomy, ab externo, with blunted suture. (Courtesy of Allen D. Beck, MD)

Video 5.4 Filtering trabeculotomy. (Courtesy of Franz Grehn, MD, PhD)

Video 5.5 Combined trabeculectomy-trabeculotomy (CTT). (Courtesy of Professor Nader Bayoumi, Alexandria University, Egypt)

Video 6.1 Pediatric trabeculectomy using the Moorfields Safer Surgery technique. (Courtesy of Maria Papadopoulos, MBBS, FRCOphth)

Video 7.1 Blunt dissection of the correct sub-tenon's plane may be started with scissors and completed with two squint hooks inserted back-to-back in this pocket and pulled gently apart. (Courtesy of Cecilia Fenerty, MD, FRCOphth and Tanya Karaconji, MD, FRANZCO)

Video 7.2 Method of inserting a tube into the anterior chamber using a blunt-tipped cannula. The tip of the cannla is firmly engaged onto the cut bevel of the tube and gently inserted through the scleral tunnel taking the tube with it. (Courtesy of Cecilia Fenerty, MD, FRCOphth and Tanya Karaconji, MD, FRANZCO)

Video 7.3 A long tunnel in the patient's native sclera created using a small mini-crescent blade (1.25 mm in width) that can be used to tunnel in the sclera up to about 2 mm posterior to the limbus, then completing the entry into the eye with a 25-gauge needle. (Coutesy of James D. Brandt, MD)

Video 7.4 Insertion of the tube of a Baerveldt glaucoma drainage device in an eye with aniridia. The lens is slightly displaced to the nasal side and insertion of the tube at a tangent avoids contact with the lens. The anterior chamber infusion maintains the anterior chamber and constant intraocular pressure throughout the procedure. (Courtesy of Cecilia Fenerty, MD, FRCOphth and Tanya Karaconji, MD, FRANZCO)

Video 8.1 Transscleral cyclophotocoagulation. The foot plate of the laser probe is placed at the limbus while laser is activated by a foot pedal and applied to the ciliary body. A pair of fine-toothed forceps helps to rotate the eye during the procedure

Video 8.2 Endoscopic cyclophotocoagulation. The tip of the endoprobe is positioned from the ciliary body such that about 4-5 ciliary processes are visible on the screen at any given time. Laser is applied to the ciliary processes until shrinkage and whitening occurs without rupture of ciliary processes or bubble formation. (Courtesy of Anna K. Junk, MD, Bascom Palmer Eye Institute, University of Miami, Miami FL, USA) (© Anna K. Junk)

Video 9.1 Bioniko eye model for simulation of angle surgery. TRAB™360 surgical technique and GATT are performed in this model.

Video 9.2 TRAB™360 surgical technique. The instrument is used to pierce the trabecular meshwork, the inner filament is threaded 180° in the Schlemm canal and then unroofed. The same procedure is performed for the remaining 180°. (Video courtesy of James D. Brandt, MD)

Video 9.3 Goniocopic assisted transluminal trabeculotomy (GATT) with the iTrack™ catheter. The catheter is grasped and directed to the opening in Schlemm canal. The catheter is then fed into the canal and then Schlemm canal is unroofed. (Courtesy of Alana L. Grajewski, MD)

Video 10.1 Surgical video with narration demonstrating optical iridectomy in Peters anomaly

Video 10.2 Ab externo 360° trabeculotomy, lysis of irido-corneal adhesions, and temporal optical sector iridectomy using illuminated catheter in a child with Peters anomaly. (Courtesy of Alana L. Grajewski, MD)

Video 11.1 Surgical technique of combined trabeculotomy-trabeculectomy in a case of primary congenital glaucoma presenting with acute corneal hydrops. (Courtesy of Anil K. Mandal, MD, FAMS, L. V. Prasad Eye Institute, Hyderabad, India)

Video 11.2 Step-by-step surgical technique for Aurolab aqueous drainage implant surgery. (Courtesy of Sirisha Senthil, MS, FRCS (Edin), L. V. Prasad Eye Institute, Hyderabad, India)

Video 11.3 Step-by-step surgical technique for Ahmed glaucoma valve surgery. (Courtesy of Sirisha Senthil, MS, FRCS (Edin), L. V. Prasad Eye Institute, Hyderabad, India)

1 Childhood Glaucoma Surgery: Perioperative Considerations

Maria Papadopoulos, Alana L. Grajewski, Elena Bitrian, and Sharon F. Freedman

Managing glaucoma in childhood is one of the greatest challenges in the field of glaucoma, especially its surgical treatment, itself a critical component of management. Most children with glaucoma will require surgery in their lifetime, often in their childhood years. The surgical repertoire for childhood glaucoma has remained relatively unchanged for many years, with most progress resulting from modifications to existing surgery. Each surgical technique has its advantages and disadvantages, with potentially good success rates when chosen appropriately and performed with meticulous attention to detail to minimize complications. The aim of surgery is to eliminate or bypass aqueous flow obstruction. The challenge of surgery is to balance greater success with fewer complications. To achieve this fine balance, the surgeon often modifies and develops a technique that is safe. Internationally, approaches to surgery for childhood glaucoma can vary, but these highly specialized operations should preferably be performed by a trained surgeon in centers with sufficient volume of patients to ensure surgical experience and skill, coupled with safe anesthesia.

Given that most children with glaucoma have normal life expectancies and may therefore need several operations to control intraocular pressure (IOP), the impact of successful surgical treatment on the patients and their families cannot be overestimated. We hope that in the new millennium, evidence from surgical trials will better guide the management of children with glaucoma and that surgical techniques will continue to evolve for greater success and safety.

Definition and Classification of Childhood Glaucoma

Childhood glaucoma is characterized by elevated intraocular pressure (IOP) and related damage to the eye, which can be caused by a diverse group of conditions. In an effort to standardize the nomenclature worldwide, the Childhood Glaucoma Research Network (CGRN) proposed a definition and validated classification for childhood glaucoma, which were presented to the international community at the World Glaucoma Association (WGA) Childhood Glaucoma Consensus in 2013. The definition and classification were adopted and are used in this book (Tables 1.1 and 1.2).

M. Papadopoulos (✉)
Glaucoma Service, Moorfields Eye Hospital, London, UK
e-mail: maria.papadopoulos@moorfields.nhs.uk

A. L. Grajewski
Samuel & Ethel Balkan International Pediatric Glaucoma Center, Bascom Palmer Eye Institute, University of Miami Miller School of Medicine, Miami, FL, USA

E. Bitrian
Department of Ophthalmology, Mayo Clinic, Rochester, MN, USA

S. F. Freedman
Department of Ophthalmology, Duke University Medical Center, Durham, NC, USA

A. L. Grajewski et al. (eds.), *Surgical Management of Childhood Glaucoma*,
https://doi.org/10.1007/978-3-319-54003-0_1

Table 1.1 Definition of childhood glaucoma and childhood glaucoma suspect

Definition of childhood glaucoma: Two or more required
IOP > 21 mmHg (investigator discretion if examination under anesthesia data alone due to the variable effects of anesthesia on all methods of IOP assessment)
Optic disc cupping: a progressive increase in cup-disc ratio, cup-disc asymmetry of ≥ 0.2 when the optic discs are of similar size, or focal rim thinning
Corneal findings: Haab striae/corneal edema or diameter ≥ 11 mm in newborn, > 12 mm in child < 1 year of age, > 13 mm any age
Progressive myopia or myopic shift coupled with an increase in ocular dimensions out of keeping with normal growth
A reproducible visual field defect that is consistent with glaucomatous optic neuropathy with no other observable reason for the visual field defect
Definition of childhood glaucoma suspect: At least one required
IOP > 21 mmHg on two separate occasions, or
Suspicious optic disc appearance for glaucoma, i.e., increased cup-disc ratio for size of optic disc, or
Suspicious visual field for glaucoma, or
Increased corneal diameter or axial length in setting of normal IOP
Based on national criteria: < 18 years of age (USA); ≤16 years of age (UK, Europe, UNICEF)

Adapted from Beck et al. [1], with permission
IOP = intraocular pressure

Table 1.2 International (CGRN/WGA) Childhood Glaucoma classification

Primary childhood glaucoma
1. **Primary congenital glaucoma** *(isolated trabeculodysgenesis)*
(a) Neonatal or newborn onset (0–1 month)
(b) Infantile onset (> 1 month–2 years)
(c) Late onset or late recognized (> 2 years)
(d) Spontaneously arrested (nonprogressive buphthalmos, Haab striae, normal IOP, and optic nerves)
2. **Juvenile open-angle glaucoma (JOAG)**
Secondary childhood glaucoma
1. **Glaucoma associated with Non-acquired Ocular anomalies** Conditions with predominantly ocular anomalies *present at birth* which may or may not be associated with systemic signs
Axenfeld-Rieger anomaly (syndrome if systemic associations)
Peters anomaly (syndrome if systemic associations)
Congenital ectropion uveae
Congenital iris hypoplasia
Aniridia
Persistent fetal vasculature (if glaucoma present before cataract surgery)
Oculodermal melanocytosis (Nevus of Ota)
Posterior polymorphous dystrophy
Microphthalmos/microcornea
Ectopia lentis
Simple ectopia lentis (no systemic associations)
Ectopia lentis et pupillae
2. **Glaucoma associated with Non-acquired Systemic Disease or Syndrome** Conditions predominantly with known syndromes, systemic anomalies, or systemic disease *present at birth* that may be associated with ocular signs
Chromosomal disorders such as trisomy 21 (Down syndrome)
Connective tissue disorders
Marfan syndrome
Weill-Marchesani syndrome
Stickler syndrome
Metabolic disorders
Homocystinuria
Lowe syndrome
Mucopolysaccharidoses
Phacomatoses
Neurofibromatosis type 1 (NF-1)
Klippel-Trenaunay-Weber syndrome
Sturge-Weber syndrome
Rubinstein-Taybi syndrome
Congenital rubella
3. **Glaucoma associated with Acquired condition** Conditions that are not inherited or present at birth but that *develop after birth*
Uveitis
Trauma (hyphemia, angle recession, ectopia lentis)
Steroid induced
Tumors (benign/malignant, ocular/orbital)
Retinopathy of prematurity
Post-surgery other than cataract surgery
4. **Glaucoma following Cataract surgery** Meets glaucoma definition only *after cataract surgery* is performed. Subdivided into three categories based upon cataract type
(a) Congenital idiopathic cataract
(b) Congenital cataract associated with ocular anomalies/systemic disease or syndrome
(c) Acquired cataract

Adapted from Beck et al. [1], with permission
CGRN/WGA Childhood Glaucoma Research Network/World Glaucoma Association, *IOP* = intraocular pressure

Childhood glaucoma is classified as primary or secondary. In *primary childhood glaucoma*, only a developmental abnormality of the anterior chamber (AC) angle exists, which is responsible for reduced aqueous outflow. In *secondary childhood glaucoma*, the condition associated with reduced aqueous outflow is classified according to whether it is present at birth (non-acquired or congenital) or acquired after birth. Non-acquired childhood glaucoma is further classified according to whether the signs are mainly ocular or systemic (Fig. 1.1).

When to Operate?

Objectives

A child should not be labeled as having glaucoma or subjected to surgery unless one is reasonably sure of the diagnosis and has excluded other conditions that may mimic glaucoma.

The objective of managing children with glaucoma is to provide a lifetime of vision. When target IOP is not achieved medically and is associated with objective evidence of ongoing ocular damage: corneal/ocular enlargement, clinical signs of uncontrolled IOP (e.g., corneal haze, photophobia, watering), optic disc progression, repeatable visual field loss, or deteriorating vision, then surgery is indicated. However, the risks associated with glaucoma surgery in children should not be underestimated, and the threshold to proceed with surgery should be high. The decision to proceed with surgery should only be made once the benefits of surgery outweigh the risks and other less risky options such as medications have been attempted.

Temporizing Measures Before Surgery

Surgery for uncontrolled glaucoma is usually preceded by medical therapy. The exact role of

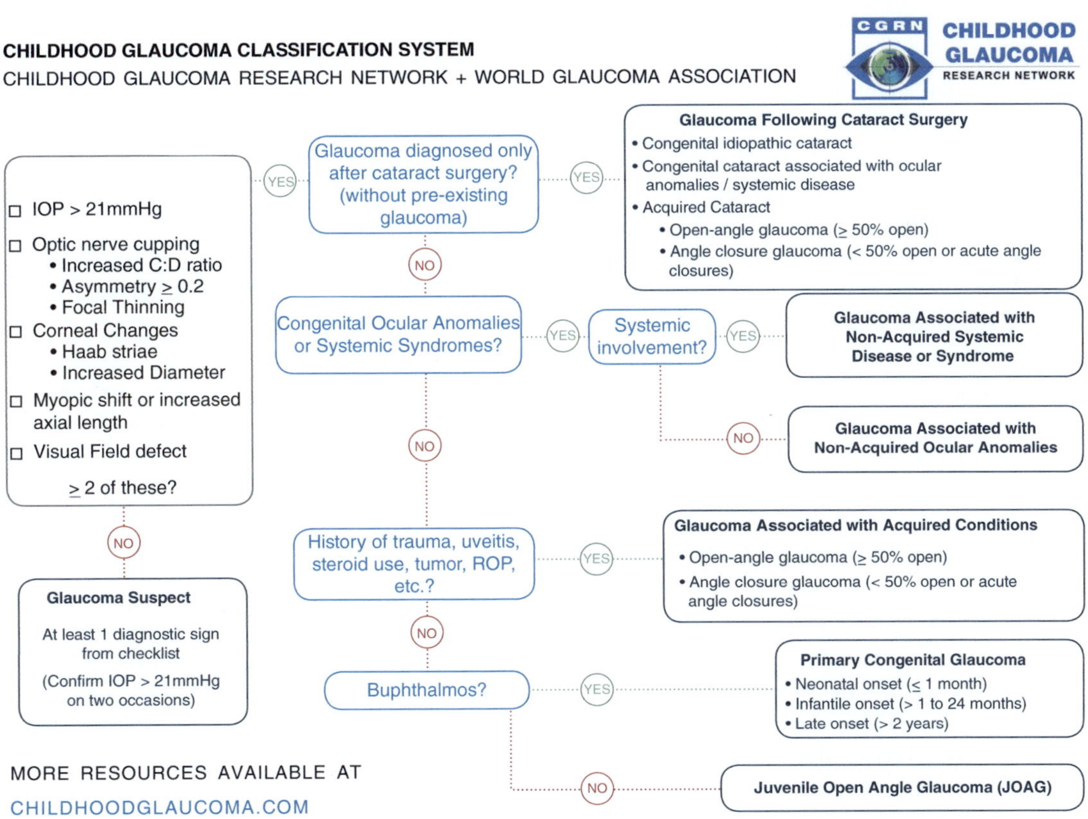

Fig. 1.1 Algorithm for Childhood Glaucoma classification. (Courtesy of the Childhood Glaucoma Research Network and the World Glaucoma Association)

medications depends largely on the type of glaucoma. For example, primary congenital glaucoma (PCG) is a surgical condition, and its diagnosis prompts surgical planning in a timely fashion in almost all cases. However, medications are useful as a temporizing measure prior to surgery to decrease the IOP and reduce corneal edema, allowing better angle visualization and the possibility of ab interno angle surgery. In most other cases of childhood glaucoma with open angles, medical treatment is first line and is escalated over time, depending on its effect in reducing IOP and achieving the desired target pressure. Medication choices and dosing must be tailored with consideration for not only the glaucoma severity but also for the age and health of the child. Infants are particularly susceptible to the systemic absorption and consequences of medications, and some medications should be used with caution (e.g., beta blockers), while others are contraindicated in small children (e.g., brimonidine). Escalation of medical therapy often occurs over many months to years. Exceptions include some cases of secondary glaucoma, e.g., glaucoma secondary to uveitis or trauma, which may present with elevated IOP that remains refractory to medical treatment and results in very rapid glaucoma progression. These cases require close monitoring and timely surgical intervention. It is important to highlight that in those cases that are poorly controlled with medications, where visual potential exists and benefits of surgery outweigh the risks, surgical intervention should not be delayed by medical management.

Consent

The relationship the physician has with the child and the parents/caregivers is very important and must be a trusting one. There is no substitute for time spent with the family especially around the time of surgery, which is quite stressful for the child and parents. This is particularly true if surgery is indicated soon after the diagnosis of glaucoma has been made. After the various options have been discussed with the parents and a decision made as to the most appropriate surgical plan, the details of the surgery should be discussed with the parents, including possible complications. It is important not to trivialize any surgery in children and to set realistic expectations regarding the outcome, the need for regular follow-up, and the possibility of unplanned surgery should problems occur. Furthermore, whenever possible, the assent of the child should be sought when making these difficult decisions.

Selecting the Appropriate Operation and Planning for Surgery

Developing a long-term surgical strategy to preserve vision in a child with glaucoma is essential due to the long life expectancy and the inevitability of repeat surgery for an incurable condition [2]. Selecting the most appropriate operation is paramount, as the first operation has the greatest chance of successfully controlling IOP [3–8]. And in eyes that have undergone multiple procedures, it is vital that the next operation be very carefully determined to maximize benefit and minimize harm and risk. However, the best surgical procedure for any particular child cannot always be determined by a preset algorithm, since it is affected by a combination of diverse factors that include glaucoma type, associated ocular and systemic features, child's age and general health, previous ocular surgery, likelihood of further ocular surgery, visual prognosis, social circumstances (i.e., likelihood of follow-up and available parental support), available local facilities and equipment, and surgeon experience. These factors, along with the absence of randomized trials to inform decision-making, result in diverse strategies to childhood glaucoma surgery internationally.

The type of glaucoma significantly influences the choice of surgery. For PCG, angle surgery is usually the procedure of choice due to its high rate of success [9]. Conversely in uveitic glaucoma, peripheral anterior synechiae make angle surgery potentially less successful [10]. Furthermore, uncontrolled uveitic glaucoma treated with transscleral diode cycloablation not only has a high failure rate but should be discouraged, as it targets an already compromised ciliary body [11]. Glaucoma following congenital cataract surgery treated with trabeculectomy is associated with poor outcomes, even when augmented with mitomycin C (MMC) [1–14]. Additionally, it may be inappropriate for children requiring contact lens refractive correction because of the potential for poor contact lens fitting in some cases and of the increased risk of infection with an avascular bleb.

Accompanying ocular anomalies and systemic disease often need to be taken into consideration. In Axenfeld-Rieger anomaly, access to angle structures may be hampered by iris attachments to Schwalbe line making angle surgery difficult. Peters anomaly associated with a significantly disorganized anterior segment may respond better to glaucoma drainage device (GDD) surgery than to trabeculectomy. In patients with Sturge-Weber syndrome and a choroidal hemangioma, a GDD with techniques to restrict flow that minimize the risk of hypotony may be preferable to trabeculectomy with its less predictable postoperative IOP and risk of hypotony. Certain surgical procedures require specific anatomic features, such as corneal clarity, which is required to perform ab interno angle surgery. However, there exist modifications to facilitate surgical procedures even when clinical features are suboptimal, for example, corneal epithelial edema can be overcome by epithelial debridement in 90% of Caucasian patients [15], and endoscopy allows a view of the angle despite corneal opacity [16]. The general health of a child may be severely compromised or limited by associated systemic disease or rare syndromes that may limit the child's tolerance for anesthesia duration and drug exposure. This influences the type of procedure toward a more temporizing or alternatively a more definitive one.

The choice of surgery is also influenced by the age at onset or presentation of glaucoma. For example, the onset of PCG less than 3 months of age, especially within the first month, is associated with a poorer prognosis for angle surgery success [17–19], as is a late presentation over the age of 2–3 years [20, 19]. However, angle surgery can still typically be the first procedure of choice in these children, given the low rate of complications.

Past surgical history and anticipated future surgical interventions (e.g., cataract extraction) may influence the decision toward GDD surgery rather than trabeculectomy, because trabeculectomy success is reduced following previous conjunctival incisional surgery and its survival with subsequent lensectomy is also less likely. Furthermore, it is vital to consider the past surgical history of the fellow eye, because if a well-performed operation is associated with a poor outcome in the fellow eye, then an alternative operation may need to be considered. Limited visual potential or a severely buphthalmic eye with compromised structural integrity, i.e., very thin sclera, may warrant less aggressive surgical intervention.

The child's social circumstances may also influence the decision regarding the most appropriate operation. If the child is likely not to attend for follow-up or follow-up is restricted due to distances required to access the tertiary care, as is often the case in the developing world, then operations such as trabeculectomy which require intensive postoperative review are best avoided. Furthermore, in the developing world, the operations available may be restricted by the availability of equipment such as GDDs due to their cost and by local surgical training and expertise.

Once the decision has been made regarding the most appropriate operation, it is incumbent on the surgeon to prepare for the operation, which includes the anticipation of potential complications and detailed consideration of how best to prevent them. Although Duke-Elder summarized the difficulties of operating on buphthalmic eyes by stating "accidents are prone to occur at the time of operation" [21], it is worth highlighting the surgical maxim that the best way to manage complications is to avoid them.

Challenges to Successful Surgery

The challenges to successful childhood glaucoma surgery are numerous and varied and include not only the surgical planning outlined above but also operative technique, a greater tendency for complications, accentuated healing response, and the potentially difficult postoperative examination and management, all of which contribute to an unpredictable outcome.

The surgical technique itself is made challenging by the thin and elastic pediatric sclera, the distorted anatomy of the buphthalmic eye, the variable anatomy of congenital ocular anomalies, and the legacy of previous surgeries. The inherent characteristics and behavior of pediatric tissues make the eye prone to complications especially likely when the surgeon lacks familiarity with buphthalmic eyes. The aggressive healing response of children is thought to hinder the success of operations dependent on external pathways of aqueous drainage from the eye.

These factors are all compounded by the difficulty of caring for children with a limited ability to cooperate and cope with the frequency of intensive anti-inflammatory postoperative medications essential to maximize success. The surgeon often faces challenges when trying to adequately examine children and perform postoperative manipulations such as suture removal. Therefore, examinations under anesthesia (EUA) may be required for this purpose, often on a repeated basis. Furthermore, significant commitment is necessary from the parents to administer the drops and attend regular postoperative follow-up, especially necessary for operations such as trabeculectomy to ensure adequate filtration and control of bleb inflammation. It is important to be mindful that these frequent visits for postoperative monitoring may impact the child's schooling and potentially the parents' ability to care for the rest of their family and their commitment to work with loss of earnings. Medical expenses when covered by the family add to the financial burden. Finally, the potential for glaucoma surgery and its complications to affect the quality of life of children and the entire family should not be overlooked [22].

When to Stop Operating?

Even though it is important to keep a child seeing for as long as possible, when the eye has limited visual potential or the fellow eye is healthy, it may be advisable to take a less aggressive approach. For example, an eye with poor vision from secondary glaucoma related to a unilateral exudative retinal detachment for which transscleral diode laser cycloablation is performed may unnecessarily place the fellow healthy eye at risk from sympathetic ophthalmia. This dilemma is more commonly faced in the developing world where resources are more limited or where treatment is funded by the family.

Inoperable Patients (What to Do with Those Who Do Not Fit Any Recognized Category)

Some children may present with congenital ocular anomalies that do not fit into any recognized category or spectrum, such as anterior segement ectasia or unclassified anterior segment anomalies. These cases can vary widely, and in some, it may not be possible to visualize the intraocular structures except with use of an anterior segment ultrasound. These children are at risk of glaucoma, as often the anterior segment anomalies are accompanied by maldevelopment of angle structures. When glaucoma occurs, the anterior segment and limbal sclera are sometimes so distorted that conventional incisional surgery is not possible, with the only choice being transscleral cycloablation.

Visual Rehabilitation and Follow-Up

The criteria for success of glaucoma surgery in children are usually IOP-related parameters and the absence of serious complications. However, the preservation of visual function is the goal in these children and the true measure of success. So, concurrent ametropic correction and amblyopia therapy, where indicated, are crucial to optimize long-term visual outcomes. Simple measures, such as protective, impact resistant lenses for monocular children are likewise critical to preserve visual function for a lifetime in these special children. Visual rehabilitation may also involve the management of corneal opacities and cataracts.

Not to be forgotten is the support these children need with regard to schooling such as the provision of low vision aids and, occasionally, with their social circumstances or mental health. There is also the care of the family as a whole, which involves not only examining siblings in certain circumstances such as autosomal dominant conditions, and offering genetic counseling, but also being sensitive to the dynamics of the family which may impact the provision of the child's care.

As these children grow up and possibly leave our practice, it is important to remember that the elevated IOP they once experienced as an infant or child may impact their ocular health as an adult. Apart from the ongoing risk of uncontrolled glaucoma at any stage for which they need lifelong follow-up [23], there is also the risk of complicated cataract surgery [24], increased risk of retinal detachment [25, 26], and corneal complications (decompensation, band keratopathy), all of which underscore the unique circumstance of high IOP in eyes at a critical time of development. It is the hope of the editors and all the contributors to this book that we can help present treatment modalities to alter the course of damage in these vulnerable eyes.

References

1. Beck A, Chang TCP, Freedman S. Definition, classification and differential diagnosis. In: Weinreb RN, Grajewski A, Papadopoulos M, Grigg J, Freedman S. (eds). Childhood Glaucoma. WGA Series-9. Amsterdam: Krugler Publications; 2013. p. 3–10.
2. Taylor RH, Ainsworth JR, Evans AR, Levin AV. The epidemiology of pediatric glaucoma: the Toronto experience. J AAPOS. 1999;3(5):308–15.
3. Inaba Z. Long-term results of trabeculectomy in the Japanese: an analysis by life-table method. Jpn J Ophthalmol. 1982;26(4):361–73.
4. Gressel MG, Heuer DK, Parrish RK 2nd. Trabeculectomy in young patients. Ophthalmology. 1984;91(10):1242–6.
5. Miller MH, Rice NS. Trabeculectomy combined with beta irradiation for congenital glaucoma. Br J Ophthalmol. 1991;75(10):584–90.
6. Dietlein TS, Jacobi PC, Krieglstein GK. Prognosis of primary ab externo surgery for primary congenital glaucoma. Br J Ophthalmol. 1999;83(3):317–22.
7. Broadway DC, Grierson I, Hitchings RA. Local effects of previous conjunctival incisional surgery and the subsequent outcome of filtration surgery. Am J Ophthalmol. 1998;125(6):805–18.
8. Papadopoulos M, Edmunds B, Chiang M, Mandal A, Grajewski AL, Khaw PT. Glaucoma surgery in children. In: Weinreb RN, Grajewski A, Papadopoulos M, Grigg J, Freedman S, editors. Childhood glaucoma, WGA consensus series 9. Amsterdam: Kugler Publications; 2013. p. 95–134.
9. Ho CL, Walton DS. Goniosurgery for glaucoma secondary to chronic anterior uveitis: prognostic factors and surgical technique. J Glaucoma. 2004;13(6):445–9.
10. Heinz C, Koch J, Heiligenhaus A. Transscleral diode laser cyclophotocoagulation as primary surgical treatment for secondary glaucoma in juvenile idiopathic arthritis: high failure rate after short term follow up. Br J Ophthalmol. 2006;90(6):737–40.
11. Beck AD, Wilson WR, Lynch MG, Lynn MJ, Noe R. Trabeculectomy with adjunctive mitomycin C in pediatric glaucoma. Am J Ophthalmol. 1998;126(5):648–57.
12. Azuara-Blanco A, Wilson RP, Spaeth GL, Schmidt CM, Augsburger JJ. Filtration procedures supplemented with mitomycin C in the management of childhood glaucoma. Br J Ophthalmol. 1999;83(2):151–6.
13. Freedman SF, McCormick K, Cox TA. Mitomycin C-augmented trabeculectomy with postoperative wound modulation in pediatric glaucoma. J AAPOS. 1999;3(2):117–24.
14. Mandal AK, Bagga H, Nutheti R, Gothwal VK, Nanda AK. Trabeculectomy with or without mitomycin-C for paediatric glaucoma in aphakia and pseudophakia following congenital cataract surgery. Eye (Lond). 2003;17(1):53–62.
15. Russell-Eggitt IM, Rice NS, Jay B, Wyse RK. Relapse following goniotomy for congenital glaucoma due to trabecular dysgenesis. Eye (Lond). 1992;6(Pt 2):197–200.
16. Bayraktar S, Koseoglu T. Endoscopic goniotomy with anterior chamber maintainer: surgical technique and one-year results. Ophthalmic Surg Lasers. 2001;32(6):496–502.
17. Lister A. The prognosis in congenital glaucoma. Trans Ophthalmol Soc U K. 1966;86:5–18.
18. Walton DS. Primary congenital open-angle glaucoma. In: Chandler PA, Grant WM, Epstein DL, editors. Chandler and Grant's glaucoma. 2nd ed. Philadelphia: Lea & Febiger; 1979. p. 329–43.
19. Akimoto M, Tanihara H, Negi A, Nagata M. Surgical results of trabeculotomy ab externo for developmental glaucoma. Arch Ophthalmol. 1994;112(12):1540–4.
20. Shaffer RN. Prognosis of goniotomy in primary infantile glaucoma (trabeculodysgenesis). Trans Am Ophthalmol Soc. 1982;80:321–5.
21. Duke-Elder S, editor. System of ophthalmology. Vol III: Normal and abnormal development. Part 2: Congenital deformities. London: Henry Kimpton Publishers; 1969. p. 562.

22. Dahlmann-Noor A, Tailor V, Bunce C, Abou-Rayyah Y, Adams G, Brookes J, et al. Quality of life and functional vision in children with glaucoma. Ophthalmology. 2017;124(7):1048–55.
23. de Silva DJ, Khaw PT, Brookes JL. Long-term outcome of primary congenital glaucoma. J AAPOS. 2011;15(2):148–52.
24. Walton DS. Chronic newborn primary congenital glaucoma with secondary lens subluxation. J Pediatr Ophthalmol Strabismus. 2009;46(4):200. 231
25. Al-Harthi E, Al-Shahwan S, Al-Turkmani S, Khan AO. Retinal detachment and congenital glaucoma. Ophthalmology. 2007;114(8):1590–1.
26. Satofuka S, Imamura Y, Ishida S, Ozawa Y, Tsubota K, Inoue M. Rhegmatogenous retinal detachment associated with primary congenital glaucoma. Int Ophthalmol. 2008;28(5):369–71.

Anesthetic Considerations in the Evaluation of Children with Glaucoma and Associated Conditions

2

Jacqueline L. Tutiven, Dorothea Kadarian-Baumgard, and Alecia L. S. Stein

Introduction

Each year in the United States, more than 6 million infants and toddlers require some form of anesthesia to facilitate a wide array of examinations, procedures, and surgeries. Unlike adults, who are able to submit to all but the most invasive examinations and diagnostic procedures awake or with mild sedation, most children are unable to tolerate all but the most minor medical procedures in an awake, non-sedated state. In this population, even detailed eye exams can be challenging without the assistance of some sedation, and in many cases general anesthesia is required to complete necessary diagnostic and treatment interventions. These sessions often occur in an ambulatory surgical environment and are not always coupled with an actual surgical intervention.

Given the importance of sedated examination in the unique setting of childhood glaucoma, this chapter is devoted to the practice of pediatric anesthesia and what every pediatric glaucoma specialist should know about bringing their smallest patients to the operating suite, including the preoperative, intraoperative, and postoperative components of a visit, a discussion of optimizing patients prior to undergoing anesthesia, and possible complications that may arise during an anesthetic. Lastly, as the breadth of practice and age range is wide in the treatment of childhood glaucoma, there are some salient points regarding the child's age and the comorbidities one will encounter in anesthetizing those with systemic syndromes that affect multiple organ systems.

J. L. Tutiven (✉)
Pediatric Anesthesia Fellowship, University of Miami
Department of Anesthesiology, University of Miami
Miller School of Medicine, Miami, FL, USA
e-mail: jtutiven@med.miami.edu

D. Kadarian-Baumgard
Division of Pediatric Anesthesia, Department of Anesthesiology, Holtz Children's Hospital at Jackson Memorial Hospital, University of Miami Miller School of Medicine, Miami, FL, USA

A. L. S. Stein
Division of Pediatric Anesthesiology, Department of Anesthesiology, Perioperative Medicine and Pain Management, University of Miami Health Centers, FL, USA

Jackson Memorial Hospital, University of Miami Miller School of Medicine, FL, USA

Preoperative Assessment

Pediatric Anesthesia in the Ambulatory Setting

Most children undergoing examination or surgical intervention with anesthesia will do so in the ambulatory setting. Each year, over 3 million children receive anesthesia care on an outpatient same-day basis, many of which occur in a freestanding facility separate from a hospital [1]. There are specific guidelines for the pediatric

A. L. Grajewski et al. (eds.), *Surgical Management of Childhood Glaucoma*,
https://doi.org/10.1007/978-3-319-54003-0_2

ambulatory setting with regard to appropriate criteria for same-day surgery, preoperative workup, and discharge. Specifically, current or recent upper respiratory tract infection, apnea risk in those with sleep apnea or in infants, and potentially undiagnosed myopathies or cardiac disease are special areas of concern during triaging pediatric cases for same-day surgery [2]. In this setting, the plan is for same-day discharge; in order to ensure that this approach is efficient and safe, short-acting drugs, multimodal pain control, and regional anesthetics when possible are utilized at every opportunity [2].

Routine management of childhood glaucoma consists of serial exams and/or surgical interventions when warranted from the time of diagnosis onward. In some cases, these children present soon after birth and thus will undergo comprehensive examinations under anesthesia (EUAs) repeatedly throughout their early childhood. Children are almost twice as likely to experience any perioperative adverse event (incidence 35%) as adults (incidence 18%) [3]. Neonates, high-risk patients (American Society of Anesthesiologists [ASA] level III and above), and children with congenital heart disease have a higher relative risk of cardiac arrest [4, 5] and subsequent mortalities, especially neonates [6], and require the specialized knowledge of pediatric anesthesiologists.

Pediatric Patient Selection and Optimization

Prior to each scheduled anesthetic session, every child must have an evaluation and clearance from an anesthesiologist to ensure that they are fit and optimized for anesthesia. The details of optimization are individualized to each child and specifically consider the presence of any additional medical problems, co-associated syndromes, cardiopulmonary dysfunction, and recent or acute illness, all of which may increase perioperative risk.

The child's medical history, birth and perinatal history, recent hospitalizations, and current post-conceptual age are factored into the above assessment to calculate risk and to formulate a plan for the anesthesiologist's approach to their flow through the perioperative day. Medical history review includes perinatal events and hospitalizations with review of relevant medical records, specifically including any pertaining to neonatal intensive care unit (NICU) or pediatric intensive care unit admissions. An assessment of functional capacity with a focused physical exam includes, at minimum, heart, lungs, and airway assessment and review of applicable laboratory values. A discussion with parents or caregivers and the patients, when applicable, addresses risks and benefits of the planned anesthesia, as well as reviewing anesthesia-related instructions for the day of the procedure [7].

A thorough risk assessment considers co-associated disease states, pervasive developmental disorders, metabolic disorders, neuromuscular disorders, muscular dystrophies, congenital syndromes, and genetic disorders when formulating the anesthesia plan. The presence of an unexplained murmur should undergo possible evaluation. Untreated congenital cardiac disease may require a pediatric anesthesiologist with subspecialty training in congenital heart disease, as these patients may exhibit cardiac physiology vulnerable to administered anesthetics. This categorical assessment of disease states will allow for a more organized preoperative assessment of anatomical dysmorphology, with special attention given to craniofacial abnormalities and metabolic and end-organ compromise [8, 9].

The patient and their caregivers will undergo this pre-anesthesia workup either in the days leading up to the scheduled procedure in an ambulatory anesthesia preoperative clinic or over the phone when indicated for otherwise healthy patients. The final details will be discussed in person on the day of the procedure with the members of the anesthesia care team.

Physical Exam and Airway Considerations

The Mallampati classification is a key component of the airway examination. It is the gradation assessment of the oral aperture and the hard and soft palate and is one of several objective findings that assist the anesthesiologist in predicting airway complications. Children who are cooperative with examination of their oropharynx will receive a Mallampati classification, but it is expected that infants and typically toddlers will not cooperate with this exam (Fig. 2.1). Neonates and infants have several anatomical differences of the mouth and airway compared to older children and adults, which should be familiar to the pediatric anesthesiologist. Briefly, this includes a large tongue in relation to the area of the mouth, obligate nose breathing for the first 3 months of life, a large oblong-shaped epiglottis, anteriorly slanted vocal cords, and a glottis opening situated higher in the neck at the level of C3–C4 of the cervical spine. These differences result in a higher incidence of obstruction and difficult mask ventilation in children less than 1 year of age. However, overall the incidence of difficult mask ventilation in children is 0.2% compared to 1.4% in adults [10–14].

Anesthesia Assessment and Plan

American Society of Anesthesiology Physical Status Classification Each patient, child and adult alike, receives a numeric score referring to the ASA physical status classification system (Table 2.1) [14–17]. The ASA status is a subjective assessment of a patient's risk of adverse cardiopulmonary complications while receiving sedation or general anesthesia. Pediatric patients who are categorized ASA I and II are considered at lower risk for procedural sedation and general anesthesia. Patients with ASA status III or higher have significant systemic dysfunction and typically are quite ill. These patients usually require careful medical optimization of their systemic conditions prior to elective surgery, and in most cases their surgeries are best performed in a hospital operating suite and not in a strictly ambulatory setting.

Preoperative Fasting, *nil* per os (NPO) Status Once appropriate review and examination have taken place, a plan for the anesthetic approach will be formulated. Patients will receive their presurgical instructions with regard to fasting times, which medications to withhold versus which to take, and any other specific orders for preparation [18]. The ASA guidelines recommend fasting times prior to surgery, which can be reviewed in Table 2.2 [19]. Pediatric patients and parents should be given specific instruction to follow fasting guidelines, which allow for clear liquids 2 h prior and breast milk 4 h prior to surgery. Infants and neonates are especially sensitive to fluid shifts and rapidly dehydrate and therefore are not able to tolerate depleted intravascular states that accompany the prolonged fasting periods expected of adults.

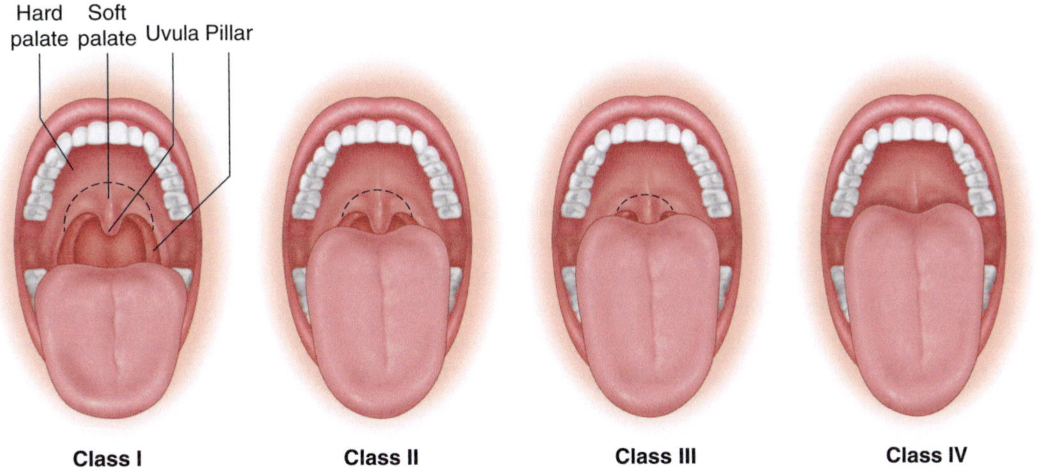

Fig. 2.1 Mallampati assessment of the oral aperture. (Courtesy of Jacqueline L. Tutiven, MD)

Table 2.1 Adapted from the American society of anesthesiologists modified ASA physical status classification system 2013 [15, 16]

Class	Physical status	Example
I	A healthy patient	A fit patient with an umbilical hernia
II	A patient with mild systemic disease	Mild diabetes and controlled hypertension
III	A patient with severe systemic disease that is a constant threat to life	Moderate to severe COPD and angina
IV	An incapacitating disease	Congestive heart failure
V	A moribund patient not expected to live	Ruptured aortic aneurysm
E	Emergency case	–

Table 2.2 American society of Anesthesiologists pre-procedure fasting guidelines

Ingested material	Minimum fasting period (h)
Clear liquids (water, pedialyte, apple juice, black coffee/tea)	2
Breast milk	4
Formula (nonhuman milk, juice with pulp, light meal)	6
Light meal (toast and clear fluid)	6
Heavy meal (high fat content)	8

Data from the American Society of Anesthesiologists Committee [19]

Aspiration Aspiration intraoperatively can be a fatal complication, and about 50% of patients who do aspirate end up developing various levels of lung injury, including aspiration pneumonia [20]. Almost all of the medications routinely used in anesthesia will decrease lower esophageal sphincter tone and potentially increase the risk of aspiration [21]. There are many predisposing conditions that can also increase the risk of aspiration; while some are anatomic abnormalities that may relate to the child's specific syndrome (Table 2.3), others include obesity, hiatal hernia, or need for emergency surgery, to name a few. For emergency surgeries, when the appropriate NPO time cannot be honored, a technique of cricoid pressure with rapid administration of induction agents and paralytics is used to secure the airway as quickly as possible after loss of lower esophageal sphincter tone and protective airway reflexes. This rapid sequence induction technique requires the use of a cuffed endotracheal tube (ETT) and avoidance of bag mask ventilation to avoid insufflation of the stomach. Therefore, no breath is delivered to the apneic patient until the ETT is secured and placement has been confirmed with inflation of the cuff in order to limit regurgitation of stomach content into the lungs.

Table 2.3 The effects of anesthetic medications and techniques on intraocular pressure

Drug or procedure	Intraocular pressure change
Induction/sedation agents	
Propofol	↓↓
Etomidate	↓↓
alpha-2 agonists—dexmedetomidine	↓
Ketamine	+/–
Benzodiazepines	
Midazolam	↓↓
Opioids	↓
Inhaled anesthetics	
Volatiles (sevoflurane)	0/↓
Nitrous oxide	↓
Neuromuscular blockade	
Depolarizing agents (succinylcholine)	↑
Non-depolarizing agents	↓
Direct laryngoscopy	↑↑
Valsalva maneuver (coughing, "bearing down")	↑↑

Delivery of Anesthesia Care and Anesthetic Technique

Sedation for Examinations and Induction of General Anesthesia

Sedation of pediatric patients should be provided by specialists who have acquired an advanced set of skills, knowledge, and certification to practice with absolute adherence to published guidelines. Risk assessment for procedural sedation should not be taken lightly. In the United States, the American Academy of Pediatrics, the American Academy of Pediatric Dentistry, the American College of Emergency Medicine, and the ASA have published revised guidelines for the procedural sedation in infants and children. Similarly, in the United Kingdom, guidelines have been produced by the National Institute for Health and Care Excellence (NICE). Irrespective of the level of sedation that is intended, pediatric sedation exemplifies a continuum. As such, it may consequentially result in respiratory depression with a loss of protective airway reflexes.

Therefore, procedural sedation must be provided within an area that provides necessary resuscitation and supportive equipment. Unexpected complications may arise, and practitioners should not be fraught with the inability of rescuing a patient due to lack of skill, appropriate resuscitation equipment, medicines, or specialized ancillary staff. Every patient is administered oxygen, via nasal cannula, while receiving intramuscular (IM) or intravenous (IV) sedation. Observation and monitoring of vital signs of a sedated pediatric patient include heart rate, pulse oximetry, respiratory rate, and blood pressure recorded at regular intervals. Because sedation is a continuum of a phase of anesthetic somnolence and analgesia, purposeful responses may wane to a point where intervention is required [22]. Infants, as opposed to older children, have greater total body volumes of distribution for certain water-soluble pharmacologic agents while less total body volume of distribution for liposoluble agents. This may present difficulty in predicting how a patient, in this case an infant, will respond to a continuum of sedation. Practitioners administering moderate to deep sedation and analgesia should be ready to rescue patients who may enter into a deeper level of sedation and analgesia. This requires specialized airway management skills. Anesthesiologists are usually best suited to administer sedation to infants and toddlers [17, 19, 23].

There are only a few drugs that are used for pediatric sedation, but more often than not, one sole agent may not be enough to provide adequate sedation. A cocktail of drugs may be needed, as some drugs suppress the ability to breathe, while others may not. Using more than one complementary agent can also decrease the narcotic dose required to maintain a deep enough level of sedation [24].

Midazolam Midazolam is a widely selected benzodiazepine, chosen for its anxiolytic effects, its amnestic properties, and its ability to decrease eye muscle tone along with minimally affecting IOP [25]. Midazolam can be administered orally, intravenously, rectally, or intranasally and is used as a premedication to encourage a child's cooperation. In addition to providing sedation, anxiolysis, and anterograde amnesia, midazolam can help combat emergence delirium after general anesthesia. The side effects of midazolam can be minor, including hiccups to paradoxical hyperactive reactions [26].

Midazolam has a rapid onset of action, within 15–20 min after oral ingestion. A brief half-life time, 1–4 h, gives it a safer margin than using chloral hydrate, for instance, which has a much longer half-life and may not be the best sedative on an outpatient basis [25, 27]. Midazolam is frequently used in conjunction with the following sedative medications, as it is usually insufficient to provide adequate sedation for examination, e.g., as part of premedication.

Ketamine A N-methyl-D-aspartate (NMDA) receptor antagonist and phencyclidine derivative, ketamine has been and continues to be a commonly used anesthetic for procedural sedation. Its pharmacokinetic profile gives it particular properties that have allowed it to be used in infants and children for noninvasive diagnostic exams and minor emergency room procedures. Ketamine is a "dissociative anesthetic," in that it provides sedation and analgesia through NMDA receptor antagonism, potassium/sodium hyperpolarization-activated cyclic nucleotide-gated channel 1 (HCN1) receptor antagonism, and a balanced modulating interplay among cholinergic, aminergic, and opioid systems. Dissociation occurs between the cerebral cortex and the limbic system, resulting in antinociception or *analgesia*, increasing levels of sedation, hypnosis, and unconsciousness with marked adrenergic sympathetic activity. Ketamine also causes cerebral excitation with evidence of seizure-like activity in susceptible individuals, transient increase in IOP [26, 28], and elevation of heart rate and systemic blood pressure.

Ketamine can be administered by IV or IM with the former being preferred, as its effects are longer-lasting. The overall incidence of severe adverse complications and events remains low as long as risk assessment for adverse events is considered and discussed prior to sedation. Green et al. pooled data from 8282 pediatric ketamine sedations in the emergency departments and demonstrated that an overall incidence of upper airway and pulmonary adverse events was 3.9% [23]. Clinical variables shown to increase risks among this age group include patients younger than 2 years of age, young adults aged 13 or older, high IV dosages greater than 2.5 mg/kg or a total dose of 5 mg/kg, and concurrent use of anticholinergic or benzodiazepines [29–31].

The potential benefit of ketamine is that there is little to no risk of apnea, as it does not interfere with breathing, in contrast to the more commonly used agent, propofol. However, it does have the potential to cause laryngospasm and rapid desaturation. Anticholinergic use, such as atropine or glycopyrrolate, can help reduce the increased laryngeal secretions associated with ketamine use. Glycopyrrolate is most often used due to its short half-life and because it does not cross the blood-brain barrier as atropine does. Hemodynamic compromise is not a concern with ketamine as it is with other agents; therefore, ketamine is considered safer to use in those with hemodynamic instability. Ketamine is generally well tolerated in the pediatric population and is sometimes the only option for sedation in those who carry too high a risk to receive agents that could cause hemodynamic or respiratory compromise [23].

Propofol Propofol is an IV sedative-hypnotic agent that, when given as a bolus, will quickly result in a loss of consciousness followed by a quick and smooth awakening. Propofol causes cardiovascular and respiratory depression, decreases cerebral metabolic uptake of oxygen, and decreases cerebral blood flow and intracranial pressure (ICP). Its depressant effect is uniformly distributed in the central nervous system, decreasing synaptic transmission, and will also act as an anticonvulsant, mediated via gamma-aminobutyric acid receptors. Changes in IOP have been noted with low-dose IV sedation with propofol. An IOP decrease of 20–25% can be expected after an initial bolus of propofol with 0.5 mg/kg and is likely due to extraocular muscle relaxation [28, 29, 31, 32].

Pain on injection is a common adverse event that can be decreased by adding lidocaine to the IV line. Anaphylaxis is rare. The incidence of airway obstruction and apnea is very high in infants and children undergoing continuous sedation with propofol; hence credentialed providers of deep sedation/anesthesia must demonstrate appropriate skills in airway rescue management. A report from the Pediatric Sedation Consortium Research group presented data on more than 49,000 sedation/anesthesia encounters utilizing propofol. Their analysis found it unlikely for propofol to yield worrisome adverse outcomes when well-motivated and appropriately supported sedation/anesthesia services are in place [33–36].

Dexmedetomidine Dexmedetomidine is an α-2-adrenergic agonist approved in the United States by the Food and Drug Administration as an IV sedative for patients intubated in the ICU and for patients requiring procedural sedation without intubation. As an off-label medication, dexmedetomidine has been used in children, in and out of the operating room, for surgical, medical, and procedural sedation in the pediatric ICU. Dexmedetomidine provides sedation, maintains respiratory drive, and attenuates analgesia, emergence delirium, and pain in the postoperative period. Notably, upper airway patency is maintained with dexmedetomidine infusions during sedation in children. This is also noted in children with obstructive sleep apnea when compared to propofol [37]. In children, 93% of IV dexmedetomidine is protein bound, and its redistribution half-life is approximately 7 min. It is biotransformed in the liver to inactive metabolites. Adrenoceptors in the central nervous system mediate the cardiovascular effects of dexmedetomidine, mainly causing systemic hypotension and bradycardia, through central sympatholysis. A slow loading infusion is recommended to attenuate the drop in blood pressure. A loading dose of 0.5 μg/kg, infused over 5 min, can give modest 10% decrease in systolic blood pressure [37, 38]. Dexmedetomidine-induced bradycardia can decrease heart rates up to 30% from awake states. Intravenous glycopyrrolate yields unexpected responses and does not attenuate the bradycardia, and transient systemic hypertension has been reported [39, 40].

Oral dexmedetomidine (2.6 μg/kg) has been used as a preoperative sedative, achieving sedation within 30 min, comparable to midazolam at 0.5 mg/kg, and has a similar recovery profile, but it is slow and unpredictable [36, 40]. Intranasal (IN) dexmedetomidine, 1 μg/kg, can provide adequate sedation in approximately 50% of children within 1 h. Preoperative anxiolysis, provided by IN dexmedetomidine, decreases heart rate by 11% within the hour and has been found to assure effective sleep in patients before they enter the operating room. Although dexmedetomidine is available and used in children, specific indications are not in place for its use in the pediatric population, and more clinical research is needed on the hemodynamic challenges, analgesia, and anesthesia recovery in infants.

Sedation may not be well tolerated in the pediatric population as incomplete anesthesia of the globe may elicit discomfort during examination, causing the patient to move, cry, and elicit higher than normal IOPs due to agitation. In contrast, general anesthesia ensures a stable airway and an akinetic globe; however, it usually lowers the IOP.

General Anesthesia

General anesthesia is most often used in preference to sedation in childhood glaucoma patients requiring a comprehensive examination (including IOP), since a procedure may follow the EUA if needed. Establishment of general anesthesia renders the patient unconscious and static in order to obtain clinical findings. Vascular access can be easier to obtain and may be required prior to advancing airway support and for surgical procedures. General anesthesia is also beneficial in that the anesthesiologist can control ventilation via various modes available for use on the ventilator and has the ability to change the respiratory rate of the patient. Hypoventilation or hyperventilation can change arterial partial pressure of carbon dioxide (P_{aCO2}) and cause changes in IOP. Therefore spontaneous ventilation can be overridden with controlled ventilation in the patient with an endotracheal tube (ETT), a laryngeal mask airway (k), or via bag mask ventilation by the anesthesia provider and with titration of anesthetic agents. The disadvantage of general anesthesia is that all volatile agents and most IV anesthetic agents will cause a change, usually a decrease, in IOP, which can lead to falsely reassuring IOPs. The exception to this is ketamine, which may potentially and transiently increase IOP.

At 6 months of age, infants under general anesthesia often need a higher minimum alveolar concentration (MAC) of volatile anesthetics to produce an optimal depth of anesthesia and avoid Bell's phenomenon (palpebral oculogyric reflex) on the eye being examined and operated on. Bell's phenomenon denotes light anesthesia and will increase IOP. Higher MAC of volatile anesthetics often results in unstable hemodynamics reflected by low mean arterial pressures. Cardiovascular changes seen in infants under general anesthesia include hypotension, tachycardia, and decrease in venous pressure. For patients who exhibit Bell's phenomenon while under an appropriate amount of general anesthetic, it is advised to consider a balanced anesthetic, protecting the airway with an ETT and adding a muscle relaxant to attenuate this reflex. This will decrease nociceptive stimulus on the eye being examined, decrease the anesthetic requirements through volatile anesthetics or IV anesthetics, and provide akinesia for surgical procedures [41, 42].

General anesthesia has been reported to cause a significant and often time-dependent decrease in IOP after anesthetic induction. The timing of IOP measurement under anesthesia is important and should be consistent with serial examinations. IOP tends to fluctuate, with the lowest IOP occurring after induction of anesthesia and prior to instrumentation of the airway and the highest IOP occurring 1 min after extubation [43].

Bag Mask Ventilation In certain scenarios (i.e., short EUAs), the patient will need to be anesthetized, but actual placement of an airway device is not necessary, and maintenance of anesthesia can be simply sustained through bag mask ventilation. This technique involves placement of a face mask over the patient's nose and mouth, with or without the use of an oral airway, to deliver anesthetic gases to patients while they breathe spontaneously. It is the least invasive but does not provide for selective entry of air into the trachea. The major disadvantage is that peak airway pressures must remain relatively low so as not to insufflate the stomach and cause regurgitation of stomach content that can be aspirated into the lungs. This decreased amount of airway pressure will not allow for adequate-sized breaths to be delivered to the patient, and hypercarbia could ensue. Light plane of anesthesia and laryngospasm remain disadvantageous to this technique in addition to possibly increasing IOP from external compression of the globe by the face mask. This method is nonetheless vital to performing inhalational induction so that venous access and future placement of an airway can be obtained. IOP may be measured once the patient has entered stage III depth of anesthesia and before IV access is obtained. One-hundred-percent oxygen is delivered prior to removing the mask. The face mask may be removed, especially in infants and children with small faces, to obtain IOP measurements, while the anesthesia provider maintains airway patency maneuvers, such as a chin lift during IOP measurement. If the mask is kept in place, the anesthesiologist avoids positive pressure ventilation through the mask during the actual IOP assessment. Once the IOP measurements are taken, IV access is secured, and an advanced airway or supraglottic airway is placed for continued EUA or surgery [42, 44].

The Supraglottic or Laryngeal Mask Airway (LMA) Supraglottic airways sit above the glottic opening and do not pass through the vocal cords. The LMA is the most commonly used supraglottic airway device in spontaneously ventilated patients. Positive airway pressure is required to perform adequate ventilation with the LMA, and it has a higher success rate with a lower complication rate than ETT [45]. The LMA remains in the supraglottic area and does not go through the vocal cords. This reduces the cough reflex seen with endotracheal intubation. Therefore, a lighter plane of anesthesia is required when compared to placement of an ETT. This has less effect on the patient's hemodynamics and preserves blood pressure, while it also avoids the sympathetic surge that follows placement of an ETT. This effect is proven by the lack of change seen in IOP from baseline after insertion of the LMA [46].

The disadvantage is similar to the bag mask ventilation technique; insufflation of the stomach can occur at high airway pressures leading to aspiration. Although the complication rate is lower than with placement of an ETT, partial airway obstruction can occur, and inadequate ventilation can ensue. Ill-fitting LMAs can induce edema of the airway, especially if used for a prolonged procedure [47, 48]. Prolonged procedures (>2 h) are typically not the ideal cases to be performed with a supraglottic airway. There are increased risk of regurgitation and increased amount of gastric volume as surgery time increases [48]. There is also a potential risk for pharyngeal ischemia when higher than recommended cuff pressures are used [49]. These complications are rare, and more recent studies and reviews are showing that even prolonged surgeries have a very low risk of the previously described complications [34]. During emergence from general anesthesia, the LMA does not protect against laryngospasm. Therefore, placement and removal should be performed when a patient is no longer in the hyper-reactive phase of their anesthetic, or phase II.

LMA failure is more likely in children with acquired or congenital airway syndromes. The LMA was designed for the normal airway anatomy. Craniofacial dysmorphology, seen in many syndromes that present for glaucoma and other eye surgeries, can alter the airway anatomy. This would predispose the patient to an ill-fitting LMA [50]. The LMA is part of the pediatric difficult airway algorithm and can be a lifesaving device in children with difficult airways. Every pediatric airway should be thoroughly examined and assessed for appropriate airway management as a case-by-case/risk to benefit ratio decision. Hence, the "best" approach to airway management will vary for all children and especially those with craniofacial abnormalities and airway anomalies.

Endotracheal Intubation Placement of an ETT involves use of a laryngoscope, which allows visualization of the patient's vocal cords and epiglottis. Placement of the ETT requires operator experience, especially in the pediatric patient with a difficult airway that can be caused by syndromic variations in anatomy. The major advantage of an ETT is that ventilation is easier to control with minimal concern for stomach insufflation and laryngospasm, as occur with light anesthesia. The cuff can also help prevent regurgitation of stomach content from being aspirated into the lungs, which the supraglottic airway devices do not prevent. Ventilation can be controlled via a pressure or volume mode of ventilation, avoiding barotrauma. Patients may still breathe spontaneously with an ETT, although a deeper plane of anesthesia may be required to avoid emerging to stage II of anesthesia, leading to coughing against the ETT, which will increase IOP and risk interfering with intraocular procedures for glaucoma. Maintaining a patient under deep anesthesia could also lead to hypoventilation and hypercarbia. The benefit of a spontaneously breathing patient is the ability to draw air into the lungs via negative pressure that will decrease central venous pressure (CVP) and allow for an IOP more similar to the patient's baseline when they are not anesthetized. Positive pressure ventilation will increase CVP and in turn increase IOP, as it limits venous drainage from the head and neck. The use of spontaneous and controlled ventilation with their advantages and disadvantages is also applicable to the LMA, while pulmonary respiratory parameters are adjusted to deliver adequate volumes [50].

Perioperative Physiology Affecting Intraocular Pressure

Intraocular pressure and its measurement can be greatly affected when a patient is anesthetized or sedated. The point at which IOP measurement occurs is essential for accurate assessment of glaucoma, and it may vary from the preinduction phase, where a patient may receive premedication of an anxiolytic, such as midazolam, to the extubation phase where coughing on an ETT can greatly raise IOP to up to 34–40 mmHg [41]. It is essential to understand how anesthesia medications—both IV agents and inhaled volatile anesthetics—as well as how the time point during an anesthetic may impact the measurement of IOP. These effects are briefly summarized in Table 2.3.

Intraocular pressure can be affected by external pressure on the eye, venous congestion, and changes in intraocular volumes. The patient, surgeon, and anesthesiologist can influence these three factors in a multitude of ways.

External Compression External pressure to the eye will increase IOP [42]. Careful attention must be paid to patient positioning. Eyes must remain free of pressure in all positions (prone, supine, or lateral). Elevation of the head, such as placing a patient in the reverse Trendelenburg position, can also ameliorate increased IOP because it allows for venous drainage [51, 52].

An increase in extraocular muscle tone can increase IOP from external compression. This has been seen with spasms, mediated by the depolarizing muscle blocker, succinylcholine [53].

Venous Congestion Venous congestion can impede drainage of the head and neck, which in turn can increase IOP and ICP. Increasing CVP can inhibit efflux from the eye and increase IOP [54, 55]. CVP can be greatly affected by patient positioning, choice of anesthetic, and parameters set on the patient ventilator. High peak airway pressures and use of high levels of positive end-expiratory pressure (PEEP) while a patient is under general endotracheal anesthesia will impede venous drainage from the head and neck due to increasing CVP. Any positive pressure application in the ventilated patient has the potential to increase CVP. This is in contrast to a patient who is breathing spontaneously, creating negative inspiratory pressures, without the assistance of the ventilator, which decreases CVP [56].

The spontaneously breathing patient has a negative airway pressure with each inspiration, thereby reducing CVP and increasing venous drainage from the head and neck, reducing IOP. Work of breathing and airway resistance plays an indirect role on IOP. Depending on the type of airway support in use, i.e., face mask, an LMA, or an ETT, and if a patient is left spontaneously breathing or on a mechanical ventilator, the IOP will be affected [56, 57]. Placement of an oral airway device to permit unobstructed flow will decrease inspiratory work of breathing and measurements of IOP in infants and children and should be performed after an appropriate depth of anesthesia is achieved and before definitive airway manipulation.

Changes in Intraocular Volume Blood volume and aqueous humor formation and drainage affect intraocular volume and IOP. The basal intraocular blood volume is determined by intraocular vessel tone, which is affected by P_{aCO2}. An increase in P_{aCO2} will increase IOP because of increasing choroidal blood volume [54]. This effect can be manipulated under anesthesia where hypoventilation results in an increase in arterial CO_2, a mild acidotic state, and vasodilation of cerebral vessels with concomitant increase in choroidal blood volume. Alternatively, hyperventilation will reduce P_{aCO2} and produce vasoconstriction of choroidal blood vessels and a lowering of IOP. Generally, arterial pressure has very little effect on IOP [55, 58, 59].

Autonomic Stimulation and Changes in Aqueous Humor Volume and Drainage Peripheral autonomic fibers from the pterygopalatine ganglion (parasympathetic) and the superior cervical ganglion (sympathetic), along with local influences from trigeminal sensory fibers, innervate structures that maintain IOP in a complex interrelated way. Aqueous humor is formed by the ciliary epithelium, and its production is increased with sympathetic stimulation and decreased with parasympathetic stimulation. The adrenergic nervous system plays a significant and complex role in the regulation of IOP. Autonomic nerve fibers innervate the ciliary processes, the trabecular meshwork, and the episcleral blood vessels. These last vessels are actually arteriovenous anastomoses. Their vascular tonicity or episcleral venous pressure (EVP) is afforded to the episcleral blood vessels via parasympathetic, sympathetic, and trigeminal fibers. This EVP needs to be overcome in order to allow for proper outflow of aqueous humor; internal adrenergic stimulation and locally applied β agonists (epinephrine) will decrease IOP. Clonidine, an α-2-adrenoreceptor agonist, will also directly decrease IOP when placed as a topical treatment. Yet, β-adrenergic antagonists can also decrease IOP. This occurs as there may be different sites of action for a β agonist (reabsorption areas) and antagonist (decreases secretion) [60, 61]. Further physiologic research may contribute to understanding the complex interrelationship of the central pathways, ascending neuromodulatory pathways, the extrinsic system, and the local autonomic nervous system (intrinsic system) on the neuromodulation affecting IOP [62, 63].

Changes in Volume of the Vitreous Humor The volume of vitreous humor is generally constant but can be affected by hydration and osmotically active agents such as mannitol, which can create a significant reduction in IOP. Preoperative dehydration, seen in infants with prolonged NPO status before being examined under anesthesia, may reflect a mild decrease in IOP [63–65].

Anesthetic Agents and Their Effect on Intraocular Pressure

Inhaled Anesthetics Volatile anesthetics that are in current use today include the halogenated agents of sevoflurane, isoflurane, and desflurane. Halothane is no longer available for use in the United States but could be found in other parts of the world. Nitrous oxide is the oldest inhaled anesthetic that is available but must be used with other halogenated agents due to its low potency [66].

Nitrous oxide requires a high minimum alveolar concentration in order to provide reliable anesthesia, but giving high concentration of nitrous oxide is limited due to its ability to cause hypoxia. Nitrous oxide has greater solubility than nitrogen and can expand in air-filled spaces, in addition to causing diffusion hypoxia when given in concentrations greater than 3:1 with oxygen. Therefore, nitrous oxide has been used as a sole agent in concentrations of 70% or less to provide anxiolysis to patients. The benefits include its rapid onset and offset, minimal changes on hemodynamics, and minimal effect on IOP [67]. When used as a sole agent, there is no concern for malignant hyperthermia or possibly even emergence delirium [68]. Nitrous oxide is controversial because of its increased risk of postoperative nausea and vomiting, its potential of inactivation of vitamin B_{12}, and the possibility of expansion of air-filled structures. This is of concern when surgeries involve the inner ear or with the use of an intraocular gas. Perfluoropropane (C_3F_8), sulfur hexafluoride (SF_6), and filtered room air are commonly used in retinal surgery, which, when coupled with the use of nitrous oxide, can expand the intraocular gas leading to increased IOP and potentially permanent visual loss. The avoidance of nitrous oxide for 3 months is recommended after ophthalmic surgery involving the use of an intraocular gas unless the intraocular gas has become completely absorbed [69].

Sevoflurane is the halogenated agent of choice for both the typical pediatric inhalational induction and for the maintenance phase of a general anesthetic, as it is fast-acting and the least irritating to the airways. Other agents are less useful in this setting; desflurane, while fast-acting, is the most pungent; isoflurane has a slower onset to achieving a deep anesthetic level and is also very unpleasant for inhalation induction. Both will induce harsh coughing and significant airway irritation in patients of all ages [70, 71]. Desflurane induces sympathetic stimulation, with transient increases in blood pressure and tachycardia [70]. However, such fluctuations are not linked to increases of IOP when compared to the use of sevoflurane. The mechanism for lowering IOP, upon the use of halogenated agents, is likely related to an increase in the outflow of aqueous humor and decreased aqueous production, along with relaxation of extraocular muscles [72]. Schäfer and colleagues described the mechanism of decreased IOP after the use of sevoflurane as being due to a decrease in heart rate and blood pressure, which would also decrease CVP and potentially choroidal blood flow [32]. Since there are many factors that can influence the IOP of a child under anesthesia, the timing of IOP measurement related to inhalational anesthesia is important. It is generally recommended that IOP should be checked immediately after inhalational induction, as IOP continues to decrease with time [32].

Intravenous Agents Intravenous agents for the induction of anesthesia include propofol, etomidate, ketamine, and thiopental (although thiopental is no longer available in the United States). Dexmedetomidine is also commonly used for the maintenance of anesthesia when volatile agents may be contraindicated. As previously described, all of these agents will decrease IOP except ketamine. Ketamine is a dissociative anesthetic that can also cause an increase in blood pressure and heart rate. Controversy exists whether or not induction dose ketamine causes an increase in IOP or has no effect at all. Older studies examined ketamine without the use of premedication, such as midazolam, and found that IOP was increased after administration possibly due to causing nystagmus and increased extraocular muscle tone [32]. More recent studies have been unable to replicate this when premedication was given and found that IOP measured under ketamine fairly accurately represents IOP in the awake state [32, 73, 74]. Ketamine has unpleasant side effects, including increased oral secretions, which could potentially cause laryngospasm (reduced with atropine or glycopyrrolate), nystagmus, and unpleasant dreams or hallucinations. The use of midazolam can help mitigate these unpleasant dreams. Premedication of atropine and midazolam given 20–30 min prior to attending the operating suite is recommended.

Propofol is the most commonly used induction agent, as its profile has fewer side effects compared with other agents. Propofol is rarely contraindicated unless there is a history of a mitochondrial disorder; prolonged exposure may lead to propofol infusion syndrome [75, 76]. Propofol formulations commonly include a soybean oil emulsion and egg lecithin, which have previously been contraindicated in patients with soy or egg allergy. Most patients with egg allergy are actually allergic to the proteins found in egg white, but not the yolk. Multiple studies have confirmed the safety of propofol use in egg or soy allergy [77]. When compared with etomidate and thiopental, all of which decrease systolic blood pressure and IOP after induction, propofol was found to decrease IOP the most and to prevent an increase in IOP when an LMA was inserted [78]. Propofol has also been found to cause a significant decrease in IOP when compared to sevoflurane alone [33].

Local Anesthetics for Analgesia

Local anesthetics (LAs) play a key role in reducing the need for opioid-based analgesia and are especially useful in ophthalmic ambulatory surgery. The application of LAs to the surface of the pediatric globe, or placement along periocular tissues, should be performed by specialty-trained physicians on children under general anesthesia, almost always by the operating surgeon in cases of childhood glaucoma. LAs are classified as either amino-esters or amino-amide compounds, both of which possess characteristics unique to their class. Common agents used in pediatric eye surgery are summarized in Table 2.4.

Amino-Esters Amino-esters are hydrolyzed by plasma cholinesterases. Cholinesterases, enzymes found ubiquitously in plasma and tissues, quickly metabolize these esters, giving them a low toxicity profile in older children. Neonates and infants have decreased levels of plasma cholinesterase and, as such, are susceptible to a buildup of toxic levels when given in summative fashion. Fortunately, ester LAs are short-lived, being metabolized within minutes. Tetracaine and proparacaine are two common ester LAs utilized in ophthalmic surgery on infants and children.

Amino-Amides Amino-amides are eliminated by hepatic enzymatic degradation. The amino-amides include lidocaine, bupivacaine, ropivacaine, and levobupivacaine. The neonatal hepatic system is immature at birth, with limited enzymatic metabolism of such agents, which increases the risk of drug buildup causing LA toxicity. Hepatic clearance of LAs approaches adult levels by 8 months of age [79]. Bupivacaine is a common agent used in infants and children eye blocks at concentrations of 0.25–0.5%. It is typically bound to plasma-binding proteins, α-1-glycoprotein and albumin. Neonatal levels of these proteins are less than those in adults, resulting in a greater free fraction of bupivacaine and other circulating highly bound drugs, thus rendering the potential cardiotoxicity a key consideration in dosing in neonates and children under general anesthesia. A single-dose slow bolus

Table 2.4 Local anesthetics commonly used in eye surgery with recommended maximal dosages

Local anesthetic	Class	Maximum dose (mg/kg)	Duration of action (min)
Procaine	Ester	10	60–90
2-Chloroprocaine	Ester	20	30–40
Tetracaine	Ester	20	30–60
Lidocaine	Amide	1.5	180–600
Bupivacaine	Amide	2–4	180–600
Ropivacaine	Amide	2–4	180–600
Levobupivacaine	Amide	2–4	180–600

Data adapted from the American Academy of Pediatrics; American Academy of Pediatric Dentistry, Coté CJ, Wilson S; Work Group on Sedation [15].

injection for ophthalmic blocks may range from 2 to 4 mg/kg. Ropivacaine is an S(−) enantiomer and a racemate of bupivacaine and exhibits fewer cardiovascular and central nervous system side effects [80].

Local Anesthetic Systemic Toxicity Local anesthetic systemic toxicity involves the cardiovascular and central nervous systems with symptoms that include tinnitus, perioral numbness, dizziness, agitation, and seizures [76]. The most feared complication involves complete circulatory arrest that does not respond to normal resuscitative efforts. The treatment of choice is a lipid emulsion 20%, with avoidance of most vasopressors and a much reduced dosage of epinephrine (<1 μg/kg) [80–82].

Postoperative Analgesia

After invasive surgery that is likely to be painful, such as glaucoma drainage device surgery or laser cyclodestruction, a long-acting local anesthetic via the sub-Tenon or peribulbar route at the end of the procedure significantly reduces postoperative pain and postoperative nausea and vomiting (PONV). The size of the globe is an important consideration for peribulbar blocks. The anteroposterior length of a typical adult globe is approximately 22–24 mm. A premature neonate may have an axial length of 15 mm, while a full-term neonate's globe is characteristically 16–17 mm in length. The globe continues to grow until reaching full size at approximately 3 years of age. A short-beveled needle or angled cannula can be used with an amide anesthetic; our institution uses ropivacaine 0.375% for an inferotemporal approach to a peribulbar block (Fig. 2.2) [83].

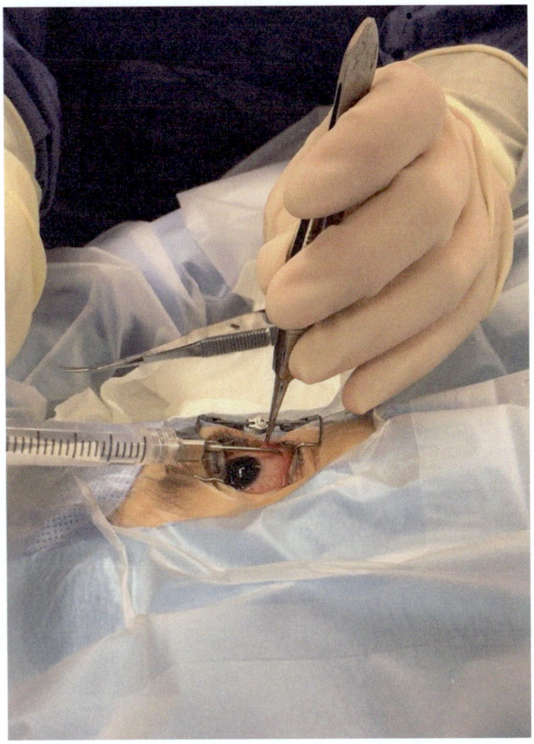

Fig. 2.2 Sub-Tenon pediatric eye block. A short-beveled needle or angled cannula can be used with an amide anesthetic; our institution uses ropivacaine 0.375% for an inferotemporal approach to a peribulbar block useful for postoperative analgesia at the end of major surgery. (Courtesy of Jacqueline L. Tutiven, MD)

Topical Anesthesia and Neonatal Intensive Care Unit Patients

Neonates and premature infants residing in NICUs do not typically require sedation for the brief measurement of IOP. Diagnostic modalities that require minimal movements can fuel discussion on how best to provide immobility in NICUs without exposure to anesthetics. Most academic centers in the United States and United Kingdom conduct *feed and swaddle* techniques for magnetic resonance imaging (MRI) and other noninvasive diagnostics, avoiding sedation altogether [84]. A topical local anesthetic, usually a very short-acting ester anesthetic eye drop, is applied, not only to decrease possible discomfort but to depress the corneal reflex upon achieved surface analgesia. Common topical preparations are lidocaine, tetracaine, and proparacaine. Studies in healthy adults have demonstrated that episcleral venous pressure is not affected by topical anesthetics [85]. Systemic absorption is increased in neonates and infants. The thin keratin layer of the newborn's skin around the eyes, conjunctiva, nasal mucosa, and gastrointestinal tract increases the systemic absorption of these and many other ocular medications, easily contributing to toxic effects of these or other ocular medications. Punctal occlusion over the nasal lacrimal canal can reduce up to 90% of this absorption. Excess medication overflow should be immediately cleaned and punctal occlusion placed for 3 min to decrease systemic absorption [85, 86].

Postanesthesia Care Unit and the Recovery Period

Monitoring and documentation of all types of anesthetic given to patients must be continued into the recovery phase within the postanesthesia care unit (PACU).

Post-extubation Croup

Small children and infants recovering from general anesthesia are at risk for post-extubation complications such as stridor and dyspnea due to laryngeal swelling. This is seen especially in children convalescing from upper respiratory infections that required an ETT during surgery. The supraglottic airway or LMA may be superior in the aspect of maintaining laryngeal airway patency with less postoperative laryngeal swelling [87].

Postoperative Nausea and Vomiting

Postoperative nausea and vomiting is a major concern following general anesthesia. The risk of PONV may also be elevated due to the type of surgery and its duration even when only sedation is involved, as with surgery on the eye. Children undergoing ocular surgery experience increased incidence of PONV, likely due to a trigeminal-medullary oculo-emetic response, especially following emergence from general anesthesia. Use of inhaled volatile anesthetics, e.g., nitrous oxide, and the inclusion of opioids for pain control are associated with a greater incidence of PONV as is a history of motion sickness. Age of onset of PONV occurs after 2 years of age and increases until puberty, and the risk of PONV in children is thought to be twice that of adults [88]. Prophylaxis against PONV is recommended for those at high risk, and it includes the use of 5-HT_3 antagonists such as ondansetron, the glucocorticoids such as dexamethasone 0.15 mg/kg, and hydration, unless there is a contraindication [88]. Other ancillary medications that can be used effectively to reduce the risk of PONV include clonidine, metoclopramide, droperidol, and substitution of general volatile anesthesia with total IV anesthesia (TIVA) using propofol or dexmedetomidine or some combination thereof.

Ophthalmic surgeries carry one of the highest risks of PONV with an elicitation of the oculocardiac reflex during surgery thought to be predictive of PONV [89]. PONV most frequently occurs in the first 3 h following general anesthesia but can occur up to 24 h after. Persistent PONV in the PACU may herald ongoing acute pressure/volume changes occurring within the eye that may need immediate attention from the surgeon or surgical team [90, 91].

Postoperative Pain

The dissection of extraocular and intraocular tissues is painful and often complicated with postoperative PONV, stressful hemodynamics (high mean arterial pressures), and increased incidence of oculocardiac reflexes (OCR) reflected in the PACU area as moderate pain scores. As mentioned above, the use of a long-acting local anesthetic given via the peribulbar or sub-Tenon route just before emergence from general anesthesia reduces surgical pain and the incidence of PONV. This is due to an effective nerve conduction block of the efferent fibers of the trigeminal nerves that disrupts the trigemino-emetic reflex.

A multimodal approach to pain control best decreases opioid requirement and possibility of PONV. Ketorolac is a nonsteroidal anti-inflammatory drug that can be used topically, via IV or via IM. Acetaminophen is also available in a wide array of formulations, including IV, rectal, pill, or liquid with a low side effect profile.

Intravenous acetaminophen is a novel analgesic for pediatric use in the perioperative period. It offers an alternative or supplement to opioid analgesia when treating surgical pain in term neonates or former preterm infants in whom the reduction of opioid-associated side effects is desirable. Neonates greater than 10 days of age and children weighing up to 33 kg can receive 15 mg/kg every 6 h without evidence of hepatotoxicity. An increase in unconjugated hyperbilirubinemia reflects a low drug clearance, which would dictate lowering the dose [92].

Malignant Hyperthermia

Malignant hyperthermia (MH) is a fatal, unless treated, complication from the use of succinylcholine or volatile anesthetics. There is a hypermetabolic response from these anesthetic triggering agents, which leads to increased intracellular calcium concentration causing an overwhelming metabolic stimulation resulting in increased carbon dioxide and lactic acidosis. This is manifested as tachycardia, tachypnea, and an elevation in body temperature being a late and ominous sign [89]. Treatment involves early recognition with the only antidote, dantrolene. Dantrolene helps to decrease intracellular calcium concentration and should be continued continuously over the next 24 h [93]. An MH reaction often occurs in the operating room but can be delayed to the recovery room after the anesthetic has been terminated. Therefore, there must always exist an index of suspicion when there is unexplained tachycardia, tachypnea, or elevated body temperature that does not respond to normal interventions. Patients that have had previous general anesthetics without an episode of MH are not immune from MH during future anesthetic sessions. Patients on average require three exposures to triggering anesthetic agents to have an MH episode [94, 95].

The suspicion for MH offers a variety of presentations, from sudden death under anesthesia in a family member or the patient may provide a vague history of a family member having an "allergy" to anesthesia. Routine testing is not recommended unless a family member had an MH episode.

The confirmation test for MH is offered only in five centers across the United States and Canada, is extremely expensive, and may not be covered by some insurance plans. The gold standard for diagnosis is the caffeine-halothane contracture test. A person is considered MH susceptible if contracture tests are positive to both caffeine and halothane, and they are considered not susceptible to MH if both tests are negative [95]. Genetic testing is also available for MH as it is autosomal dominant, and the mutation can result de novo. Even if a patient has a negative mutation result, they may still have a positive muscle contracture test deeming them MH susceptible as there are at least 30 causal mutations for MH [96].

Therefore, a diagnosis of MH prior to the operating room is extremely rare unless the patient personally has had a previous reaction. Due to the insidious onset of MH, and difficulty in diagnosis, there is a 24-hour hotline available to anesthesia providers to offer advice regarding symptoms and treatment. If there is a high suspicion for MH, the patient should be scheduled as the first case of the day, and anesthesia machine should be prepared. The vaporizers should ideally be removed from the anesthesia machine, and fresh gas flow should be kept at 10 liters per minute for at least 10 to >90 min depending on the machine. The carbon dioxide canister, breathing circuit, and fresh gas hoses should be new. Each anesthesia machine has different recommendations regarding preparation for a malignant hyperthermia-susceptible patient [96]. Total IV anesthesia (TIVA) should be used to avoid anesthetic vaporizers, and depolarizing muscle relaxants, succinylcholine, should be avoided.

Special Considerations

Many of the children who require anesthesia in the management of childhood glaucoma are healthy and otherwise free of systemic disease such that most anesthesiologists may manage their anesthesia. However, there are those that will require the specialized knowledge of a pediatric anesthesiologist. The following section summarizes the approach to the more complex patients who may exhibit physiologic and/or anatomic abnormalities that occur with various etiologies of secondary glaucoma and present added risk during induction, airway management, and emergence and postoperatively.

Anesthetic Considerations of Pediatric Glaucoma in the Neonate

Primary congenital glaucoma is the commonest glaucoma seen in infants; however many will develop increased IOP secondary to manifestations of syndromes and systemic disease or as a consequence of prematurity [97]. Neonates share a unique physiology that is shifting from that which is adapted to an in utero environment to life outside the uterus, which requires close and careful intraoperative management. Despite vast improvements, perioperative complication rates, morbidity, and mortality remain disproportionately high in neonates undergoing general anesthesia [3, 5, 97, 98]. The incidence of perioperative neonatal (less than 30 days of life) mortality after cardiac arrest is estimated to be 144.7 per 10,000 anesthetics (0.014%) compared to 2.1 deaths per 10,000 anesthetics (0.00021%) in children aged greater than 10 years (overall mortality 6.8 per 10,000 anesthetics) [5]. Factors which contribute to higher mortality rates include level of preoperative illness, neonatal/infant physiology with depressed cardiopulmonary reserves, and surgical complexity. Neonates, infants, and preterm infants are at an increased risk of apnea due to immaturity of their respiratory center, underdeveloped chemoreceptor responses to CO_2 levels in the blood, and delayed laryngeal reflexes.

While glaucoma surgery in the neonate is considered low risk for adverse cardiopulmonary events, carrying the neonate through an anesthetic brings to the forefront several issues of concern which are unique to the population and include intracardiac shunting with patent foramen ovale or ductus arteriosus open, immature cardiopulmonary physiology that is heart rate dependent, tendencies toward rapid desaturation, and a narrow range of temperature and glucose homeostasis. Furthermore, immature renal function with decreased glomerular filtration rates, compared to adults, impacts many administered anesthetic drugs and sensitivity to opioids and inhaled agents. Anatomical differences of the airway lend to difficult intubation and ventilation in the inexperienced provider, and finally a large percentage of these neonates will have associated congenital anomalies requiring increased vigilance and care [99].

Neurotoxicity and the Neonate Newborns are very susceptible to anesthetics, and the requirement needs to be measured carefully against the urgency, type, and length of surgery. For the past decade, anesthesia-related neurotoxicity risks in newborns and infants have been a topic of interest worldwide. Although epidemiological evidence has not been consistent, it does appear to indicate that neurotoxicity may result after prolonged or repeated exposures to anesthetics early in life [99, 100]. The decision to subject a child to an EUA should not be taken lightly and should be performed with the view to aiding clinical decision-making. Concerns of neurotoxicity should be considered in the context of a disease, which is potentially blinding if not adequately assessed or managed.

Programmed cell death, apoptosis, is an important factor during the development and remodeling of all multicellular organisms, in this case, neuronal tissue. Commonly used anesthetic agents increase neuro-apoptosis and have neurodegenerative effects after exposure in the neonatal period of rodents [99]. Systematic reviews of preclinical and clinical studies have suggested a strong indication of increased neuronal apoptosis after general anesthesia exposure in piglets and nonhuman primates. Studies on rodents and primates support a causal relationship between anesthesia and neonatal neurotoxicity [101]. Retrospective clinical human data in epidemiologic studies saw 10,450 siblings born in 1999, enrolled in the New York State Medicaid program, and found that the incidence of behavioral and developmental problems was 128.2 diagnosis per 1000 person-years for the exposed group compared to 56.3 diagnosis per 1000 non-exposed group. The FDA gave a safety alert advisory to health-care professionals. Health-care professionals are to "balance the benefit of appropriate anesthesia in young children and pregnant women against the risks." This is markedly important for cases that may run longer than 3 h or when multiple procedures are required in one patient less than 3 years of age.

These studies were compromised by methodological issues and have been deemed important but nonconclusive. The GAS study (general anesthesia vs. spinal) and the PANDA study (Pediatric Anesthesia and Neurodevelopmental Assessment study) were able to support that a single short anesthetic exposure was not associated with neurodevelopmental compromise [102, 103]. Thoughtful consideration should be given to brain developmental stages. General anesthetics may have an impact on future cognitive and behavioral milestones in humans.

Anesthetic Implications of Childhood Glaucoma Associated with Systemic Disease

A majority of childhood glaucoma cases presenting to the operating suite can be considered to be primary glaucoma with defects limited to one or both eyes and no systemic syndrome or disease. Secondary childhood glaucoma occurs when an independent disease process impairs the ocular filtration system [104–106] which results from an impressive array of clinical conditions, some of which are associated with systemic abnormalities affecting one or more organ systems.

The classification of childhood glaucoma has undergone multiple iterations [99–101], with the latest system as that proposed by the Childhood Glaucoma Research Network and validated by the World Glaucoma Association Consensus on Childhood Glaucoma [107]. Regardless of classification method, it is apparent that a significant proportion of childhood glaucoma is an ocular manifestation of systemic disease. Upward of 36% of all eyes with the diagnosis of childhood glaucoma have secondary glaucoma, i.e., glaucoma associated with non-acquired systemic disease/syndrome, or have an association with an acquired condition [96], and over 45 unique syndromes have been linked to childhood glaucoma [104]. As such, it is imperative for the diagnosing clinician as well as the consultant pediatric anesthesiologist to recognize associated systemic disease or syndromes because of the potential problems for those who require anesthesia, surgery, or intensive acute care management. Children born with these rare syndromes may have problems associated with cardiopulmonary disease and congenital malformations, facial dysmorphisms resulting in difficulties with intubation and/or ventilation, and neurologic effects such as seizure disorders and increased ICPs [108]. These phenotypic manifestations present significant risk during general anesthesia and require careful planning and specific modifications to the anesthetic technique to ensure safe perioperative care. Several of the most common disorders and conditions associated with childhood glaucoma are summarized in Table 2.5 [109–116].

The Cardiopulmonary System in a Syndromic Child Congenital heart disease is a prevalent finding in this cohort of syndromic children. Because the association is so strong, neonates born with dysmorphic features and heart murmur undergo detailed cardiac evaluation and imaging to rule out congenital cardiac disease [117]. A typical childhood glaucoma practice will encounter infants and children who carry structural and functional cardiac defects because many of the syndromes associated with non-acquired glaucoma carry strong associations with congenital cardiac defects, as well. For example, trisomy 13 (Patau syndrome) and trisomy 21 (Down syndrome) each are at high risk for cardiac involvement; in fact, 80% and 50% of afflicted children will have significant congenital cardiac involvement, respectively [115, 116].

The presence of congenital heart disease alone adds considerable perioperative risk and increases perioperative mortality by twofold [118, 119]. Accordingly, children with congenital heart

Table 2.5 Systemic effects and corresponding anesthetic considerations of several common etiologies of secondary childhood glaucoma

Systems affected						
	Cardiovascular	Respiratory	HEENT/airway	Neurologic/ neuromuscular	Metabolic/endocrine	Anesthetic considerations
Glaucoma associated with non-acquired systemic disease or syndrome						
Phacomatoses (64%)						
Sturge-weber (involves the brain, skin, and eyes; ipsilateral vascular anomalies of meninges [leptomeningeal angioma], port-wine stain)	Coarctation of the aorta, visceral/ intraoral angiomatoses, cutaneous hemangiomata, possible AV shunting and HF	–	Hemangiomas of the lips, buccal mucosa, macrocheilia, palate and tongue involvement	Seizures beginning in infancy, intracranial calcifications, leptomeningeal angiomas (98%), hemiparesis, hemianopia, cerebral cortex atrophy	–	Evaluate neurological function closely (EEG imaging), and evaluate heart and airway for malformation presence. Baseline blood and coagulation lab values. Intraoperatively, consider oral vascular involvement and potential for bleeding when planning for intubation. Avoid regional anesthesia due to meningeal hemangioma. Pulse oximetry may be difficult due to capillary anomalies. Avoid medications that reduce seizure threshold, continue anti-epileptic medications up to surgery, and consider neurology consultation for seizure management in severe cases
Klippel-Trenaunay-weber (port-wine stain, abnormal overgrowth of soft tissues and bones, and vein malformations)	Venous and cutaneous capillary malformation, lymphatic abnormalities	Vein malformations → risk of DVT and PE	–	Cerebral aneurysms, spinal cord AVM	Soft tissues/bony hyperplasia	80% of spinal cord lesions rupture/bleed at some point. Avoid cough/Valsalva maneuvers. Baseline blood lab values should be obtained. Obtain neurologic evaluation to localize malformations and avoid perioperative hypertension. Blunt hemodynamic responses to laryngoscopy/surgical stimulation and extubation. Central neuraxial techniques are contraindicated. Avoid triggers and institute prevention techniques for PONV

Neurofibromatosis (skin pigmentation [cafe au lait spots] and benign nerve tumor growth along the skin, brain, and other parts of the body)	Possible thoracic/ abdominal aorta coarctation, renal artery stenosis → HTN	–	Macrocephaly, possible laryngeal/pharyngeal neurofibromas → difficult ventilation/ intubation	Multiple neurofibromas of the skin and nerves, scoliosis, seizures. Frequent involvement of spinal cord	Possible association with pheochromocytoma/ MEN IIB	Consider reviewing MRI to r/o tumor formation in the cervical spine, brain stem, airway or anterior mediastinum. Avoid neuraxial techniques because of possible spinal column involvement. Nerve monitoring is essential, and one may need to tailor the use of muscle relaxants
Chromosomal disorders						
Trisomy 13 (specific midline dysmorphic features, severe intellectual disability, and abnormalities affecting multiple body systems)	Highly associated (80%), VSD/ ASD, aortic coarctation, PDA, cardiomyopathy, dextrocardia	Apneic episodes possible. Bi-lobed lung	Cleft lip (60–80%) +/– palate, deafness, airway and nose abnormalities, choanal atresia	Severe development delay, motor seizures, microcephaly, microphthalmia, absent corpus callosum, spina bifida	Feeding difficulties, failure to thrive	Evaluation of cardiac, urologic, neurological function and anatomy for potential airway difficulties. Challenging mask ventilation. Latex precautions with spina bifida. Consider postoperative inpatient observation. Death often occurs before 6 months of life
Trisomy 21 (associated with intellectual disability, a characteristic facial appearance, and hypotonia in infancy)	Congenital heart disease (50%): VDS, ASD, AV canal defect, endocardial cushion defect	Recurrent lung infections	Microphthalmia, macroglossia, pharyngeal hypotonia, subglottic stenosis, obstructive sleep apnea, midface hypoplasia, high narrow arch	Atlantoaxial instability, cognitive and motor delay with hypotonia	Congenital hypothyroidism, immune deficiency	Anticipate difficult intravenous access. Potential for perioperative airway obstruction. Cervical instability may cause post-intubation subluxation. If symptomatic, cervical spine films and smaller endotracheal tube should be used for intubation. Preoperative cardiac evaluations should be considered in view of potential bradycardia on inhalation inductions. Consider post-op observation or admission if airway difficulties/obstruction exists

(continued)

Table 2.5 (continued)

Systems affected						
	Cardiovascular	Respiratory	HEENT/airway	Neurologic/ neuromuscular	Metabolic/endocrine	Anesthetic considerations
Connective tissue disorders						
Stickler syndrome (progressive arthro-ophthalmology condition affecting eyes, face, and joints)	Mitral valve prolapse (50%)	–	Flat distinctive face, sensorineural deafness (10%), myopia, PRS (10%) → retrognathia, glossoptosis, airway obstruction +/–cleft palate	Intracranial calcifications, normal intellect	Bony enlargement of joints at birth, hypermobility	Cardiac evaluation preoperatively. PRS strongly associated—Prepare for difficult intubation. Examine joint mobility, and position carefully. Consider regional anesthetic
Marfan syndrome (generalized connective tissue disorder with weakness of the connective tissues)	Valvular (MVP, TR, MR) or aortic root dissection (progressive into adulthood)	Intrinsic lung involvement—Emphysema, bronchogenic cysts → spontaneous/ tension pneumothoraces, restrictive lung disease from vertebral/chest wall deformities	Temporomandibular joint at risk of subluxation or dislocation → difficult intubation	High-arched palate	Hyperextensible joints, disproportionately long extremities, pectus excavatum, kyphoscoliosis	Cardiopulmonary evaluation. Careful mechanical ventilation to avoid barotrauma-induced pneumothoraces. Careful positioning and protection of joints. Control blood pressure and lung pressures under anesthesia. Neonatal/infantile form: Lax skin, scoliosis, adducted thumbs, extremity contractures, micrognathia, muscle hypoplasia, ectopia lentis, severe cardiac valve insufficiency/aortic dilatation resulting in early death
Craniofacial						
Rubinstein-Taybi (short stature; moderate/severe developmental delay distinctive facial features; broad thumbs and first toes; and other cardiac, digestive and respiratory malformations)	33% cardiac defects (PDA, ASD, or VSD)	Frequent respiratory infections, asthma	Characteristic facies (100%)—Microcephaly (84%), micrognathia (100%), choanal atresia, narrow mouth/palate, frontal bossing, hearing loss/low-set ears; feeding/swallowing difficulties	Significant development delay (100%), corpus callosum agenesis, hypotonia, hyperreflexia, seizures. Association with neurological tumors (neuroblastoma, meningioma)	Short stature (94%), scoliosis	Evaluate cardiac function and thorough airway examination. Risk of pulmonary aspiration due to GI anomalies. Difficult laryngoscopy with facial malformations

Glaucoma associated with non-acquired ocular conditions						
Rieger syndrome/ SHORT syndrome (short stature, hyperextensibility of joints or hernia or both, ocular depression, Rieger anomaly, and teething delay) when *without* dental/skeletal defects	–	–	Maxillary > mandibular hypoplasia, midface hypoplasia, dental hypoplasia	Myotonic dystrophy (rare reports with Rieger syndrome), sensorineural deafness, development and speech delays	Pituitary deficiencies: Adrenal insufficiency, short stature, low birth weight dwarfism, lipoatrophy, DM	Perioperative glucose monitoring—Fasting and glucose/ insulin requirements will depend on severity of DM. Hyperextensible joints—Manipulate the neck and joints during positioning with care. Look out for low birth weights in neonatal period. Cautious use of NDNMB due to unpredictable paralytic response. Dental and craniofacial abnormalities may lead to difficult airway
Glaucoma associated with acquired conditions						
Retinopathy of prematurity (common blinding disease in neonates associated with delayed retinal vascular growth and hypoxia-induced pathological growth)	Immature sympathetic nervous system, proclivity of bradycardia	Apnea of prematurity risk with anemia and GA, BPD, history of prolonged intubation secondary to lung immaturity	Anatomic variation of the neonatal airway	Intravertebral hemorrhage, seizures in the extreme prematurity	Possible hypotonia, immature glucose regulation, immature hepatic metabolism of medications	Avoid hypoxemia. May require overnight stay if outpatient procedure. EUA may be done at bedside in NICU if inpatient

(continued)

Table 2.5 (continued)

Systems affected						
	Cardiovascular	Respiratory	HEENT/airway	Neurologic/ neuromuscular	Metabolic/endocrine	Anesthetic considerations
Intraocular neoplasms						
Retinoblastoma (familial malignant ocular tumor of the retina caused by defect in specific Rb regulatory gene)	–	–	–	Potential local invasion or into optic nerve	Late disease with bone metastasis	Can be associated with other primary malignancies (leukemia, lymphoma, pinealoma, Ewing or osteogenic sarcoma) and 13q syndromes. Caution during administration of laser therapy (safety risk) and during intra-arterial chemotherapy → a severe bronchospastic reaction (autonomic cardiorespiratory reflex) and hemodynamic instability, which requires treatment with epinephrine). Children undergo many anesthetics and likely develop significant associated anxiety

ASD Atrial septal defect, *AV Arteriovenous, AVM Arteriovenous malformation, BPD* Bronchopulmonary dysplasia, *CHD* Congenital heart disease, *DM* Diabetes mellitus, *DVT* Deep vein thrombosis, *EEG* Electroencephalography, *EUA* Examination under anesthesia, *GA* General anesthesia, *GI* Gastrointestinal, *HEENT* Head, ears, eyes, nose, throat, *HF* Heart failure, *HTN* Hypertension, *MEN* Multiple endocrine neoplasia, *MR* Mitral regurgitation, *MRI* Magnetic resonance imaging, *MVP* Mitral valve prolapse, *NDNMB* Non-depolarizing neuromuscular blockade, *NICU* Neonatal intensive care unit, *PDA* Patent ductus arteriosus, *PE* Pulmonary embolism, *PONV* Postoperative nausea and vomiting, *PRS* Pierre Robin sequence, *SHORT* Mnemonic for short stature, hyperextensibility, ocular depression (deeply set eyes), Rieger anomaly, and teething delay, *TR* Tricuspid regurgitation, *VSD* Ventral septal defect

Note: For neurofibromatosis type 1, Klippel-Trenaunay syndrome, Sturge-Weber syndrome, trisomy 13, Down syndrome, and Stickler syndrome, see also the US Dept. of Health and Human Services, US National Library of Medicine, Genetics Home Reference. https://ghr.nlm.nih.gov/about

disease must undergo careful evaluation and optimization prior to entering the perioperative setting, which will include detailed records of the structural and functional anatomy. Additionally, all procedural and surgical history—palliative versus corrective—and current cardiac function should be provided for review and appropriate risk assessment [120].

Several factors will impact the plan for the anesthetic care of these patients. The nature, complexity, and status of surgical repair, as well as the presence of significant intracardiac shunting of blood, will determine whether the additional expertise of pediatric anesthesiologists with subspecialty training in congenital cardiac anesthesia will be necessary. Furthermore, the choice of anesthesia medications, IV access location, and need for invasive monitoring in those with limited hemodynamic reserve and careful choosing of location of perioperative care (i.e., choosing a hospital operative setting rather than outpatient ambulatory surgery center) which should be at a pediatric center with those familiar with the care of these individuals will be tailored accordingly [121]. After anesthesia exposure or surgical intervention, some of these children may require extended observation in the postanesthesia recovery unit or inpatient admission for close continuous monitoring. With appropriate and complete preoperative evaluation, experienced anesthesiologist care, appropriate use of agents, techniques, and invasive monitoring, anesthetic care in children with congenital heart disease can be safe and effective during the bulk of noncardiac surgeries.

References

1. Cullen KA, Hall MJ, Golosinskiy A. Ambulatory surgery in the United States, 2006. Natl Health Stat Report. 2009;11:1–2.
2. August DA, Everett LL. Pediatric ambulatory anesthesia. Anesthesiol Clin. 2014;32(2):411–29.
3. Cohen MM, Cameron CB, Duncan PG. Pediatric anesthesia morbidity and mortality in the perioperative period. Anesth Analg. 1990;70(2):160–7.
4. Bhananker SM, Ramamoorthy C, Geiduschek JM, Posner KL, Domino KB, Haberkern CM, et al. Anesthesia-related cardiac arrest in children: update from the Pediatric Perioperative Cardiac Arrest Registry. Anesth Analg. 2007;105(2):344–50.
5. Flick RP, Sprung J, Harrison TE, Gleich SJ, Schroeder DR, Hanson AC, et al. Perioperative cardiac arrests in children between 1988 and 2005 at a tertiary referral center: a study of 92,881 patients. Anesthesiology. 2007;106(2):226–37. quiz 413–4
6. Ramamoorthy C, Haberkern CM, Bhananker SM, Domino KB, Posner KL, Campos JS, Morray JP. Anesthesia-related cardiac arrest in children with heart disease: data from the Pediatric Perioperative Cardiac Arrest (POCA) registry. Anesth Analg. 2010;110(5):1376–82.
7. Committee on Standards and Practice Parameters, Apfelbaum JL, Connis RT, Nickinovich DG, American Society of Anesthesiologists Task Force on Preanesthesia Evaluation, Pasternak LR, Arens JF, Caplan RA, et al. Practice advisory for preanesthesia evaluation. An updated report by the American Society of Anesthesiologists Task Force on Pre-anesthesia Evaluation. Anesthesiology. 2012;116(3):522–38.
8. Bryson GL, Chung F, Finegan BA, Friedman Z, Miller DR, van Vlymen J, et al. Canadian Ambulatory Anesthesia Research Education group. Patient selection in ambulatory anesthesia - an evidence-based review: part I. Can J Anaesth. 2004;51(8):768–81. Review
9. Bryson GL, Chung F, Cox RG, Crowe MJ, Fuller J, Henderson C, et al. Canadian Ambulatory Anesthesia Research Education group. Patient selection in ambulatory anesthesia - an evidence-based review: part II. Can J Anaesth. 2004;51(8):782–94. Review
10. Heinrich S, Birkholz T, Ihmsen H, Irouschek A, Ackermann A, Schmidt J. Incidence and predictors of difficult laryngoscopy in 11,219 pediatric anesthesia procedures. Paediatr Anaesth. 2012;22(8):729–36.
11. Heinrich S, Birkholz T, Ihmsen H, Irouschek A, Ackermann A, Cesnjevar R, Schmidt J. Incidence and predictors of poor laryngoscopic view in children undergoing pediatric cardiac surgery. J Cardiothorac Vasc Anesth. 2013;27(3):516–21.
12. Mirghassemi A, Soltani AE, Abtahi M. Evaluation of laryngoscopic views and related influencing factors in a pediatric population. Paediatr Anaesth. 2011;21(6):663–7.
13. Crosby ET, Cooper RM, Douglas MJ, Doyle DJ, Hung OR, Labrecque P, et al. The unanticipated difficult airway with recommendations for management. Can J Anaesth. 1998;45(8):757–76. Review
14. Kumar HV, Schroeder JW, Gang Z, Sheldon SH. Mallampati score and pediatric obstructive apnea. J Clin Sleep Med. 2014;10(9):985–90.
15. American Academy of Pediatrics, American Academy of Pediatric Dentistry, Coté CJ, Wilson S, Work Group on Sedation. Guidelines for monitoring and management of pediatric patients during and

after sedation for diagnostic and therapeutic procedures: an update. Pediatrics. 2006;118(6):2587–602.
16. American Society of Anesthesiologists. ASA physical status classification system. Last approved by the ASA House of Delegates on 15 Oct 2014. https://www.asahq.org/resources/clinical-information/asa-physical-status-classification-system. Accessed 17 Jun 2017.
17. Motas D, McDermott NB, VanSickle T, Friesen RH. Depth of consciousness and deep sedation attained in children as administered by nonanesthesiologists in a children's hospital. Pediatri Anaesth. 2004;14(3):256–0.
18. American Academy of Pediatrics, American Academy of Pediatric Dentistry. Guideline for monitoring and management of pediatric patients during and after sedation for diagnostic and therapeutic procedures. Pediatr Dent. 2008–2009;30(7 Suppl):143–59.
19. Practice guidelines for preoperative fasting and the use of pharmacologic agents to reduce the risk of pulmonary aspiration: application to healthy patients undergoing elective procedures. An updated report by the American Society of Anesthesiologists Taskforce on Preoperative Fasting and the Use of Pharmacologic Agents to Reduce the Risk of Pulmonary Aspiration. Anesthesiology. 2017;126(3):376–93.
20. Olsson GL, Hallen B, Hambraeus-Jonzon K. Aspiration during anaesthesia: a computer-aided study of 185,358 anaesthetics. Acta Anaesthesiolo Scand. 1986;30(1):84–92.
21. Benington S, Severn A. Preventing aspiration and regurgitation. Anesth Intensive Care Med. 2007;8(9):368–72.
22. Malviya S, Voepel-Lewis T, Tait AR, Merkel S, Tremper K, Naughton N. Depth of sedation in children undergoing computed tomography; validity and reliability of the University of Michigan Sedation Scale (UMSS). Br J Anaesth. 2002;88(2):241–5.
23. Green SM, Mason KP, Krauss BS. Ketamine and propofol sedation by emergency medicine specialists: mainstream or menace? Br J Anaesth. 2016;116(4):449–51.
24. Dial S, Silver P, Bock K, Sagy M. Pediatric sedation for procedures titrated to a desired degree of immobility results in unpredictable depth of sedation. Pediatr Emerg Care. 2001;17(6):414–20.
25. Oberacher-Velten I, Prasser C, Rochon J, Ittner KP, Helbig H, Lorenz B. The effect of midazolam on intraocular pressure in children during examination under sedation. Br J Ophthalmol. 2011;95(8):1102–5.
26. Fazi L, Jantzen EC, Rose JB, Kurth CD, Watcha MF. A comparison of oral clonidine and oral midazolam as preanesthetic medications in the pediatric tonsillectomy patients. Anesth Analg. 2001;92(1):56–61.
27. Gobeaux D, Sardinal F. Midazolam and flumazenil in ophthalmology. Acta Anaesthesthiol Scand Suppl. 1990;92:35–8.
28. Nagdeve NG, Yaddanapudi S, Pandav SS. The effect of different doses of ketamine on intraocular pressure in anesthetized children. J Pediatr Ophthalmol Strabismus. 2006;43(4):219–23.
29. Kim KS, Kwak HJ, Min SK, Lee SY, Kim KM, Kim JY. The effect of ketamine on tracheal intubating conditions without neuromuscular blockade during sevoflurane induction in children. J Anesthesia. 2011;25(2):195–9.
30. Morris C, Perris A, Klein J, Mahoney P. Anesthesia in haemodynamically compromised patients: does ketamine represent the best choice of induction agent? Anesthesiology. 2009;64(5):532–9.
31. Sator-Katzenschlager S, Deusch E, Dolezal S, Michalek-Sauberer A, Grubmüller R, Heinze G, Wedrich A. Sevoflurane and propofol decrease intraocular pressure equally during non-ophthalmic surgery and recovery. Br J Anaesth. 2002;89(5):764–6.
32. Schäfer R, Klett J, Auffarth G, Polarz H, Völcker HE, Martin E, Böttiger BW. Intraocular pressure more reduced during anesthesia with propofol than with Sevoflurane: both combined with remifentanil. Acta Anaesthesiol Scand. 2002;46(6):703–6.
33. Neel S, Deitch R Jr, Moorthy SS, Dierdorf S, Yee R. Changes in intraocular pressure during low dose intravenous sedation with propofol before cataract surgery. Br J Ophthalmol. 1995;79(12):1093–7.
34. Lauretti GR, Lauretti CR, Lauretti-Fihlo A. Propofol decreases ocular pressure in outpatients undergoing trabeculectomy. J Clin Anaesth. 1997;9(4):289–92.
35. Cravero JP, Beach ML, Blike GT, Gallagher SM, Hertzog JH, Pediatric Sedation Research Consortium. The incidence and nature of adverse events during pediatric sedation/anesthesia with propofol for procedures outside the operating room: a report from the Pediatric Sedation Research Consortium. Anesth Analg. 2009;108(3):795–804.
36. Asserhøj LL, Mosbech H, Krøigaard M, Garvey LH. No evidence for contraindications to the use of propofol in adults allergic to egg, soy or peanut. Br J Anaesth. 2016;116(1):77–82.
37. Mahmoud M, Gunter J, Donnelly LF, Wang Y, Nick TG, Sadhasivam S. A comparison of Dexmedetomidine with propofol for magnetic resonance imaging sleep studies in children. Anesth Analg. 2009;109(3):745–53.
38. Deutsch E, Tobias JD. Hemodynamic and respiratory changes following dexmedetomidine administration during general anesthesia: sevoflurane vs desflurane. Pediatr Anesth. 2007;17(5):438–44.
39. Mason KP, Zgleszewski S, Forman RE, Stark C, DiNardo JA. An exaggerated hypertensive response to glycopyrrolate therapy for bradycardia associated with high dose dexmedetomidine. Anesth Analg. 2009;108(3):906–8.
40. Mason KP, Lerman J. Dexmedetomidine in children: current knowledge and future applications. Anesth Analg. 2011;113(5):1129–42.

41. Termühlen J, Gottschalk A, Eter N, Hoffmann EM, Van Aken H, Grenzebach U, Prokosch V. Does general anesthesia have a clinical impact on intraocular pressure in children? Paediatr Anaesth. 2016;26(9):936–41.
42. Bhargava AK, Setlur R, Sreevastava D. Correlation of bispectral index and Guedel's stages of ether anesthesia. Anesth Analg. 2004;98(1):132–4.
43. Blumberg D, Congdon N, Jampel H, Gilbert D, Elliott R, Rivers R, et al. The effects of sevoflurane and ketamine on intraocular pressure in children during examination under anesthesia. Am J Ophthalmol. 2007;143(3):494–9.
44. Korenfeld MS, Dueker DK. Review of external ocular compression: clinical applications of the ocular pressure estimator. Clin Ophthalmol. 2016;10:343–57.
45. Verghese C, Brimacombe JR. Survey of laryngeal mask airway usage in 11,910 patients: safety and efficacy for conventional and nonconventional usage. Anesth Analg. 1996;82(1):129–33.
46. Bhardwaj N, Yaddanapudi S, Singh S, Pandav SS. Insertion of laryngeal mask airway does not increase the intraocular pressure in children with glaucoma. Paediatr Anesth. 2011;21(10):1036–40.
47. Stillman PC. Lingual oedema associated with the prolonged use of an inappropriately large laryngeal mask airway (LMARM) in an infant. Paediatr Anaesth. 2003;13(7):637–9.
48. Akhtar TM, Street MK. Risk of aspiration with a laryngeal mask airway. Br J Anaesth. 1994;72(4):447–50.
49. Marjot R. Pressure exerted by the laryngeal mask airway cuff upon the pharyngeal mucosa. Br J Anaesth. 1993;70(1):25–9.
50. Mathis MR, Haydar B, Taylor EL, Morris M, Malviya SV, Christensen RE, et al. Failure of the Laryngeal Mask Airway Unique™ and Classic™ in the pediatric surgical patient: a study of clinical predictors and outcomes. Anesthesiology. 2013;119(6):1284–95.
51. Berdahl JP, Fautsch MP, Stinnett SS, Allingham RR. Intracranial pressure in primary open angle glaucoma, normal tension glaucoma, and ocular hypertension: a case-control study. Invest Ophthalmol Vis Sci. 2008;49(12):5412–8.
52. Ozcan MS, Praetel C, Bhatti MT, Gravenstein N, Mahla ME, Seubert CN. The effect of body inclination during prone positioning on intraocular pressure in awake volunteers: a comparison of two operating tables. Anesth Analg. 2004;99(4):115–8.
53. Chiu CL, Jaais F, Wang CY. Effect of rocuronium compared with succinylcholine on intraocular pressure during rapid sequence induction anesthesia. Br J Anaesth. 1999;82(5):757–60.
54. Murphy DF. Anesthesia and intraocular pressure. Anesth Analg. 1985;64(5):520–30.
55. Cymbor M, Knapp E, Carlin F. Idiopathic elevated episcleral venous pressure with secondary glaucoma. Optom Vic Sci. 2013;90(7):e213–7.
56. Teba L, Viti A, Banks DE, Fons A, Barbera M, Hshieh PB. Intraocular pressure during mechanical ventilation with different levels of positive end-expiratory pressure. Crit Care Med. 1993;21(6):867–70.
57. Cunningham AJ. Intraocular pressure – physiology and implications for anesthetic management. Can Anaesth Soc J. 1986;33(2):195–208.
58. Okafor KC, Brandt JD. Measuring intraocular pressure. Curr Opin Ophthalmol. 2015;26(2):103–9.
59. Mamikonian VR, Galoian NS, Sheremet NL, Kazarian EE, Kharlap SI, Shmeleva-Demir OA, et al. Peculiarities of ocular blood flow in ischemic optic neuropathy and normal tension glaucoma. Vestn Oftalmol. 2013, 129(4):3–8. *(Article in Russian)*
60. Singleton CD, Robertson D, Byrne DW, Joos KM. Effect of posture on blood and intraocular pressures in multiple system atrophy, pure autonomic failure and baroreflex failure. Circulation. 2003;108(19):2349–54.
61. Nathanson JA. Adrenergic regulation of intraocular pressure: identification of beta-2-adrenergic-simulated adenylate cyclase in ciliary process epithelium. Proc Natl Acad Sci U S A. 1980;77(12):7420–4.
62. McDougal DH, Graham PD. Autonomic control of the eye. Compr Physiol. 2015;5(1):439–73.
63. Kreiglstein CK, Langham ME, Leydhecker W. The peripheral and central neural action of clonidine in normal and glaucomatous eyes. Invest Ophthalmol Vis Sci. 1978;17(2):149–58.
64. Oltulu R, Satirtav G, Ersan I, Soylu E, Okka M, Zengin N. Effect of dehydration and fasting on corneal biomechanical properties and intraocular pressures. Eye Contact Lens. 2016;42(6):392–4.
65. Hunt AP, Feigl B, Stewart IB. The intraocular pressure response to dehydration: a pilot study. Eur J Appl Physiol. 2012;112(5):1963–6.
66. Mikhail M, Sabri K, Levin AV. The effect of anesthesia on intraocular pressure measurement in children. Surv Ophthalmol. 2017;62(5):648–58.
67. Lalwani K, Fox EB, Fu R, Edmunds B, Kelly LD. The effect of nitrous oxide on intra-ocular pressure in healthy adults. Anaesthesia. 2012;67(3):256–60.
68. Shibata S, Shigeomi S, Sato W, Enzan K. Nitrous oxide administration during washout of sevoflurane improves post anesthetic agitation in children. J Anesth. 2005;12(2):160–3.
69. Lee EJ. Use of nitrous oxide causing severe visual loss 37 days after retinal surgery. Br J Anaesth. 2004;93(3):464–6.
70. TerRiet MF, DeSouza GJ, Jacobs JS, Young D, Lewis MC, Herrington C, Gold MI. Which is more pungent: isoflurane, sevoflurane or desflurane? Br J Anaesth. 2000;85(2):305–7.
71. Eber TJ, Muzi M. Sympathetic hyperactivity during desflurane anesthesia in healthy volunteers. A comparison with isoflurane. Anesthesiology. 1993;79(3):444–53.

72. Part TJ, Lim HK, Jang KY Um DJ. The effects of desflurane and sevoflurane on the intraocular pressure associated with endotracheal intubation in pediatric ophthalmic surgery. Korean J Anesthesiol. 2013;64(2):117–21.
73. Yodhikawa K, Murai Y. The effect of ketamine on intraocular pressure in children. Anesth Analg. 1971;50(2):199–202.
74. Jones L, Sung V, Lascaratos G, Nagi H, Holder R. Intraocular pressure after ketamine and sevoflurane in children with glaucoma undergoing examination under anesthesia. Br J Ophthalmol. 2010;94(1):33–5.
75. Vanlander AV, Okun JG, de Jaeger A, Smet J, De Latter E, De Paepe B, et al. Possible pathogenic mechanism of propofol infusion syndrome involves coenzyme Q. Anesthesiology. 2015;122(2):343–52.
76. Vanlander AV, Jorens PG, Smet J, De Paepe B, Verbrugghe W, Van den Eynden GG, et al. Inborn oxidative phosphorylation defect as risk factor for propofol infusion syndrome. Acta Anaesthesiol Scand. 2012;56(4):530–5.
77. Molina-Infante J, Arias A, Vara-Brenes D, Prados-Manzano R, Gonzalez-Cervera J, Alvarado-Arenas M, Lucendo AJ. Propofol administration is safe in adult eosinophilic patients sensitized to egg, soy or peanut. Allergy. 2014;69(3):388–94.
78. Alipour M, Derakhshan A, Pourmazar R, Abrishami M, Ghanbarabadi VG. Effects of propofol, etomidate and thiopental on intraocular pressure and hemodynamic responses in pharmacoemulsification by insertion of laryngeal mask airway. J Ocul Pharmacol Ther. 2014;30(8):665–9.
79. Besunder IB, Reed MD, Blumer IL. Principles of drug bio disposition in the neonate. A critical evaluation of the pharmacologic-pharmacodynamic interface (Part I). Clin Pharmacokinet. 1998;14(4):189–216.
80. Mulroy MF. Systemic toxicity and Cardiotoxicity from local anesthetics: incidence and preventative measures. Reg Anesth Pain Med. 2002;27(6):556–61.
81. Litz RJ, Roessel T, Heller AR, Stehr SN. Reversal of central nervous system and cardiac toxicity after local anesthetic intoxication by lipid emulsion injection. Anesth Analg. 2008;106(5):1575–7.
82. Weinberg GL. Lipid emulsion infusion: resuscitation for local anesthetic and other drug over dose. Anesthesiology. 2012;117(1):180–7.
83. Patel Z, Palte HP, Tutiven J. Postoperative analgesia and infant vitreoretinal surgery. Paediatr Anaesth. 2012;22(12):1225–6.
84. Tocchio S, Kline-Fath B, Kanal E, Schmithorst VJ, Panigrahy A. MRI evaluation and safety in the developing brain. Semin Perinatol. 2015;39(2):73–104.
85. Malihi M, MaLaren JW, Sit AJ. Effect of topical anesthesia on episcleral venous pressure in normal human subjects. Invest Ophthalmol Vic Sci. 2015;56(5):2968–70.
86. Guidelines for the ethical conduct of studies to evaluate drugs in pediatric populations. Committee on drugs, American Academy of Pediatrics. Pediatrics. 1995;95(2):286–94.
87. Tanaka A, Isono S, Ishikawa T, Sato J, Nishino T. Laryngeal resistance before and after minor surgery: endotracheal tube versus laryngeal mask airway. Anesthesiol. 2003;99(2):252–8.
88. Sayed JA, F Riad MA, M Ali MO. Comparison of dexmedetomidine or intravenous fluids or combination of both on postoperative nausea, vomiting and pain in pediatric strabismus surgery. J Clin Anaesth. 2016;34:136–42.
89. Allen LE, Sudesh S, Sandramouli S, Cooper G, McFarlane D, Willshaw HE. The association between the oculocardiac reflex and post-operative vomiting in children undergoing strabismus surgery. Eye (Lond). 1998;12(Pt 2):193–6.
90. Villeret I, Laffon M, Duchalais A, Blond MH, Lecuyer AI, Mercier C. Incidence of postoperative nausea and vomiting in paediatric ambulatory surgery. Paediatr Anaesth. 2002;12(8):712–7.
91. Gupta N, Kumar R, Kumar S, Sehgal R, Sharma KR. A prospective randomized double blind study to evaluate the effect of peribulbar block or topical application of local anaesthetic combined with general anaesthesia on intraoperative and postoperative complications during paediatric strabismus surgery. Anaesthesiol. 2007;62(11):1110–3.
92. Palmer GM, Atkins M, Anderson BJ, Smith KR, Culnane TJ, McNally CM, et al. I.V. Acetaminophen pharmacokinetics in neonates after multiple doses. Br J Anaesth. 2008;101(4):523–30.
93. Hopkins PM. Malignant hyperthermia: advances in clinical management and diagnosis. Br J Anaesth. 2000;85(1):118–28.
94. Krause T, Gerbershagen MU, Fiege M, Weisshorn R, Wappler F. Dantrolene—a review of its pharmacology, therapeutic use and new developments. Anaesthesia. 2004;59(4):364–73.
95. Rosenberg H, Pollock N, Schiemann A, Bulger T, Stowell K. Malignant hyperthermia: a review. Orphanet J Rare Dis. 2015;10:93.
96. Kim TW, Nemergut ME. Preparation of modern anesthesia workstations for malignant hyperthermia-susceptible patients: a review of past and present practice. Anesthesiology. 2011;114(1):205–12.
97. Hoguet A, Grajewski A, Hodapp E, Chang TC. A retrospective survey of childhood glaucoma prevalence according to Childhood Glaucoma Research Network classification. Indian J Ophthalmol. 2016;64(2):118–23.
98. van der Griend BF, Lister NA, McKenzie IM, Martin N, Ragg PG, Sheppard SJ, Davidson AJ. Postoperative mortality in children after 101,885 anesthetics at a tertiary pediatric hospital. Anesth Analg. 2011;112(6):1440–7.
99. Houck CS, Vinson AE. Anaesthetic considerations for surgery in newborns. Arch Dis Child Fetal Neonatal Ed. 2017;102(4):F359–63.

100. Jevtovic-Todorovic V. General anesthetics and neurotoxicity: how much do we know? Anesthesiol Clin. 2016;34(3):439–51.
101. Zhang X, Liu F, Slikker W Jr, Wang C, Paule MG. Minimally invasive biomarkers of general anesthetic-induced developmental neurotoxicity. Neurotoxicol Teratol. 2017;60:95–101.
102. Andropoulos DB, Greene MF. Perspective: Anesthesia and developing brains-implications of the FDA warning. N Engl J Med. 2017;376(10):905–7.
103. Alam A, Suen KC, Hana Z, Sanders RD, Maze M, Ma D. Neuroprotection and neurotoxicity in the developing brain: an update on the effects of dexmedetomidine and xenon. Neurotoxicol Teratol. 2017;60:102–16.
104. Yeung H, Walton D. Clinical classification of childhood glaucoma. Arch Ophthalmol. 2010; 128(6):680–4.
105. Hoskin H, Shaffer R, Hetherington J. Anatomical classification of the developmental glaucoma. Arch Ophthalmol. 1984;102(9):1331–6.
106. Roy FH. Comprehensive development glaucoma classification. Ann Ophthalmol. 2005;37(4):237–44.
107. Beck A, Chang TCP, Freedman S. Definition, classification, differential diagnosis. In: Weinreb RN, Grajewski A, Papadopoulos M, Grigg J, Freedman S, editors. Childhood glaucoma, World Glaucoma Association Consensus Series 9. Amsterdam: Kugler Publications; 2013. p. 3–10.
108. Tutiven J. Anaesthetic consideration for syndromic children undergoing eye surgery. Curr Anaesth Crit Care. 2006;17(3–4):207–13.
109. Bissonnette B, Luginbuehl I, Marciniak B, Dalens B, editors. Syndromes: rapid recognition and perioperative implications. New York: McGraw Hill; 2006.
110. Chen J, Smith LE. Retinopathy of prematurity. Angiogenesis. 2007;10(2):133–40.
111. Ichhpujani P, Singh R. Pediatric genetic diseases causing glaucoma. J Pediatr Genet. 2014;3(4):209–18.
112. Klumpp S, Jorge LM, Aziz-Sultan MA. Hemodynamic instability induced by superselective angiography of the ophthalmic artery. Case Rep Anesthesiol. 2013;2013:408670.
113. Smith DW, Patau K, Therman E, Inhorn SL. A new autosomal trisomy syndrome: multiple congenital anomalies caused by an extra chromosome. J Pediatr. 1960;57:338–45.
114. Stevens CA. Rubinstein-Taybi Syndrome. 30 Aug 2002 [Updated 7 Aug 2014]. In: Adam MP, Ardinger HH, Pagon RA, et al., editors. GeneReviews® [Internet]. Seattle: University of Washington; 1993–2017. Available from: https://www.ncbi.nlm.nih.gov/books/NBK1526/. Accessed 19 Dec 2017.
115. Pollard R, Beasley J. Anaesthesia for patients with trisomy 13 (Patau's syndrome). Paediatr Anaesth. 1996;6(2):151–3.
116. Cladis FP. Appendix D: Index of syndromes and their pediatric anesthetic implications. In: Davis PJ, Cladis FP, Motoyama EK, editors. Smith's anesthesia for infants and children. 8th ed. Philadelphia: Mosby; 2011.
117. Wren C, Richmond S, Donaldson L. Presentation of congenital heart disease in infancy: implications for routine examination. Arch Dis Child Fetal Neonatal Ed. 1999;80(1):F49–53.
118. Hoffman J. Incidence of congenital heart disease, part I: postnatal incidence. Pediatr Cardiol. 1995;16(3):103–13.
119. Baum V, Barton D, Gutgesell HP. Influence of congenital heart disease on mortality after noncardiac surgery in hospitalized children. Pediatrics. 2000;105(2):332–5.
120. Sümpelmann R, Osthaus W. The pediatric cardiac patient presenting for noncardiac surgery. Curr Opin Anaesthesiol. 2007;20(3):216–20.
121. White M. Approach to managing children with heart disease for noncardiac surgery. Paediatr Anaesth. 2011;21(5):522–9.

3 Pediatric Examination Under Anesthesia

Mahmoud A. Fayed, Teresa C. Chen, Oscar Albis-Donado, and Elena Bitrian

Introduction

Pediatric examination under anesthesia (EUA) remains an essential part of the diagnosis and treatment of infants and children with glaucoma. Figure 3.1 shows an algorithm of a suggested approach to the evaluation of a child with glaucoma or glaucoma suspect [1]. After the initial clinical presentation, the EUA can be used to confirm the diagnosis and to establish the severity of the disease if this is not possible in the clinic setting and in many cases to also initiate treatment. As the management of childhood glaucoma often requires multiple anesthetic events, in an effort to decrease the burden and risk of anesthetic exposure, the ophthalmologist performing the EUA should be prepared to proceed with glaucoma surgery if necessary. Similarly, the ophthalmologist who plans to do the EUA should be familiar with and prepared for each of the possible components of the examination needed for the diagnosis and assessment of glaucoma.

Components of the EUA can include assessment of any combination of the following:

- General appearance
- Intraocular pressure (IOP)
- Anterior segment
  - Gonioscopy
- Central corneal thickness (CCT)
- Posterior segment
- Refraction
- Ultrasonography: amplitude scan (A-scan) and brightness scan (B-scan) or ultrasound biomicroscopy (UBM)
- Specialized imaging: optical coherence tomography (OCT) and intravenous fluorescein angiography (IVFA)

Preparation for Examination under Anesthesia

It is important to explain to the parents and, in an age-appropriate manner, to the patient what to expect during the EUA. It is also essential to discuss with the family what other interventions for treatment during this anesthetic session may be necessary, depending on the findings of the examination. Obtaining as much information as possible

M. A. Fayed
Glaucoma Service, Massachusetts Eye and Ear Infirmary, Harvard Medical School, Boston, MA, USA

T. C. Chen
Department of Ophthalmology, Massachusetts Eye and Ear Infirmary, Harvard Medical School, Boston, MA, USA

O. Albis-Donado
Department of Glaucoma, Instituto Mexicano de Oftalmolgía IAP, Querétaro, Mexico

E. Bitrian (✉)
Department of Ophthalmology, Mayo Clinic, Rochester, MN, USA

A. L. Grajewski et al. (eds.), *Surgical Management of Childhood Glaucoma*, https://doi.org/10.1007/978-3-319-54003-0_3

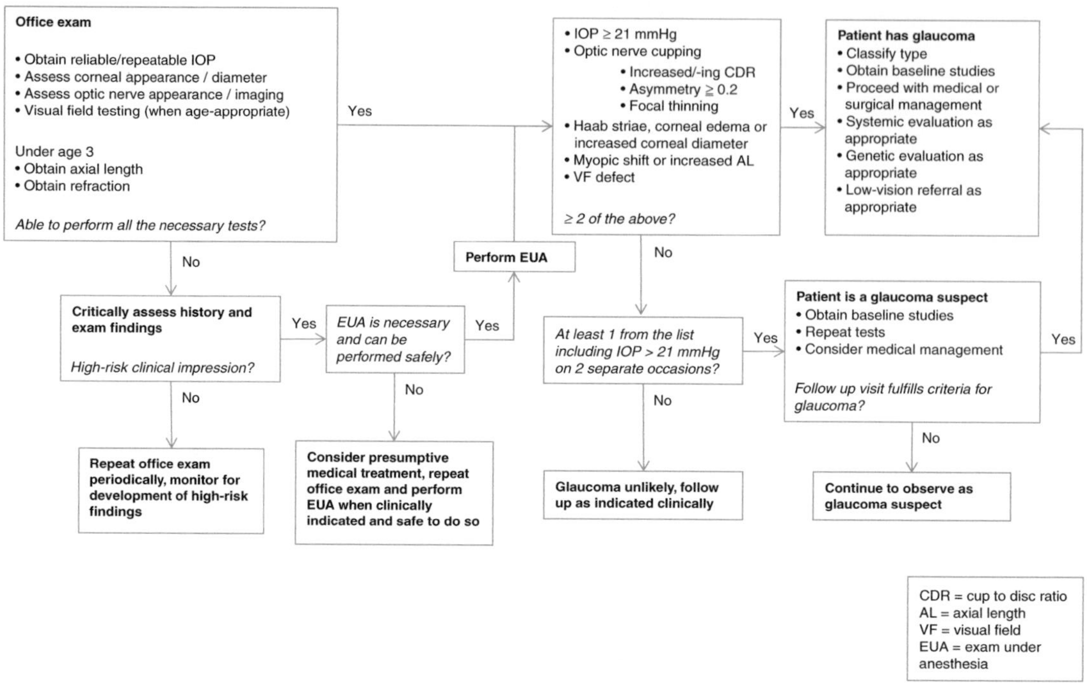

Fig. 3.1 Algorithm of a suggested approach to evaluate children with glaucoma or glaucoma suspects. (From Papadopoulos et al. [1], with permission)

before the EUA is of value both for counseling the parents and for developing a clinical management plan. The level of suspicion or certainty that a child has glaucoma, to be confirmed at the time of the EUA, also opens the door for discussion of treatment options, risks, and benefits. Even if uncertainty exists preoperatively, appropriate consent for possible procedures should be obtained.

Preoperative Care

Mild sedation may be given to the patients in the preoperative area to decrease the level of anxiety, and this may allow for an IOP check using the ICare® rebound tonometer (ICare Finland Oy, Vantaa, Finland), in the child uncooperative with clinic tonometry, which may then be able to be correlated to the IOP measurement taken during the EUA by other tonometric methods. For EUA with ketamine, agents that reduce bronchial secretions leading to laryngeal spasm (e.g., atropine or glycopyrrolate) should also be considered.

Many children benefit from having their parents escort them to the operating room and stay with them until the anesthesia is initiated. This may significantly decrease the level of anxiety for the child, allowing them to be more relaxed when the anesthesia is induced and therefore facilitating a more accurate IOP measurement.

Examination

General Appearance

Before the child undergoes general anesthesia, visual behavior should be assessed both in clinic and in the preoperative area. An external assessment is also useful looking for ocular asymmetry, face abnormalities, gait, and general level of development. Some of the external exam may be completed once the child is asleep and documentation obtained with external photography.

Measurement of IOP

Intraocular pressure in normal eyes of children tends to be lower than in normal adult eyes and typically increases with advancing age [2]. An accurate IOP measurement is an important part of the exam and influences both diagnosis and management. Unlike other elements of the eye exam, IOP measurement can be directly affected by anesthesia and is discussed extensively in Chapter 2. All inhalational anesthetics decrease the IOP. For this reason, some surgeons prefer intravenous (IV) induction with ketamine or use of succinylcholine. Whatever the method chosen, it is important to have a consistent approach with serial EUA and a good working relationship with the anesthesia team so that they fully appreciate the variables which potentially affect IOP measurement.

While IOP is an important finding to be collected during the EUA, it may be altered by many factors related to the anesthetic session itself and not just the type of anesthesia. Hence it should be considered within the context of the remaining findings of the examination.

Methods of IOP Assessment in the Operating Room

There are several methods to measure IOP, but only some of these can be used in the operating room setting with a recumbent patient. The tonometers most frequently used are Tono-Pen®, Perkins applanation tonometer, pneumatonometry, and Schiøtz indentation tonometry. Others methods such as Goldmann applanation, ICare® rebound tonometer, and noncontact tonometers are not used in the operating room setting and so will not be discussed here. However, it is worth noting that the ICare® PRO can measure IOP in a supine patient but is not currently approved for use in the United States [3].

Tono-Pen® The Tono-Pen® (Reichert Technologies, Depew NY, USA) is a portable electronic applanation device, which uses batteries as a power source. This device applanates a small area of the cornea and is useful in eyes with localized corneal scars or edema, which can be avoided [4–10]. Because it is portable, it can also be used in the office setting.

The Tono-Pen® takes multiple readings, after which the mean IOP and the standard deviation are displayed. Measurements with standard deviations of 5 or less are considered acceptable [4, 5].

It is critical that the Tono-Pen® be held vertically for calibration. When the eye pressure is outside of the normal range, the concordance between Goldmann applanation and Tono-Pen® applanation is variable, with some studies suggesting that Tono-Pen® pressures can be lower, higher, or similar [5, 11]. Tono-Pen® and Goldmann applanation pressures are more similar for IOPs between 10 and 20 mmHg [5, 6]. However, in general, the Tono-Pen® tends to overestimate IOPs, with pressures of 1.4–12.1 mmHg higher than Goldmann readings [8–10].

Perkins Applanation Tonometry The main advantage of the Perkins applanation tonometer (Haag-Streit, Bern, Switzerland) is that it is a handheld portable device, which allows for measuring IOP in both the upright and supine positions [12]. Therefore, Perkins tonometry is ideal for examining babies, children, and uncooperative patients, as well as anesthetized and bedridden patients. Similar to the Goldmann applanation tonometer, Perkins tonometry is based on the "Imbert-Fick Law," which states that the pressure (P) inside an ideal, dry, thin-walled sphere equals the force (F) needed to flatten its surface. Applanation tonometry measures the force needed to flatten the corneal surface area (A) with a diameter of 3.06 mm, or $P = F/A$ [13].

One important potential source for inaccurate applanation tonometry measurements for a child in the operating room would be inadvertent pressure on the eye, corneal irregularities (i.e., scarring, high astigmatism), and, possibly, corneal thickness values greater or less than average, just to name a few [14, 15]. Although much has been written about CCT and its influence upon measured IOP in adults, the recorded IOP in children should never be adjusted based solely upon the CCT, but rather, the target IOP may be changed based upon an unusually thin (lowered) or thick but nonedematous (raised) CCT [16, 17].

Pneumatonometer The pneumatonometer is a pressure-sensing device, which can be useful for patients with corneal scars or corneal edema. It is a gas-filled chamber covered by a Silastic diaphragm. The gas in the chamber escapes through an exhaust vent. As the diaphragm touches the cornea, the gas vent is reduced in size and the pressure in the chamber rises. A portion of the gas flow pushes the outer part of the tonometer tip against the cornea and depresses the corneal surface, and another portion maintains the pressure required to balance the pressure on the other side of the tip membrane (i.e., the IOP) [18]. The small 5 mm fenestrated membrane at the end of the device is the part that touches the cornea.

Pneumatonometry readings tend to be higher than Goldmann IOP readings and can even be much as 8.6 mmHg higher [19–21].

Schiøtz Tonometer The Schiøtz tonometer (Sklar Instruments, West Chester PA, USA) is an indentation tonometer that measures the corneal indentation produced by a known weight from 5.5 to 7.5 gm. It is portable and low cost. The contact point of the Schiøtz device is a rounded cup that matches the shape of the cornea. A central hole in the cup permits a central cylindrical weight to impinge on the cornea and therefore can be used during an EUA with the patient in the supine position [18]. The main problem with Schiøtz tonometry is that it is affected by ocular rigidity, and the pediatric eye may be relatively "elastic."

Schiøtz indentation tonometry tends to give higher readings than any of the applantation tonometers, with higher readings up to 16.5 mmHg more [18, 19].

In general, most surgeons have moved away from the use of the Schiøtz tonometry as other more reliable methods for measuring pressure have been developed.

Other

Other specialized testing less frequently performed during an EUA include tonometry with Ocular Response Analyzer® (Reichert Technologies) or Corvis® (Oculus, Arlington WA, USA) [22, 23] and specular microscopy.

Anterior Segment Evaluation

As elevated IOP affects an infant's or child's eye with resultant changes to the anterior segment that may be dramatic, they should be documented initially and then serially evaluated during EUA sessions. Hence, the measurement and inspection of the cornea, anterior chamber (AC), iris, angle, and lens all constitute portions of the EUA.

While the corneal diameter is usually measured with a caliper held against a ruler for confirmation to the nearest 1/4 mm, the remaining anterior segment evaluation is usually performed with a handheld slit lamp and by some clinicians with the operating microscope.

The cornea should be examined for the presence of corneal edema, opacities, and "breaks" in Descemet membrane (Haab striae). Other distinguishing findings such as the presence of posterior embryotoxon should be recorded.

Corneal enlargement secondary to elevated IOP is usually seen before the age of 3 years, so corneal diameter is important to establish the diagnosis and to monitor treatment effect and/or glaucoma progression. The normal horizontal neonatal diameter is around 10 mm and increases by about 1 mm during the first year. Corneal diameter greater than 11 mm in a newborn and 12 mm in an infant less than 1 year of age is suggestive of glaucoma. A measurement of greater than 13 mm is abnormal at any age. These findings along with other indicators of the effect from elevation IOP such as Haab striae are diagnostic of elevated IOP at some time before 3 years of age. The corneal diameter is measured with calipers from limbus to limbus, both horizontal and vertical, and checked with a graduated ruler. The exact location of the limbus is not always easy to determine. The superior limbus may have pannus and the entire limbus is often stretched. This makes the normal distinct landmarks blurred, but this is still a valuable part of evaluating change over time. Comparison of the two corneal diameters for asymmetry is also useful.

The AC, if visible, should be assessed for depth. In the normal neonate, the AC is somewhat shallow, and in a neonate or young infant with an enlarged cornea, there is a relatively deeper AC.

Examining the iris and pupil for abnormalities may suggest a secondary cause of glaucoma. Iris abnormalities such as peripheral corneal adhesions should be noted and recorded. In some secondary glaucomas such as Axenfeld-Rieger anomaly, the pupil and iris adhesions may rarely change over time. Other distinguishing iris details should be noted: stromal hypoplasia, loss of iris crypts, peripheral scalloping of posterior pigment, and prominent iris vessels. Each of these details may help distinguish the type of glaucoma, whether it is primary congenital glaucoma (PCG) with normal iris and peripheral stromal atrophy or diffuse iris atrophy, which may indicate congenital iris hypoplasia or a variant of aniridia. Sectoral iris atrophy may indicate a partial coloboma.

Evaluation of the lens for coexistent congenital cataract may suggest a secondary glaucoma diagnosis such as in Lowe syndrome or congenital rubella syndrome. Abnormal size or shape of the lens or configuration should also be noted during the EUA.

Gonioscopy is an important element of an EUA, both for diagnosis of the cause of glaucoma and to help plan the most appropriate treatment. Most types of childhood glaucoma will have anomalies in the angle that should be identified and documented in the examination. Normal angle development has been shown using electron microscopy to occur by the posterior sliding of the ciliary body from Schwalbe line (fifth month) to the scleral spur (ninth month) and then to a location behind the scleral spur (postnatally) due to differential growth rates of the corneoscleral coat compared to the uveal tract [24]. Inhibited sliding of the uveal tract to reveal angle structures is thought to occur in PCG. This generally results in an anterior position of the ciliary body and peripheral iris covering the trabecular meshwork and an immature angle appearance, similar to the late fetal position. However, the angle appearance depends on the timing of the arrest in angle maturation. The earlier, the more immature the angle appearance and the less angle structures visible and vice versa. So it may sometimes be difficult to distinguish a PCG angle from the normal infant angle. In the normal newborn eye, the peripheral iris and ciliary body have usually recessed to the level of scleral spur or even posterior to scleral spur, but the trabecular meshwork is poorly pigmented and can be difficult to identify (Fig. 3.2a). Looking for the "corneal wedge" with the portable slit lamp is often useful in identifying the trabecular meshwork. The scleral spur is also a key landmark that can be identified as a whitish band. In PCG the iris insertion is usually higher than normal, and the scleral spur may not be visualized (Fig. 3.2b). The level of insertion can vary in different areas of the angle. Even in unilateral glaucoma, the angle of the fellow eye may not be completely normal, and both eyes should be always examined. Other anomalies can be observed on gonioscopy, like iridocorneal adhesions in Axenfeld-Rieger syndrome (Fig. 3.2c) or blood in Schlemm's canal in Sturge-Weber syndrome.

To perform gonioscopy, a certain degree of corneal transparency is needed. Both direct and indirect gonioscopies can be performed. Direct gonioscopy is performed using a Koeppe lens and a Barkan light with a handheld binocular microscope or handheld portable slit lamp (Fig. 3.3). Any isotonic solution (such as natural tears) may be used as the interface between the cornea and the gonioscopic lens. The angle structures of the two eyes may be compared by placing a gonioscopic lens on each eye and then moving the slit lamp between them sequentially. While direct gonioscopy affords a beautiful stereo view of the angle, the angle may also be evaluated using the operating microscope and a gonioprism to perform direct gonioscopy (Fig. 3.4).

Gonioscopy photographs may be taken using the microscope's camera, if present, and the surgeon may simultaneously evaluate the visualization of the angle for possible surgery. Gonioscopic photographs may also be easily taken using the RetCam digital imaging system (Natus Medical, Pleasanton CA, USA) and the 130° lens, with a mound of viscous coupling

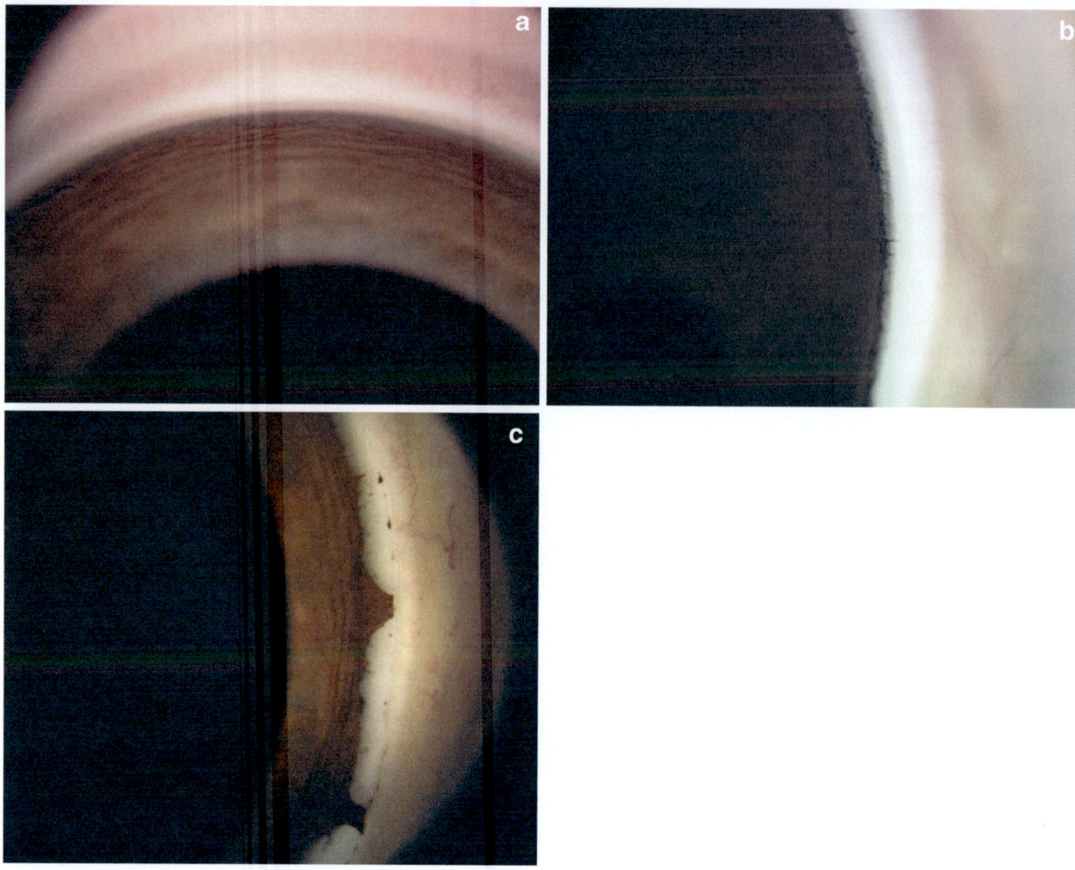

Fig. 3.2 (**a**) Normal angle appearance in a child without glaucoma; (**b**) angle appearance in primary congenital glaucoma; (**c**) gonioscopic view of angle adhesions in a patient with Axenfeld-Rieger syndrome. (Courtesy of Ta Chen Peter Chang, MD, Department of Ophthalmology, Bascom Palmer Eye Institute, Miami, Florida, USA)

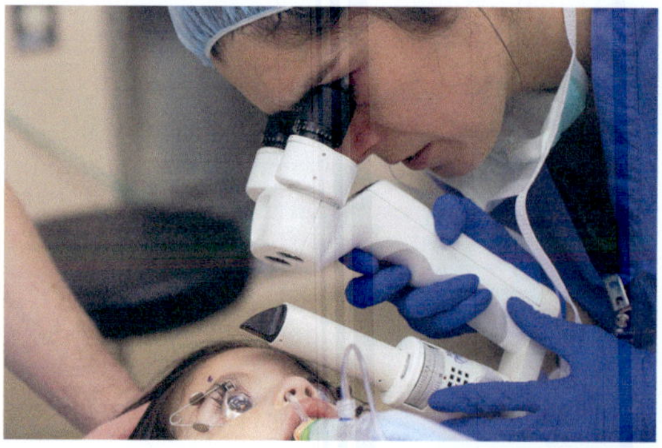

Fig. 3.3 Examination of the angle structures with a Koeppe lens and a portable slit lamp during examination under anesthesia

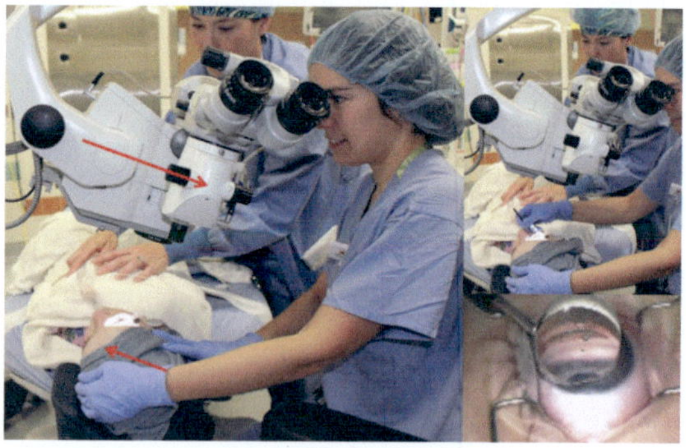

Fig. 3.4 Gonioscopic examination using the operating microscope in a 30° tilted position and a Swan-Jacob lens

agent (aqueous-based lubrication ointment seems ideal) on the smooth concave surface of the lens tip as an optical bridge between the lens and the cornea, affording a direct angle view. The process can be thought of as building a Koeppe lens at the tip of the camera. For direct imaging of the angle, the camera has to be at a slight tilt and the

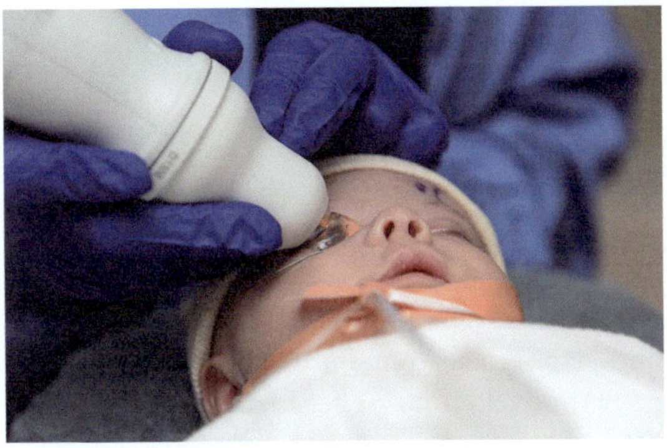

Fig. 3.5 The RetCam and a wide-angle lens can be used to take pictures of the angle in children with glaucoma

coupling of the gel is placed at the opposite limbus and directed toward the opposite angle with the wide-angle lens held obliquely (Fig. 3.5). UBM can also provide an image of the angle especially when the view of the angle is obscured by cornea edema or scar [25].

Measurement of Central Corneal Thickness

The role of central corneal thickness (CCT) in the evaluation of the measured IOP in childhood glaucoma is complex. CCT affects the accuracy of all applanation IOP measurement devices (Goldmann, Perkins, and Tono-Pen®). In general, thinner corneas tend to underestimate IOP, and thicker corneas tend to overestimate the IOP compared to the actual value. While this may be true, other considerations in infants and children affect the role of pachymetry in the overall evaluation of child with glaucoma or suspected glaucoma [26].

CCT in normal infants increases with age from 1–11 years. White and Hispanic normal infants of 1 year old had CCT 553 microns at the 50th percentile. African-American children had thinner corneas than White and Hispanic children by approximately 20 microns [27]. Children with PCG and juvenile open-angle glaucoma have thinner central corneas than normal subjects. Children with glaucoma following cataract surgery and children with glaucoma associated with some non-acquired ocular anomalies such as aniridia have thicker CCT than normal [28–30].

While CCT should be measured during the EUA in all children with glaucoma or suspected glaucoma, it should not be used to adjust the IOP [26].

Also of note in the setting of evaluation of a child with glaucoma, corneal edema can be associated with falsely low IOP readings, because IOP readings can also be affected by corneal hysteresis or the relative stiffness of the cornea. Tactile estimation of IOP in these cases is often useful.

Posterior Segment Evaluation: Optic Nerve and Fundus

Dilated fundoscopy is performed during the EUA once the IOP has been measured and the anterior segment examination completed. If angle surgery is contemplated, then dilated fundoscopy may be performed prior to the EUA in the office or deferred. However, given the importance of the appearance and documentation of the optic nerve, it is probably best to complete this portion of the exam and instill a fast-acting miotic (acetylcholine chloride intraocular solution, or Miochol-E [Bausch & Lomb, Bridgewater NJ, USA]) before angle surgery. If, however, the view is compromised due to corneal edema or scar and surgery is planned, it is not worth the additional risk of trauma to intraocular structures to dilate the pupil prior to surgery because the posterior segment examination and attempted photograph are unlikely to prove helpful.

The posterior segment is best visualized by binocular indirect ophthalmoscopy using a 28D or 20D lens. A 20D lens will provide higher magnification. The purpose of the fundoscopy is to rule out other pathology as well as to identify retinal findings consistent with other ocular or systemic syndromes. The optic nerve can also be visualized in detail with a direct ophthalmoscope through a Koeppe lens. Using the RetCam and the 130° lens, it is possible to document all of the retina and the periphery.

The appearance of the optic disc is of singular importance both in the diagnosis of glaucoma and in determining severity and progression. The disc appearance (size of the nerve, degree of cupping, focal loss, color, presence of hemorrhage, noted abnormality) should be carefully recorded and photographed whenever possible for comparison to detect optic disc change on subsequent EUA. Photographs can be obtained with a variety of cameras, including the RetCam, using the 30° or 80° lens for disc photos. If the RetCam is not available, the optic disc can be photographed using the surgical microscope and a fundus flat contact lens or the central mirror of a three-mirror Goldmann lens.

Refraction

While cycloplegic refraction is usually done in the outpatient setting, there are indications for retinoscopy during an EUA, especially if the clinic evaluation is impeded by poor cooperation or other ocular features such as opacities in the visual axis. The spherical equivalent can also be useful in the sense that increasing myopic refraction can be a surrogate for (and also corroborate) axial length (AL) elongation in the face of poorly controlled IOP.

Ultrasound Amplitude Scan (A-Scan) and Brightness Scan (B-Scan)

Axial length measurements determined by A-scan biomicroscopy is one of the key objective findings obtained as part of the EUA. It is a quantitative measurement between both eyes and also a measurement of the change in axial growth over time. The measurement is not affected by confounding variables such as anesthesia. The normal ocular axial growth curve is greatest within the first year, followed by a gradual increase in globe elongation during the next 4–5 years and then a plateau by 6–7 years of age. The rapid change in ocular axial growth in childhood glaucoma is based on the distensibility of the eye in response to increase in IOP.

Measurement of AL can be used in the baseline assessment for diagnosis of glaucoma, but even more importantly, the serial measurements of AL can be used to confirm stability or to suggest progression. Normative data for axial lengths in the pediatric population can be used in comparison, based on the age of the child (Fig. 3.6 [1, 31, 32]). In general, axial length after 3 years of age is not of comparison value.

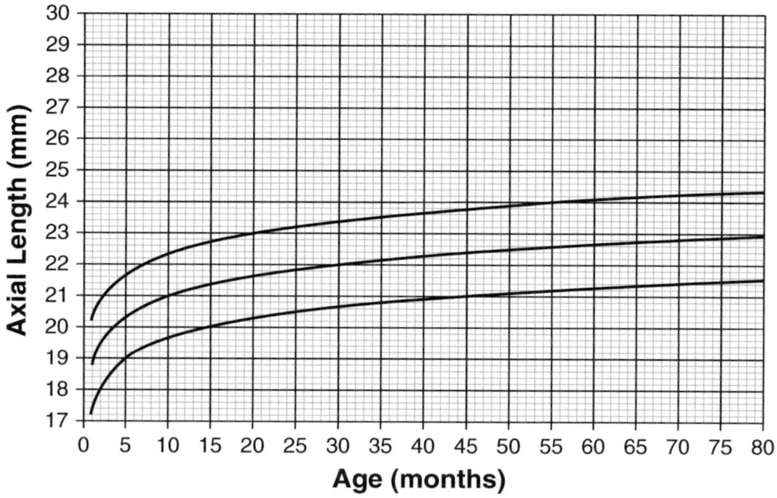

Fig. 3.6 Axial length in millimeters plotted against the age in months. The *middle line* represents the mean axial length of normal eyes, and the *upper and lower lines* represent the standard deviations. (From Papadopoulos et al. [1] and Law et al. [31], with permission. Graph is based on the formula of the curve in Sampaolesi and Caruso [32])

B-scan ultrasonography helps to evaluate the posterior segment in those eyes where the view is limited by corneal, lenticular, or other pathologies or when the pupil is small and dilation is contraindicated due to the likely surgery to follow the EUA. The screening B-scan can eliminate gross pathology and help to identify retinal detachments, choroidal detachments, and – when extreme – optic nerve cupping. Additionally, the B-scan ultrasound is helpful in confirming a fluid-filled bleb overlying a glaucoma drainage device in children [33].

Specialized Imaging

The EUA does afford an opportunity to obtain some specialized testing that would be difficult or impossible to complete in the outpatient setting, depending on the temperament and/or age of the patient. Anterior and posterior segment OCT, UBM, and IVFA are all supplemental investigations that may help to elucidate and document the anatomy and pathology present at the time of the exam. This is especially valuable when other sections of the exam are limited by lack of clarity of the cornea and disrupted anatomy.

Optical Coherence Tomography (OCT)

Anterior and posterior segment OCT with the use of portable units such as the Bioptigen Envisu™ SDOCT (Leica Microsystems, Buffalo Grove IL, USA) and iVue (Optovue, Fremont CA, USA) can offer additional perspectives on the anatomy of both the normal and abnormal structures detected during the EUA. The limitation in utility of some of these measurements is the lack of normative data of some of these measurements in children. In particular, optic disc imaging and retinal nerve fiber layer (RNFL) have no normative databases for children.

Ultrasound Biomicroscopy (UBM)

There are those patients whose anatomy poses challenges, in particular those who present with advanced disease or extremely disrupted anatomy: opaque cornea, stretched buphthalmic eye, and uncertain previous treatments. In these cases, UBM can be of great value in helping with diagnosis and surgical decision-making (Fig. 3.7a, b).

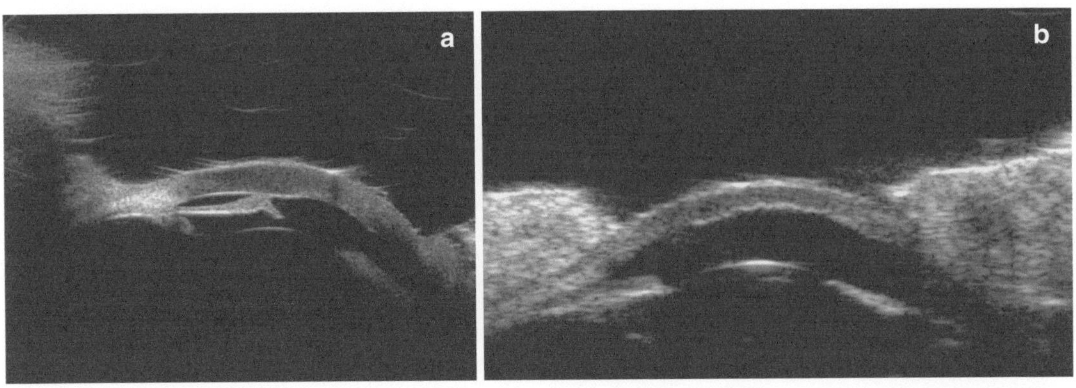

Fig. 3.7 (**a**) Ultrasound biomicroscopy (UBM) performed in a patient with Peters anomaly shows adhesions of the iris to corneal endothelium in preoperative picture; (**b**) postoperative UBM in the same patient after lysis of the iridocorneal adhesions

Intravenous Fluorescein Angiography (IVFA)

Intravenous fluorescein angiography (IVFA) can be of value if abnormalities are noted on fundus exam. This is done during the EUA with the RetCam (or similar wide-field imaging camera). Typically, to perform the fluorescein angiogram, the 130° lens is used on the RetCam, the dosage of fluorescein is 8 mg per kilo, and the dye concentration is 10% in a 5 ml sterile vial. Color photos are taken first, followed by red-free images and then fluorescein images. The fluorescein is given by the anesthesiologist following a bolus flush in the port of the IV closest to the patient [34]. The IV push of fluorescein is done at the same time that the photographer indicates he or she is ready, and the photos are completed as they would be in the outpatient manner (Fig. 3.8).

Minimizing the Need for EUA

While they are often invaluable, EUAs should be limited to an absolute minimum in order to avoid repeated anesthetic exposure in infants and young children. Rebound tonometry, obviating topical anesthetic, has decreased the frequency of EUAs in managing childhood glaucoma [35]. Additionally, all aspects of the office/clinic examination should be tailored to making the infant and child with glaucoma as comfortable as possible, thereby increasing the yield of the clinic exam for the examiner. For example, bringing an infant to the clinic when hungry will allow breast- or bottle-feeding as a distraction, while a toddler may respond to toys, videos, or other games for distraction.

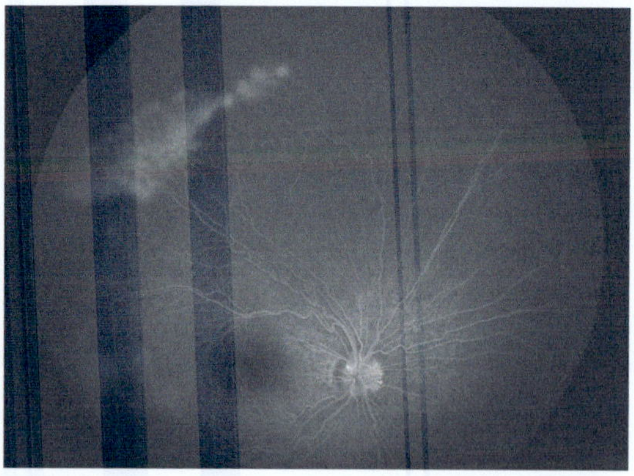

Fig. 3.8 Fluorescein angiography performed in primary congenital glaucoma shows decreased vasculature in peripheral retina with ridge of neovascularization and abnormal truncation of vessels

Given the risk, the expense, and the importance of the EUA, it should be emphasized that it should occur with all the components for a thorough examination in place and with the surgeon ready to follow the EUA with surgery, if needed, at the same session.

References

1. Papadopoulos M, Brandt JD, Sugiyama K, Khaw PT, Chua J, Law S, et al. Establishing the diagnosis and determining glaucoma progression. In: Weinreb RN, Grajewski A, Papadopoulos M, Grigg J, Freedman S, editors. Childhood glaucoma, WGA consensus series 9. Amsterdam: Kugler Publications; 2013. p. 15–42.
2. Sihota R, Tuli D, Dada T, et al. Distribution and determinants of intraocular pressure in a normal pediatric population. J Pediatr Ophthalmol Strabismus. 2006;43(1):14–8. quiz 36–7
3. Lambert SR, Melia M, Buffenn AN, Chiang MF, Simpson JL, Yang MB. Rebound tonometry in children: a report by the American Academy of Ophthalmology. Ophthalmology. 2013;120(4):e21–7.
4. Mok KH, Wong CS, Lee VW. Tono-Pen tonometer and corneal thickness. Eye (Lond). 1999;13(Pt 1):35–7.
5. Tonnu PA, Ho T, Sharma K, White E, Bunce C, Garway-Heath D. A comparison of four methods of tonometry: method agreement and interobserver variability. Br J Ophthalmol. 2005;89(7):847–50.
6. Christoffersen T, Fors T, Ringberg U, Holtedahl K. Tonometry in the general practice setting (I): Tono-Pen compared to Goldman applanation tonometry. Acta Ophthalmol. 1993;71(1):103–8.
7. Hessemer V, Rossler R, Jacobi KW. Comparison of intraocular pressure measurements with the Oculab Tono-Pen vs manometry in humans shortly after death. Am J Ophthalmol. 1988;105(6):678–82.
8. Kao SF, Lichter PR, Bergstrom TJ, Rowe S, Musch DC. Clinical comparison of the Oculab Tono-Pen to the Goldmann applanation tonometer. Ophthalmology. 1987;94(12):1541–4.
9. Kooner KS, Cooksey JC, Barron JB, Zimmerman TJ, Gupte RK, Wall JL. Tonometry comparison: Goldmann versus Tono-Pen. Ann Ophthalmol. 1992;24(1):29–36.

10. Levy J, Lifshitz T, Rosen S, Tessler Z, Biedner BZ. Is the Tono-Pen accurate for measuring intraocular pressure in young children with congenital glaucoma? JAAPOS. 2005;9(4):321–5.
11. Yilmaz I, Altan C, Aygit ED, Alagoz C, Baz O, Ahmet S, et al. Comparison of three methods of tonometry in normal subjects: Goldmann applanation tonometer, non-contact airpuff tonometer, and Tono-Pen XL. Clin Ophthalmol. 2014;8:1069–74.
12. Arora R, Bellamy H, Austin M. Applanation tonometry: a comparison of the Perkins handheld and Goldmann slit lamp-mounted methods. Clin Ophthalmol. 2014;26(8):605–10.
13. Markiewitz HH. The so-called Imbert-Fick law. Arch Ophthalmol. 1960;64:159.
14. Jamal KN, Gürses-Ozden R, Liebmann JM, Ritch R. Attempted eyelid closure affects intraocular pressure measurement in open-angle glaucoma patients. Am J Ophthalmol. 2002;134(2):186–9.
15. Lam AK, Lam CH. Effect of breath-holding on pulsatile ocular blood flow measurement in normal subjects. Optom Vis Sci. 2004;81(8):597–600.
16. Doughty MJ, Zaman ML. Human corneal thickness and its impact on intraocular pressure measures: a review and meta-analysis approach. Surv Ophthalmol. 2000;44(5):367–408.
17. Jaafar MS, Kazi GA. Normal intraocular pressure in children: a comparative study of the Perkins applanation tonometer and the pneumatonometer. J Pediatr Ophthalmol Strabismus. 1993;30(5):284–7.
18. Whitacre MM, Emig M, Hassanein K. The effect of Perkins, Tono-Pen, and Schiötz tonometry on intraocular pressure. Am J Ophthalmol. 1991;111(1):59–64.
19. Rao VJ, Gnanaraj L, Mitchell KW, Figueiredo FC. Clinical comparison of ocular blood flow tonometer, Tonopen, and Goldmann applanation tonometer for measuring intraocular pressure in postkeratoplasty eyes. Cornea. 2001;20(8):834–8.
20. Eisenberg DL, Sherman BG, McKeown CA, Schuman JS. Tonometry in adults and children. A manometric evaluation of pneumatonometry, applanation, and TonoPen in vitro and in vivo. Ophthalmology. 1998;105(7):1173–81.
21. Currie BD, Bagga H, Rademaker AW, Tanna AP. Effect of instrument orientation on the accuracy of intraocular pressure measurements in human cadaveric eyes: manometric evaluation of the model 30 classic Pneumatonometer and Tono-Pen XL. J Glaucoma. 2011;20(8):465–9.
22. Herr A, Remky A, Hirsch T, Rennings C, Plange N. Tonometry in corneal edema after cataract surgery: dynamic contour tonometry versus Goldmann applanation tonometry. Clin Ophthalmol. 2013;7:815–9.
23. Garcia-Feijoo J, Martinez-de-la-Casa JM, Morales-Fernandez L, Saenz Frances F, Santos-Bueso E, Garcia-Saenz S, Mendez-Hernandez C. New technologies for measuring intraocular pressure. Prog Brain Res. 2015;221:67–79.
24. Anderson DR. The development of the trabecular meshwork and its abnormality in primary infantile glaucoma. Tans Am Ophthalmol Soc. 1981;79:458–85.
25. Gupta V, Jha R, Srinivasan G, Dada T, Sihota R. Ultrasound biomicroscopic characteristics of the anterior segment in primary congenital glaucoma. J AAPOS. 2007;11:546–50.
26. Pediatric Eye Disease Investigator Group, Bradfield YS, Melia BM, Repka MX, Kaminski BM, Davitt BV, Johnson DA, et al. Central corneal thickness in children. Arch Ophthalmol. 2011;129(9):1132–8.
27. Brandt JD, Beiser JA, Kass MA, Gordon MO. Central Corneal Thickness in the Ocular Hyoertension Treatment Study (OHTS). Ophthalmology. 2001;108(10):1779–88.
28. Wygnanski-Jaffe T, Barequet IS. Central corneal thickness in congenital glaucoma. Cornea. 2006;25(8):923–5.
29. Brandt JD, Casuso LA, Budenz DL. Markedly increased central corneal thickness: an unrecognized finding in congenital aniridia. Am J Ophthalmol. 2004;137(2):348–50.
30. Muir KW, Duncan L, Enyedi LB, Wallace DK, Freedman SF. Central corneal thickness: congenital cataracts and aphakia. Am J Ophthalmol. 2007;144(4):502–6.
31. Law SK, Bui D, Caprioli J. Serial axial length measurements in congenital glaucoma. Am J Ophthalmol. 2001;132(6):926–8.
32. Sampaolesi R, Caruso R. Ocular echometry in the diagnosis of congenital glaucoma. Arch Ophthalmol. 1982;100(4):574–7.
33. Baig NB, Lin AA, Freedman SF. Ultrasound evaluation of glaucoma drainage devices in children. J AAPOS. 2015;19(3):281–4.
34. Henry CR, Hodapp E, Hess DJ, Blieden LS, Berrocal AM. Fluorescein angiography findings in phacomatosis pigmentovascularis. Ophthalmic Surg Lasers Imaging Retina. 2013;44(2):201–3.
35. Kageyama M, Hirooka K, Baba T, Shiraga F. Comparison of ICare rebound tonometer with noncontact tonometer in healthy children. J Glaucoma. 2011;20(a):63–6.

Angle Surgery: Goniotomy

4

David S. Walton and Elizabeth Hodapp

History

Otto Barkan performed the first goniotomy in 1935 on a 55-year-old man, and he reported a series of 11 adults in 1936 [1]. His procedure added direct visualization via a gonio lens to a technique described in 1893 by De Vincentiis. He reasoned that typical open-angle glaucoma was caused by an "impervious trabeculum" and that his procedure could restore "the physiologic function of Schlemm's (*sic*) canal" [1]. Long-term results in adults proved disappointing, but Barkan also applied the procedure with great success to congenital glaucoma, which was at the time virtually untreatable. He described the procedure as "intraocular microsurgery" that required detailed preoperative gonioscopy. Motivated by the importance of precise localization of the goniotomy incision in the trabecular meshwork, Barkan designed operating goniotomy lenses, a designated goniotomy knife, and a head-mounted binocular device that was arguably the first ophthalmic operating microscope [2].

Barkan published his first paper on goniotomy for congenital glaucoma in 1942 [3], and he discussed his surgical refinements and cumulative pediatric goniotomy results in San Francisco in November 1951, when he presented the Jackson Memorial Lecture at the 37th annual clinical congress of the American College of Surgeons [4]. Although the procedure remains much as described by Barkan, techniques and indications have evolved over the decades, and additional drainage angle procedures – collectively known as MIGS (minimally invasive glaucoma surgery) – have been developed. Goniotomy is now used in both primary and selected secondary glaucomas in children [5–7].

Indications and Contraindications

PCG is the most common indication for goniotomy. When chosen, it is generally performed as the initial procedure. Additional favorable diagnoses are listed in Table 4.1. Prophylactic goniotomy is sometimes performed in non-glaucomatous aniridic eyes with early angle closure to prevent further closure and secondary glaucoma [8].

A satisfactory view of the angle –which the surgeon can determine by doing intraoperative gonioscopy – is necessary to safely perform goni-

Electronic Supplementary Material The online version of this chapter (https://doi.org/10.1007/978-3-319-54003-0_4) contains supplementary material, which is available to authorized users.

D. S. Walton
Department of Ophthalmology, Massachusetts Eye and Ear Infirmary, Boston, MA, USA

E. Hodapp (✉)
Bascom Palmer Eye Institute, Department of Ophthalmology, University of Miami Miller School of Medicine, Miami, FL, USA
e-mail: ehodapp@med.miami.edu

A. L. Grajewski et al. (eds.), *Surgical Management of Childhood Glaucoma*,
https://doi.org/10.1007/978-3-319-54003-0_4

Table 4.1 Some favorable diagnoses for goniotomy

Primary congenital glaucoma (PCG)
Infantile and late onset better than neonatal onset
Previously controlled PCG
Glaucoma associated with non-acquired ocular anomalies
Aniridia with open-angle or limited angle closure[a]
Congenital iris hypoplasia (if open angle)
Congenital ectropion uveae (if open angle)
Glaucoma associated with non-acquired systemic disease or syndrome
Sturge-weber syndrome (infantile onset)
Klippel-Trenaunay-weber syndrome
Glaucoma associated with acquired condition
Uveitic glaucoma (if open angle)
Steroid-induced glaucoma
Glaucoma following cataract surgery
Infantile onset (if open angle)

[a]Surgery is extremely technically challenging and is viewed more as prophylaxis against glaucoma from angle closure rather than therapeutic as treatment once glaucoma has developed

otomy. If corneal epithelial edema is present, the epithelium may be removed (described below). If the corneal stroma is not clear, another procedure, often a trabeculotomy *ab externo*, either partial (with a Harms trabeculotome) or 360° (with a suture or illuminated microcatheter), is generally a better choice.

Advantages and Disadvantages

Goniotomy is faster and less traumatic compared to trabeculotomy. Circumferential treatment (360°) is not possible with a single goniotomy, and there is a lower success with goniotomy compared to circumferential trabeculotomy [9]. However, the success rate for one goniotomy is high, and the shorter operating time limits the patient's anesthetic exposure. Unlike *ab externo* trabeculotomy, the surgical limbus including conjunctiva remains intact with goniotomy. And unlike *ab interno* trabeculotomy, there is minimal intraocular manipulation.

Disadvantages of goniotomy include the fact it is technically demanding and requires considerable surgical experience to master. Furthermore, special instrumentation along with specific patient and microscope positioning are necessary. All angle surgery, goniotomy or *ab interno* trabeculotomy, requires a clear view of the angle. So while there are specific advantages to goniotomy and *ab interno* angle surgery, it does affect patient selection. If epithelial debridement is required, the child may experience significant postoperative discomfort.

Preoperative Considerations and Preparation

In most hospitals and surgical centers, goniotomy is performed less frequently than other glaucoma procedures. It is essential that the operating room staff is informed of the necessary supplies, instruments (Table 4.2), and equipment in a timely fashion and that everything needed is in the operating room to allow an uninterrupted presurgical examination and successful goniotomy procedure. Preparation for an external trabecu-

Table 4.2 Surgical instruments and supplies for goniotomy surgery

Instruments
Operating microscope
Speculum (nasal or temporal depending on approach)
Operating gonioscopy lenses
Goniotomy knife or 23- or 25-g needle on a syringe
Fine tying forceps
Fine scissors
Needle holder appropriate for small needle
Optional instruments
Locking fixation forceps
Supplies
Balanced salt solution
Pilocarpine HCl 1%
Viscoelastic agent, Healon, or similar
10-0 absorbable suture (Vicryl, Ethicon, Somerville NJ, USA)
Antibiotic ointment
Eye pad
Eye shield sized appropriately for patient
Optional supplies
30G irrigation cannula
#15 bard-Parker blade
70% isopropyl alcohol
Apraclonidine 0.5%

lotomy, described later in this chapter, is always advisable when planning for a goniotomy in case of an unsatisfactory view of the angle.

Depending on the specific clinical situation, glaucoma medications may be continued or discontinued. For example, if a patient's cloudy cornea cleared promptly with ocular hypotensive treatment, then the medication should not be stopped preoperatively so as to allow for a clear view of the surgical site. However, if the untreated intraocular pressure (IOP) level is crucial to surgical decision-making, then topical glaucoma medications are stopped 1 or 2 days before surgery. If acetazolamide is being taken, it is discontinued 12 h prior to surgery. Topical bacitracin/polymyxin ointment or other antibiotic may be administered to both eyes preoperatively at the discretion of the surgeon.

Operation

Intraoperative Preparation

Goniotomy, like all other surgical procedures, should be performed only by adequately trained individuals. The techniques of MIGS procedures, such as intraoperative gonioscopy and transcameral device placement, do translate to goniotomy. However, the nuances of goniotomy surgery, such as the ideal patient head and eye position, operating lens management, instrument selections, intraocular knife/needle management, and postoperative care, are best learned by direct observation and surgical assisting [10].

Prior to the operative procedure, an examination under anesthesia (EUA) of both eyes is performed. This operating room assessment includes tonometry, corneal diameter measurement, axial length determination if equipment is available, gonioscopy, handheld slit lamp examination, and fundoscopy (usually recommended only through an undilated pupil of a phakic eye, to avoid additional exposure of the crystalline lens during subsequent goniotomy surgery). With gonioscopy, the quality of the angle view is appraised, and the trabecular meshwork is studied to determine the site of the planned surgery.

The appropriate microscope position can be determined during the EUA, as can the best head position for the patient. In general, the light source should be about 40° from vertical, and the patient's head should be turned about 30° away from the surgeon [11, 12]. The surgeon sits facing the angle to be treated, and the assistant is seated opposite.

Apraclonidine HCl 0.5% may be administered as a drop during the EUA or on a microsurgical sponge to the limbus where the goniotomy will be performed to lessen reflux of blood during the expected period of hypotony that follows the withdrawal of the goniotomy knife or needle. Unlike brimonidine, apraclonidine rarely causes side effects in children [13]. Pilocarpine 1% or 2% is often instilled to constrict the pupil and decrease the risk of lens trauma. It should be instilled as soon as the decision to operate is made. If the pupil remains large at the time of surgery, intracameral acetylcholine may be administered immediately before the goniotomy.

Surgical Technique

If the view of the angle is limited by corneal epithelial edema and the surgeon has determined that goniotomy is still the best surgical choice, a segment of epithelium should be removed to create a clear window. This can be done by applying absolute alcohol or 70% isopropyl alcohol on a sponge to about one-fourth of the cornea 180° away from the angle to be treated. As the initial surgery is usually done in the nasal angle, the temporal cornea is usually treated. Epithelial debridement should not be done in aniridic patients, and in all patients, one should scrupulously avoid the limbal stem cells when using alcohol. After about 10 s, residual alcohol should be thoroughly blotted. The epithelium is then debrided with a #15 Bard-Parker® blade (Aspen Surgical/Hill-Rom, Ashby-de-la-Zouch, Leicestershire, UK), taking care to avoid trauma to Bowman membrane [11, 12]. If removal of the epithelium is not desired or unlikely to improve the angle view, then convert to *ab externo* trabeculotomy, either segmental, using the Harms trabeculotome, or circumferential, using a suture or iScience fiber-optic filament (iScience Interventional, Menlo Park CA, USA).

The following description refers to goniotomy performed with a Barkan goniotomy lens and a standard Swan or Barkan non-irrigating goniotomy knife. Variations based on the choice of instrument and goniotomy lens are briefly described in the next section. In particular, many surgeons use a disposable needle (23 or 25 gauge) mounted on a syringe instead of a goniotomy knife.

After preparation of the sterile surgical field and, if necessary, repositioning of the patient, the lashes are secured with tape or a surgical drape to prevent contact with the knife and to facilitate unimpeded suturing of the cornea. An appropriate lid speculum that will not interfere with the surgery is inserted.

Some surgeons will place locking forceps posteriorly on the vertical muscle insertions to allow the assistant to manipulate the eye without inducing corneal distortion and to facilitate entry of the goniotomy instrument through the cornea adjacent to the limbus. The selected magnification, device, and illumination source are adjusted to provide an optimal view of the angle. The operating gonio lens should leave about 2 mm of the exposed cornea to permit the comfortable entry of the knife (goniotomy knife or microvitreoretinal [MRV] blade) or needle (23 or 25 gauge) away from the gonio lens and to avoid elevating the gonio lens during the procedure. The surgeon's preferred surgical goniotomy lens is placed onto the cornea with either a balanced salt solution or viscoelastic under the lens acting as a fluid bridge. Some surgeons prefer to place a mound of viscoelastic either on the undersurface of the lens or onto the central cornea on which the gonio lens will sit. The goniotomy lens is usually held in place with the surgeon's nondominant hand.

The corneal incision is made with the knife or needle about 1 mm beyond the limbus and 180° from the center of the expected goniotomy incision. The assistant may need to use the forceps to gently move the eye toward the surgeon as counterpressure to facilitate entry. Once the knife is in the eye, the surgeon redirects his or her view from the limbus to the view through the operating gonio lens of the knife, which is passed across the anterior chamber (AC) under direct visualization, ideally over the iris rather than the central pupil opening.

The tip of the knife engages the middle to anterior trabecular meshwork, and the knife is passed in one direction as far as the corneal wound and view permit (Figs. 4.1 and 4.2). Then the knife returns to the middle and is passed in the other direction. Alternatively, the surgeon may engage the meshwork at one end of the site and make a single continuous incision. In either of these cases, the assistant may rotate the eye in the direction opposite to the direction of the surgeon's incision to allow more of the angle to be treated. The incision is superficial, and the surgeon should feel virtually no resistance. A distinct white line can usually be seen in the wake of the cutting instrument as it progresses circumferentially (Fig. 4.3). The knife is then withdrawn on a path over the iris, not over the pupil. The AC is deepened, and the corneal stroma around the incision is hydrated with balanced saline to maintain the IOP and discourage reflux bleeding into the AC. Typically no additional AC irrigation is done. Some surgeons use a filtered air bubble in the AC as well, to facilitate determination of the chamber integrity the following morning. If the

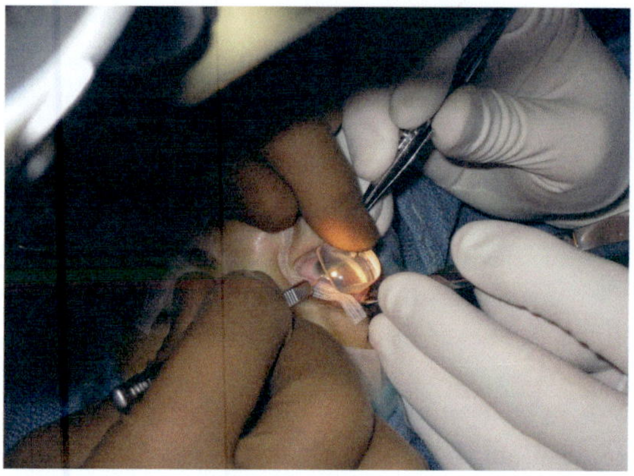

Fig. 4.1 Goniotomy in progress. The assistant stabilizes the globe using locking forceps on the vertical recti muscles, and the surgeon positions the gonio lens and performs the incision. The goniotomy is being performed at the temporal angle, so the surgeon works across the patient's nose. The surgeon in this photo is wearing surgical loupes, but most surgeons prefer to use the operating microscope which allows the assistant to view the angle and allows increased magnification if desired

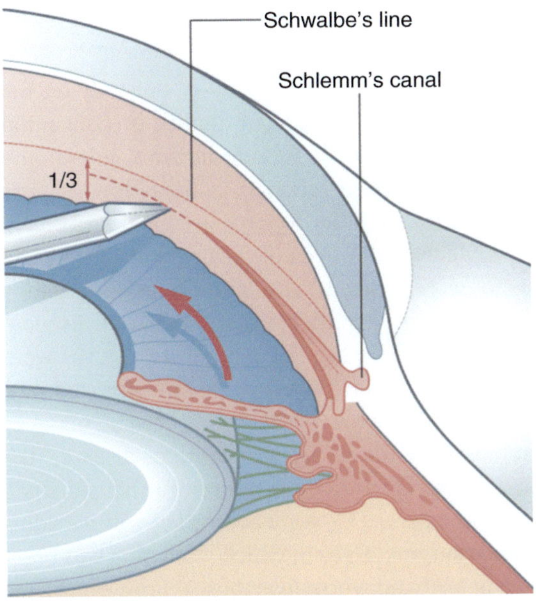

Fig. 4.2 Diagram of knife/needle engaging the anterior trabecular meshwork during goniotomy surgery. (From Chen and Walton [12], with permission)

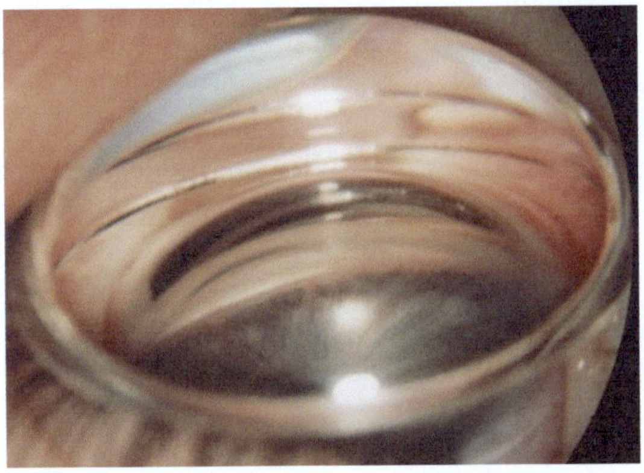

Fig. 4.3 The goniotomy cleft is easily visible as a bright white line on the left, just above the iris insertion

corneal wound is not self-sealing, it is secured with a buried 10-0 vicryl suture, which is often necessary (children may rub the eye). A 10-0 nylon suture can also be used and removed at a subsequent EUA. The operated eye is protected with a patch and shield. Topical prednisolone acetate 1%, apraclonidine HCl 0.5%, and an antibiotic subconjunctival injection and/or ointment may be administered.

If bilateral surgery is being performed, the surgical instruments should be entirely replaced or re-sterilized, the operative team should rescrub, and the second eye should be prepped and draped in the usual sterile fashion.

Videos demonstrating the various techniques for goniotomy, type of lens, with or without assistant, and with or without viscoelastic, are included (Videos 4.1, 4.2, and 4.3).

Potential Modifications

Multiple variations to the procedure described above exist and include the following:

- Locking forceps may be placed at the tenon insertion superiorly and inferiorly rather than at the muscle insertions.
- The globe may be stabilized using traction sutures rather than locking forceps or not stabilized at all.
- An irrigating goniotomy knife attached to balanced salt solution may be used.
- A 23- or 25-gauge needle may be used instead of a goniotomy knife, and it may be attached to a syringe filled with either balanced salt solution or viscoelastic (Video 4.2).
- A 23-gauge MVR blade can be used instead of a goniotomy knife.
- Viscoelastic may be injected into the AC prior to passing the surgical instrument into the angle. If used, it must be thoroughly irrigated out at the end of the case.
- A Swan-Jacob gonio lens or modified Swan-Jacob gonio lens (Ocular Instruments, Bellevue WA, USA), which is held by a handle, may be used and is generally placed onto the eye after the surgical instrument has passed across the pupil and the lens.
- A Glaukos lens with a clip (such as used in the placement of iStents) (Precision Lens, Bloomington MN, USA) can also be used, which allows lens movement.
- Atropine may be instilled at the end of the case to pull the lens posteriorly.
- Alternatively, pilocarpine may be instilled at the end of the case to pull the iris away from the incision and continued for a short time postoperatively.

Postoperative Management

Parents are advised to keep the infant/child's head elevated while sleeping to discourage additional blood reflux. Apraclonidine HCl 0.5% may be given twice daily for a few days when continued postoperative reflux of blood is observed. If a corneal suture is present, topical antibiotics are administered daily for at least a week; ointment is often more soothing than drops. Topical steroid use varies among surgeons and often depends on the presence or absence of a hyphema. In a very quiet eye, topical corticosteroids may be used for as little as a week. Often they are used on a decreasing schedule for several weeks. Some surgeons treat the eye with pilocarpine, some with atropine, and some with neither.

Postoperatively, corneal clarity and intraocular pressures are assessed to ascertain the success of the procedure, which can take up to 4–6 weeks.

Complications

Hyphema is the most common complication of goniotomy. If bleeding occurs during the procedure, it may limit the amount of angle treated. Most postoperative hyphemas resolve spontaneously, although rarely a total hyphema complicated by increased IOP requires an AC washout or other procedure.

Injury to the iris and lens may occur, particularly if the AC shallows. This occurs very rarely if the surgeon has extensive experience and is unlikely to occur if an irrigating knife or a needle is used. AC shallowing can generally be avoided by use of intracameral viscoelastic.

An iridodialysis or cyclodialysis may be created if the incision is made too posteriorly. If the incision is made too deep, the surgical instrument may perforate the limbus. These complications are extremely unlikely if the surgeon is familiar with the anterior segment and angle structures, has a satisfactory view, and practices meticulous surgical technique.

Outcomes

The success rate of goniotomy depends on the severity of the angle abnormality or congenital anomaly. If PCG is present at birth, goniotomy success has been reported to be as low as 10% [14], although other reports are much less bleak. A review of 335 eyes of 210 patients with PCG who were treated with goniotomy in infancy found that 1 year after surgery, 71% of eyes were controlled with one procedure and 93.5% were controlled with one or more procedures. Following review of up to 30 years, 62 eyes relapsed (defined as progressive disease, the institution of medical therapy, or further surgery), but at 5 years, 93% were controlled without additional surgery. Eyes in which glaucoma was present at birth did worse than those whose symptoms appeared in the first 3 months of life (36% relapse compared to 15%) [15].

Good results have been reported following goniotomy in childhood uveitis. The specific definition of success varies among studies, but IOP control with one or more goniotomies and without other glaucoma surgery is about 70% [5, 6]. A small series (five patients) noted 100% success in patients with steroid-induced glaucoma [7]. Reported results vary in patients with Sturge-Weber syndrome. In a group of patients who received one or two goniotomies and were first operated at an average age of 4 months, the pressure was <22 without medication in 6 of 12 patients with follow-up of 2–12 years [16]. However, a review of 43 patients with glaucoma related to the Sturge-Weber syndrome found long-term failure in 98% (Walton DS, Yeung HH, unpublished data).

Options After Failed Surgery

If a single goniotomy does not control the patient's glaucoma, the procedure may be repeated in a different area of the drainage angle. (Fig. 4.1 shows a procedure on the temporal angle.) Goniotomy may interfere with circumferential trabeculotomy, but it does not preclude treatment of the untreated angle by either an *ab externo* or *ab interno* procedure.

If angle surgery is not successful, medical treatment is generally resumed. If necessary, a glaucoma drainage device may be placed or a trabeculectomy may be performed. Because the conjunctiva and sclera are not incised, goniotomy is unlikely to affect the success rates of these procedures, although good data are lacking.

References

1. Barkan O. A new operation for chronic glaucoma. Am J Ophthalmol. 1936;19(11):951–66.
2. Barkan O. Microsurgery in chronic simple glaucoma. Am J Ophthalmol. 1938;21(4):403–5.
3. Barkan O. Operation for congenital glaucoma. Am J Ophthalmol. 1942;25(5):552–68.
4. Barkan O. Present status of goniotomy. The Jackson Memorial Lecture. Am J Ophthalmol. 1953;36(4):445–53.
5. Ho CL, Walton DS. Goniosurgery for glaucoma secondary to chronic anterior uveitis. J Glaucoma. 2004;13(6):445–9.
6. Bohnsack BL, Freedman SF. Surgical outcomes in childhood uveitic glaucoma. Am J Ophthalmol. 2013;155(1):134–42.
7. Choi EY, Walton DS. Goniotomy for steroid-induced glaucoma: clinical and tonographic evidence to support therapeutic goniotomy. J Ped Ophthalmol Strab. 2015;52(3):183–8.
8. Chen TC, Walton DS. Goniosurgery for prevention of aniridic glaucoma. Arch Ophthalmol. 1999;117(9):1144–8.
9. Neustein RF, Beck AD. Circumferential trabeculotomy versus conventional angle surgery: comparing long-term surgical success and clinical outcomes in children with primary congenital glaucoma. Am J Ophthalmol. 2017;183:17–24.
10. Yeung HH, Walton DS. Pediatric glaucoma: angle surgery and glaucoma drainage devices. In: Giaconi JA, Law SK, Nouri-Mahdavi K, Coleman AL, Caprioli J, editors. Pearls of glaucoma management. Berlin Heidelberg: Springer-Verlag; 2016. p. 487–94.
11. Walton DS. Goniotomy. In: Thomas JV, editor. Glaucoma surgery. St. Louis: Mosby-Year Book, Inc.; 1992. p. 107–21.
12. Chen T, Walton DS. Goniotomy. In: Chen T, editor. Glaucoma surgery, Surgical techniques in ophthalmology series. Philadelphia: Saunders; 2008. p. 153–63.
13. Wright TM, Freedman SF. Exposure to topical apraclonidine in children with glaucoma. J Glaucoma. 2009;18(5):395–8.
14. Walton DS, Katsavounidou G. Newborn primary congenital glaucoma: 2005 update. J Pediatr Ophthalmol Strab. 2005;42(6):333–41.
15. Russel-Eggitt IM, Rice NS, Barrie J, Wyse RK. Relapse following goniotomy for congenital glaucoma due to trabecular dysgenesis. Eye. 1992;6(Pt 2):197–200.
16. Olsen KE, Huang AS, Wright MM. The efficacy of goniotomy/trabeculotomy in early-onset glaucoma associated with the Sturge-weber syndrome. J AAPOS. 1998;2(6):365–8.

Angle Surgery: Trabeculotomy

5

Beth Edmunds, Allen D. Beck, Esther Hoffmann, and Franz Grehn

History

Following in the footsteps of Barkan [1], two other pioneers of angle surgery proposed a different approach to Schlemm canal (SC), via a scleral cutdown, and this became known as trabeculotomy. Both involved conjunctival and scleral dissection to access SC. The technique was further refined and popularized for the treatment of primary congenital glaucoma. In particular, trabeculotomy offered an advantage over goniotomy when corneal clouding precluded a safe gonioscopic view of the angle required for goniotomy.

Goniotomy and trabeculotomy enjoyed similar success rates in similar types of patients [2–5]. As each of these surgeries typically treated 60–120° degrees of the angle circumference, consecutive surgeries on untreated sections of the angle extended the reach of the procedure with additional IOP lowering. In 1995, Beck and Lynch [6] proposed treating the full 360° of angle circumference in one surgery, using a polypropylene suture filament and an ab externo approach. The advantage of the circumferential approach is that the full extent of the angle is treated during one surgery, potentially lessening the number of anesthetics in the subset of children that would have required more than one surgery.

The advent of an illuminated microcatheter, initially reported in the adult literature, was not wasted on pediatric glaucoma surgeons. Sarkisian [7] reported an ab externo technique akin to conventional trabeculotomy with a superficial scleral flap and underlying radial deep scleral cutdown into SC. After circumferential advancement of the microcatheter, traction is applied to the two ends of the catheter so that the noose is tightened and the catheter cheese-wires through the TM to open SC to the AC for the extent of its cannulation, similar to the original blunted polypropylene suture approach described a decade before [6]. Given the explosion of interest in adult angle surgery since then, it was not long before this was

Electronic Supplementary Material The online version of this chapter (https://doi.org/10.1007/978-3-319-54003-0_5) contains supplementary material, which is available to authorized users.

B. Edmunds (✉)
Casey Eye Institute, Oregon Health and Science University, Portland, OR, USA
e-mail: edmundsb@ohsu.edu

A. D. Beck
Department of Ophthalmology, Emory University, Atlanta, GA, USA

E. Hoffmann
Department of Ophthalmology, Childhood Glaucoma Center, University Medical Center Mainz, Mainz, Germany

F. Grehn
Department of Ophthalmology, University Hospitals Würzburg, Würzburg, Germany

A. L. Grajewski et al. (eds.), *Surgical Management of Childhood Glaucoma*,
https://doi.org/10.1007/978-3-319-54003-0_5

modified to an internal approach, published as gonioscopy-assisted transluminal trabeculotomy (GATT) by Grover et al. [8]. This can be performed with either the illuminated microcatheter or a blunted polypropylene suture. At this point, these surgeries in fact become more akin to traditional goniotomy performed circumferentially, rather than trabeculotomy, as they are performed ab interno and require a clear cornea.

In populations where children present with more severe forms of PCG, complex childhood glaucomas, or in advanced stages of disease, combining trabeculotomy with a full-thickness external filtration procedure, such as trabeculectomy, has been advocated [9–18]. Combined trabeculotomy-trabeculectomy (CTT) creates a dual outflow pathway for aqueous, by addressing the barrier to aqueous flow responsible for the disease (the trabeculotomy portion) and by providing external filtration into a bleb (the trabeculectomy portion). This allows for IOP lowering beyond the limits of episcleral venous pressure, provides a planned backup procedure should the execution of the trabeculotomy portion of the surgery be inadequate (SC is not identified in up to 15% of cases [19] or in only one direction [20, 21]), and in the longer term provides for some remaining efficacy if one portion of the procedure fails [16]. Refinements in this technique too have been proposed, such as use of mitomycin C (MMC) [14, 22], 5FU, and releasable sutures [18, 23], as for trabeculectomy alone.

Other combined approaches are also of interest, though there is less literature available. For example, with filtering trabeculotomy (FTO), conventional trabeculotomy is combined with a modification of deep sclerectomy in which the deep scleral flap is removed [24]. In this way, addressing the trabecular barrier to aqueous flow is coupled with the benefits of an external filtration system but without the risks of full-thickness penetration into the AC, as in CTT. In both viscotrabeculotomy [25] and combined viscotrabeculotomy-trabeculectomy [26], the trabeculotomy portion is supplemented by viscodilation of SC, as well as other maneuvers.

Indications and Contraindications

The most common indication for trabeculotomy, whether it be ab interno, ab externo, traditional, circumferential, or combined with filtration, is PCG. These various iterations of trabeculotomy have also been successful in other open-angle childhood glaucomas such as juvenile open-angle glaucoma (JOAG), glaucoma following cataract extraction (previously termed "aphakic" glaucoma), early-onset glaucoma associated with Sturge-Weber syndrome, and glaucoma associated with steroid use, uveitis, and angle recession, though are not as effective in these conditions as in PCG.

An absolute contraindication to an internal approach is a poor gonioscopic view of the angle structures. The surgeon should be comfortable with the surgical demands of appropriate patient positioning and microscope tilting, holding a goniolens in one hand (unless using a "hands-free" goniolens) while working in the eye with the other, and the anatomy of the angle. Corneal opacities, edema, and hyphema will also compromise the view. Trabeculotomy ab externo or combined with external filtration would be contraindicated if the condition of the conjunctiva or sclera precluded safe wound closure. Many surgeons would also avoid an angle approach in glaucomas associated with non-acquired conditions such as Axenfeld-Rieger, in more severe forms of Peters anomaly, in those aniridia cases in which the angle is narrowed or closed, and in other angle-closure situations. Although angle surgery is performed in early-onset cases of glaucoma associated with Sturge-Weber syndrome [27], it may be prudent to avoid a circumferential approach in these cases given reports of prolonged hyphema and no improvement in success compared to traditional angle surgery [28]. Prior surgeries that have violated SC, including prior trabeculotomy, are likely to produce scarring that may obstruct circumferential cannulation. However there have been reports of successful circumferential trabeculotomy after prior angle surgery [28, 29].

Combined procedures may be indicated in more severe disease and are more popular in certain populations. The choice and indications for type of surgery in different situations are influenced by the surgeon's experience and familiarity with the techniques available.

Advantages and Disadvantages

Table 5.1 provides a comparison of the main techniques.

Preoperative Considerations and Preparation

In cases of children with glaucoma requiring bilateral surgery, a decision has to be made whether to operate on both eyes during the same surgical episode or sequentially. The advantage of simultaneous bilateral surgery is quicker treatment of the fellow eye, potentially a reduction in number of anesthetics required, and quicker visual rehabilitation. The disadvantages are that both eyes are surgically unstable, there is not the opportunity to adjust the surgical approach based on the postoperative experience of the first eye, and it prolongs the duration of anesthesia.

All instruments should be in the operating room (OR) or easily accessible, and equipment, such as the lighting source for the illuminated microcatheter, checked before committing to surgery (Fig. 5.1). Furthermore, even though a circumferential approach may be planned, backup instruments (at a minimum a metal trabeculotome) should be available in case conversion to a more traditional angle surgery, or even trabeculectomy, is required. See Table 5.2 for a list of instruments.

Intraoperative Preparation

The location of the surgical site is an important consideration. In general, for trabeculotomy alone, a temporal approach is preferred. For ab interno surgeries, this provides the easiest access to the angle, avoiding awkward manipulation of instruments over other parts of the patient's face. In ab externo approaches, an inferior or temporally sited cutdown allows sparing of the superior conjunctiva and sclera for future trabeculectomy in which surgically naïve tissue is clearly linked to better trabeculectomy outcomes. This needs to be weighed against the surgeon's confidence in achieving watertight scleral wound closure as inadvertent bleb formation in the interpalpebral fissure is highly undesirable. For the same reason, trabeculotomy combined with external

Table 5.1 Advantages and disadvantages of the angle-based surgeries

Approach	Skill	Surgical time	Special equipment	Visits to OR	Treatment extent (°)	Scleral incisions
Conventional goniotomy	+++	+	Goniotomy knife (or needle), tilting microscope, goniolens	++	90–180	–
Conventional trabeculotomy	+++	++	Metal trabeculotome	++	70	++
Internal circumferential	++++	+++	Goniolens, tilting microscope, blunted polypropylene suture, or illuminated microcatheter	+	Potentially 360	–
External circumferential	++++	++++	Blades for scleral flap, blunted polypropylene suture (and goniolens), or illuminated microcatheter	+	Potentially 360	++ – +++ depending on size of flaps
Combined with external filtration	++++	++++	Scleral punch, anti-scarring agents, anterior chamber maintainer	++++	70 + bleb	++++ at 12 o'clock position

OR operating room

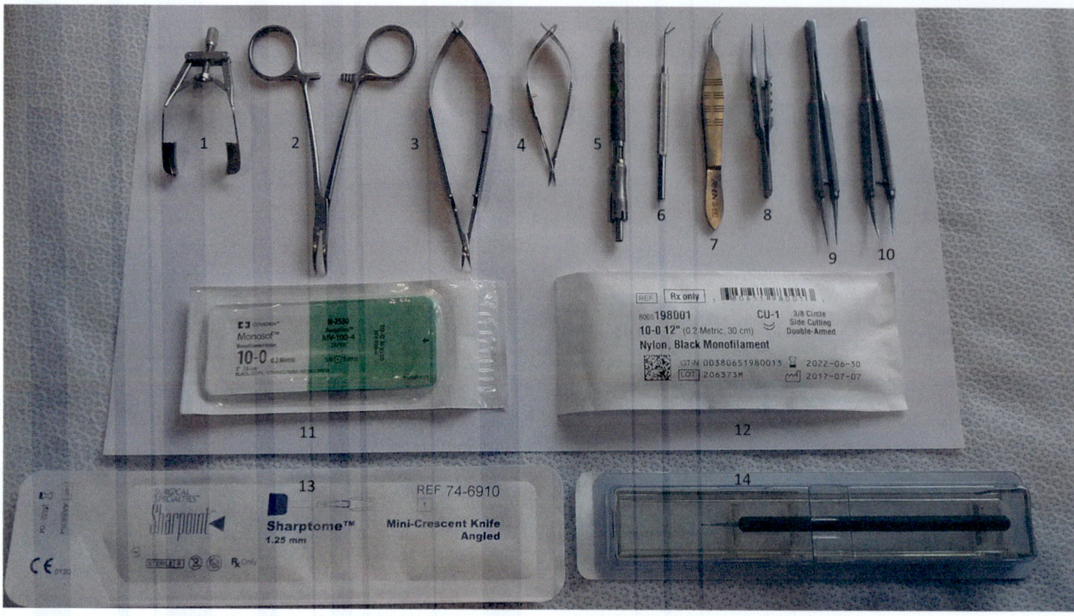

Fig. 5.1 Basic surgical instrument set for trabeculotomy. (Courtesy of Deborah Carter, RN, OHSU Casey Eye Institute, Portland OR, USA). (1) Bladed lid speculum. (2) Mosquito forceps (attaching traction suture to drape). (3) Westcott scissors. (4) Mini-Westcott scissors. (5) Diamond knife with depth-calibrated blade. (6) Ink marker for 5 × 5 parabola-shaped superficial scleral flap. (7) Lasik forceps (for manipulating illuminated microcatheter – rounded tips avoid inadvertent Descemet membrane perforation). (8) Small grooved Hoskins forcep. (9) Straight tying forcep. (10) Curved tying forcep. (11) 10/0 nylon on non-cutting needle (for delicate tissue). (12) 10/0 nylon on spatulated needle. (13) Mini-crescent knife for superficial and deep flap dissection. (14) Crescent blade for deep flap and scleral spur dissection

Table 5.2 Surgical instruments

Basic set
Sterile drape
Bladed Lieberman lid speculum
Epinephrine in 1 ml w/27 g cannula
6/0 vicryl suture for traction
Mosquito forcep for traction suture
Mini-Westcott scissors
Vannas scissors
Pierce-Hoskins notched forceps
18ga cautery
Weck-Cel sponges
30 ml bottle BSS with tip
3 cc syringe BSS with 27ga cannula
75 blade
69 blade
Crescent blade for superficial scleral flap
Miostat on 30ga cannula
Healon on 27ga cannula
Curved lasik flap forceps (Rhein 08-16163)
10/0 nylon suture on CU-1 cutting needle
Tennant tying forceps
3 cc sterile air 30ga cannula

Table 5.2 (continued)

Double-flap technique (for deep scleral flap)
Angled mini crescent blade (Rhein 03-6452)
Micro-toothed forceps (0.06 g)
Weck-Cel sponges – Damp
Choices of trabeculotomy instruments
Metal trabeculotome
Harms – Hairpin-like instrument with two bent arms; the same instrument can be used for both left and right sides. It is grasped and turned by a needle holder or between surgeon's thumb and index finger (see Fig. 5.1a)
Neuhann (Geuder Inc., Heidelberg, Germany) – Similar to Harms trabeculotome but with longer arms and a small plate to grasp and rotate the instrument (see Fig. 5.1b)
Mackensen trabeculotome – Single arm attached to a vertical handle at 90°. A pair is needed, one for the left and one for right side. The advantage is that it can be more easily turned into the AC by the handle than the Harms probe (see Fig. 5.6c)
McPherson trabeculotome – Hairpin-like instrument with two bent arms attached to a handle. A pair is needed, one for the left and one for right side. The advantage is that the direction of the inner probe can be controlled by the parallel outer arm (see Fig. 5.1a)
Microcatheter approach
iLUMIN system with iTRACK 250A microcatheter (Ellex) (see Fig. 5.5)
Microcatheter alone (Glaukos)
Blunted suture approach
6/0 polypropylene suture – Prepared by holding cautery close to tip to melt it into a small, blunted, mushroom shape (see Fig. 5.6)
Useful extras
10/0 nylon round-bodied needle
5 × 5 parabolic ink marker (Rhein 08-08233)
Stegmann PHDII micro crescent diamond knife (Mastel)

filtration, which is dependent on intentional bleb formation, should be performed superiorly.

Another vital pre- and ongoing intraoperative assessment includes a judgment of corneal clarity as this determines whether an ab interno trabeculotomy can be performed safely. The positioning of the patient and microscope and surgical view of the angle should also be checked with a goniolens prior to incising the eye. The quality of the view can also be impacted by the quality of the goniolens, the surgeon's skill, and the intraoperative developments such as hyphema.

In terms of the surgical preparation of the eye, topical miotics (pilocarpine 1–2%) can be given preoperatively, and acetylcholine chloride can be injected into the AC to draw iris over the crystalline lens to protect it from intraoperative trauma. If there is mild corneal clouding, the strategies discussed in the goniotomy section may allow sufficient clearing for an ab interno approach.

Trabeculotomy Alone

Conventional Trabeculotomy (with Metal Trabeculotome)

In this approach to trabeculotomy, an external cutdown through sclera is made (ab externo), and a metal trabeculotome is used to cannulate and tear through a section of the inner wall of SC and trabeculum into the AC. It is sometimes referred to as metal or rigid probe trabeculotomy.

Operation (Video 5.1)

Surgical Technique. Following preparation of a sterile field, a corneal traction suture is placed and the globe rotated away from the surgeon to achieve adequate exposure of the surgical site. Either fornix- or limbus-based conjunctival flaps may be used though access is easier using a fornix-based approach. Conjunctiva and Tenon capsule are dissected off the globe, and the episclera is cleaned with a blade. Gentle cautery may be required.

Most surgeons use a rectangular superficial scleral flap of 1/2 to 2/3 scleral thickness or a triangular flap. The size of the rectangular flap is usually 3 × 3 or 4 × 4 mm. Once the superficial flap has been dissected into clear cornea anteriorly and it is reflected, a small radially oriented incision at the transition zone between the sclera and cornea is made with a blade. This incision is slowly and carefully dissected deeper under high magnification, examining the depth of the incision until SC is identified, often by a small trickle of blood or aqueous from the cut ends. Care must be taken not to dissect any deeper to avoid perforation. The landmarks can be difficult to identify because of limbal stretching characteristic of buphthalmos and the pale TM characteristic of a child. Gentle probing may help confirm an ostium into the canal as the probe should enter easily without resistance. However this should be performed very gently as false passages are easily created into the suprachoroidal space behind the scleral spur or into the AC. When SC is identified, a small amount of viscoelastic can be injected to dilate the openings, and/or the outer wall can be slit open further with a blade or by snipping with Vannas scissors in a limbus-parallel direction into the lumen of the canal. This can widen the entry into SC though care needs to be exercised to ensure this is performed anterior to the scleral spur as the potential space behind SC opens easily and may be mistaken for the canal.

A valuable alternative method of reaching SC using a double scleral flap technique is described in the modifications section below.

Two examples of metal trabeculotome probes can be seen in Fig. 5.2. The trabeculotome is introduced into the canal and rotated into the AC, cutting through the internal wall of SC and TM, on each side, as in Fig. 5.3 [30]. It is helpful to stabilize the limbus at the area of the probe tip from outside with forceps (such as Kolibri) because the plane of rotation is then better defined. When the goal is trabeculotomy only (without filtration), care must be taken not to break the trabecular-Descemet membrane at the site of the deep flap. During rotation of the probe into the AC, attention should be directed to the axis of rotation. It may be helpful to gently press the angle of the probe against the scleral edge to anchor the point of rotation. It is not necessary to rotate the probe 90° into the AC, because the TM can be adequately torn while pulling out the probe with a lateral movement. If the trabecular-Descemet membrane at the site of the deep flap is preserved, there is no gross filtration of aqueous, and the risk of hypotony is low. Another advantage of the preservation of the trabecular-Descemet membrane is reduced risk of iris prolapse, and so no iridectomy is needed. Avoiding iridectomy may reduce the risk of hemorrhage and long-term cataract formation.

After the trabeculotomy is completed, the scleral incisions and/or flaps are closed with a

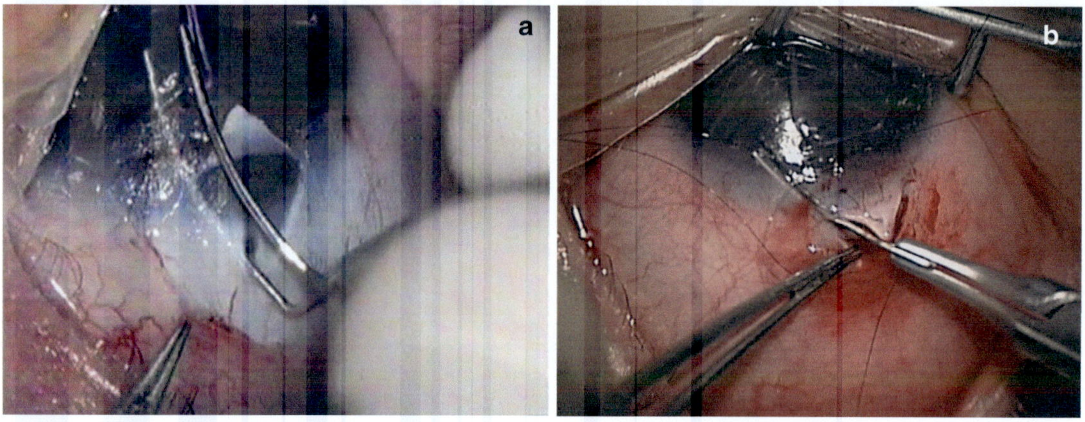

Fig. 5.2 Metal trabeculotome probes. (**a**) Harms trabeculotome. (**b**) Thomas Neuhann U-shaped trabeculotome with no handle. (Courtesy of Professor Nader Bayoumi, Alexandria University, Egypt)

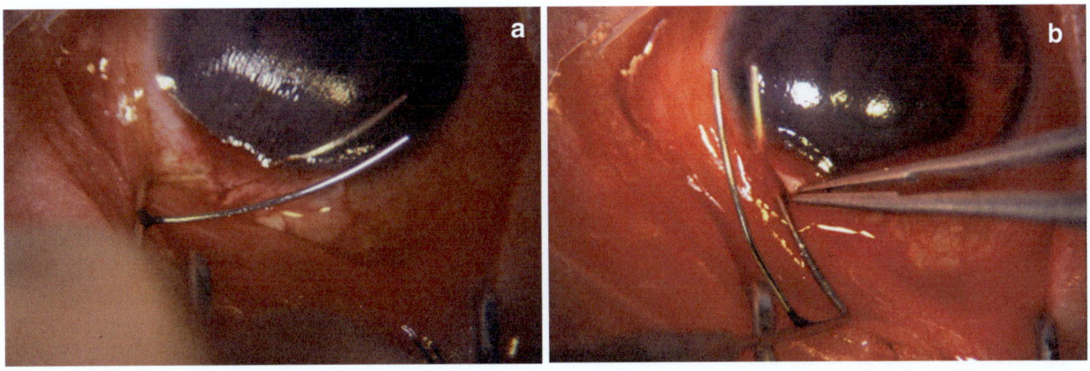

Fig. 5.3 Conventional trabeculotomy with Harms metal trabeculotome. (**a**) Trabeculotome rotating from Schlemm canal into the anterior chamber, left direction. (**b**) Trabeculotomy completed, right direction. (From Iowa Glaucoma Curriculum [29] with permission) (© University of Iowa. Courtesy of Wallace L.M. Alward, MD, Department of Ophthalmology and Visual Sciences, University of Iowa Carver College of Medicine, Iowa City, Iowa, USA)

sufficient number of watertight sutures to avoid any drainage. 10/0 nylon is preferred as it maintains its tension, while other surgeons report success with 10/0 polyglactin sutures which dissolve. Lamellar scleral sutures will avoid leakage around needle tracks. In very delicate tissue, round-bodied non-cutting needle profiles may be helpful if suture tracks leak. If the double-flap technique has been used, ensure the deep flap has watertight closure before closing the superficial flap over it. Special attention should be paid to good closure in the limbal area to avoid leaks, staphylomas, and inadvertent anterior bleb formation, which can be very difficult to repair at a later stage. Conjunctival closure should ensure a smooth limbus with well-buried sutures to avoid any irritation that would prompt eye rubbing by the child. The conjunctiva is closed by interrupted 10/0 nylon or polyglactin mattress sutures at the limbus (fornix-based conjunctival approach) or by an 8/0 or 10/0 polyglactin running suture (limbus-based conjunctival approach). Suturing the paracentesis also helps avoid hypotony, iris prolapse, or incarceration.

Once the eye is secure, postoperative subconjunctival injections of steroid and antibiotic are given and pilocarpine 2% drops instilled to maintain miosis, which is believed to keep iris from adhering to the newly incised trabecular cleft. The eye is then patched to maintain lid closure and a protective shield placed such that accidental pressure or trauma would be transmitted to the surrounding orbital bones rather than the globe.

Problem-Solving

Finding SC. The commonest reason for failing to identify SC is insufficient depth of dissection. Using high magnification and slow careful downward dissection in the anatomical location of SC, the incision can be deepened until the tell-tale trickle of blood from the cut ends of SC is seen. If no blood reflux is seen, despite correct location, the surgeon may gently probe the area with a polypropylene suture or probe. If there is any sense of forcing the probe, it is unlikely to be in SC, and continued probing will lead to false canals or perforation into the AC. If dissection has been difficult, the edges of the incision may be ragged with wayward tissue filaments impeding introduction of the probe, even though blood reflux is visible. Making an adjacent second incision to the depth of the first (facilitated by using a fresh knife or diamond blade) will create cleaner edges to allow the probe to slip into the canal more easily. In the authors' experience, the double-flap technique is a more reliable approach in locating SC, especially when the limbal anatomy is stretched and landmarks uncertain. Providing the deep flap is indeed deep enough, it will incise the outer wall of SC along its length and deroof it.

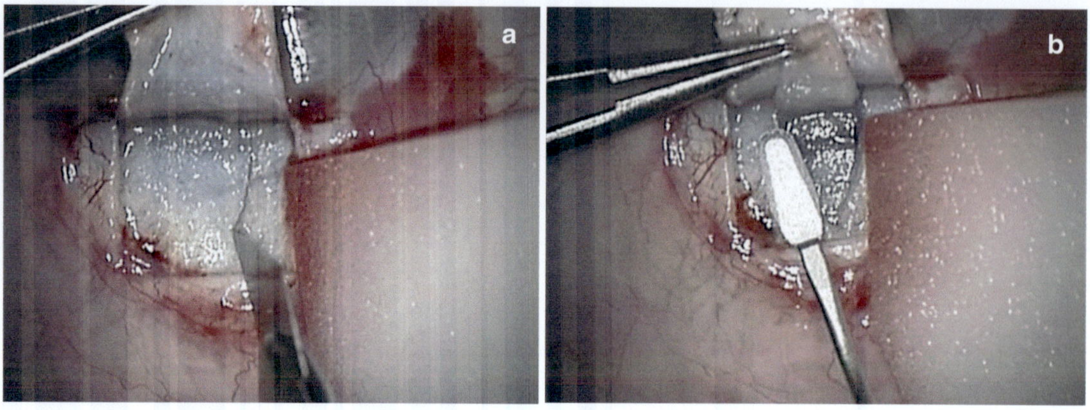

Fig. 5.4 Double scleral flap technique. (**a**) Deep scleral flap (double flap technique). (**b**) Deroofing Schlemm canal. (Courtesy of Franz Grehn, MD, PhD)

Potential Modifications

Traction Suture. In a severely buphthalmic eye and/or when it is difficult to achieve adequate exposure with a limbal traction suture, one or two transconjunctival rectus muscle traction sutures may provide safer and better exposure of the surgical site.

Double Scleral Flap (Superficial and Deep) Approach. A valuable alternative to the deep radial scleral cutdown approach to locating SC is derived from deep sclerectomy (Fig. 5.4 shows this approach as part of filtering trabeculotomy). A superficial half-thickness scleral flap is dissected anteriorly into clear cornea. This flap may be rectangular, triangular, or paraboloid and approximately 4 × 4 mm in size. Either a caliper can be used, or an inked marker, to delineate the dimensions of this superficial flap. The dimensions of a second, smaller, deep scleral flap are scored with a sharp blade to lie 1 millimeter within the borders of the superficial flap. The base of the deeper flap should be fashioned in the plane just above the choroid. At the beginning of the development of this flap, the posterior margin/apex is carefully deepened until the grayness of underlying uveal tissue is apparent. The flap is then dissected anteriorly maintaining this plane just above the ciliary body. This is best done with the microscope on high magnification and high illumination. Fine-toothed forceps (0.06 gauge) for gentle flap retraction, and a fresh sharp crescent blade, are helpful to achieve clean incisions without tearing tissue in the delicate flap base. If this depth is maintained as the flap is developed anteriorly, it will deroof SC as it reaches the limbal area. The thus exposed inner wall of SC has a smooth, white, glistening appearance compared to the texture of the scleral dissection, and there is usually a trickle of blood refluxing from the freshly cut ends of the canal.

Circumferential 360 Trabeculotomy (Illuminated Microcatheter or Blunted Suture Approaches)

This group of surgeries treats the full or almost full circumferential extent of the angle by cannulating SC by either an illuminated microcatheter or a blunted polypropylene suture. The catheter or suture can be introduced into SC via an external scleral cutdown (ab externo) or from within the AC via an internal TM incision (ab interno). Only the ab externo approach is described in the chapter. For the ab interno approach, which is more akin to goniotomy, please refer to Chap. 8.

Illuminated Microcatheter (Ab Externo) Operation (Video 5.2)

Surgical Technique. A corneal traction suture is placed and the globe rotated away from the surgeon to achieve adequate exposure of the surgical site. A 5–6 mm fornix-based conjunctival flap is dissected from the limbus posteriorly with an inferior radial relaxing incision. Conjunctiva and

Tenon capsule should be dissected completely off the underlying sclera to allow clean scleral incisions. Cleaning episcleral tissue off the globe with strokes of a curved blade (e.g., Beaver blade) and gentle cautery also help prepare the surgical site.

A half-thickness, 5 × 5mm (or slightly smaller in some surgeon's methods) superficial scleral flap is fashioned. SC is identified either using a radial scleral cut down in the area over the suspected region of SC or a 3 × 3-mm-deep scleral flap (double-flap technique as in Fig. 5.4). Both flaps are slightly larger than for the blunted suture approach as the microcatheter is stiffer than the suture and may kink with excessive bending.

Once SC has been reached, a small paracentesis may be made to decompress the eye a little, acetylcholine chloride injected if the pupil is not yet miotic, and a small amount of viscoelastic injected to maintain the AC. Avoid overinflating the eye as this can compress SC and make introduction and threading of the catheter more difficult and/or predispose to Descemet membrane prolapse which is then more vulnerable to rupture or perforation by instruments.

The illuminated microcatheter may be primed with viscoelastic (Ellex version) and set on blinking mode (Ellex or Glaukos). Dimming the room and microscope lights allows better identification of the blinking tip as it travels through SC. Reducing the magnification of the microscope allows the entire limbal area of the globe to be visualized. The catheter must be handled with smooth-tipped forceps so as not to damage it, and blunt-tipped forceps are also helpful in avoiding inadvertent piercing of DM while working with the catheter. If the catheter becomes kinked, it will not travel safely through SC.

The catheter should be positioned so that its approach is in the horizontal plane of the limbus. The tip can then be introduced into SC opening with as little distortion as possible. Either use an assistant or secure the catheter to the drape to keep it in the appropriate plane. The catheter is then fed into SC in small increments, avoiding pushing too hard if obstruction is encountered as this will distort the catheter; there is usually minimal or slight resistance. Its course around the limbus in SC can be verified by visualizing the illuminated tip at all times, as in Fig. 5.5a. If the light is not visible, withdraw the catheter until it is seen blinking again in an appropriate position (considering that the limbal anatomy is stretched in buphthalmic eyes and typical landmarks may not be as reliable). The tip may have inadvertently been inserted into the AC (a clue to this is twitching of the iris as the catheter is advanced) or diverted into a collector channel or tracked into the suprachoroidal space if introduced behind the scleral spur rather than into SC. If the catheter has become misdirected and is not in SC, one can attempt to withdraw and re-advance it, but usually

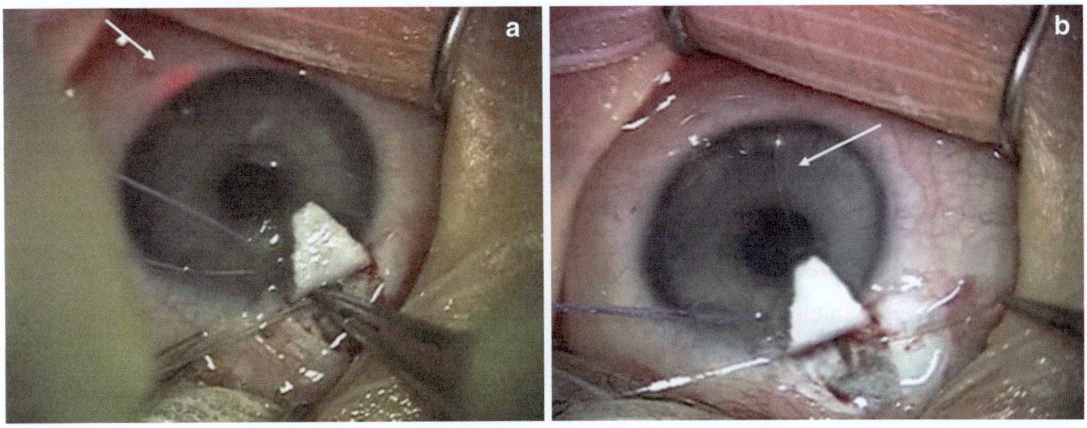

Fig. 5.5 Circumferential trabeculotomy with illuminated microcatheter. (**a**) Threading microcatheter into Schlemm canal, arrow showing illuminated tip. (**b**) Microcatheter tearing through trabeculum into anterior chamber, arrow showing microcatheter loop. (From Sarkisian [7], with permission)

it is not able to be redirected into the proper trajectory. It must be removed (unless it has almost completed its circumferential path, in which case a cutdown can be made over the blinking light to retrieve the far end of the catheter; see below under "obstruction") and reintroduced into the other cut end of SC in the opposite direction.

Once the catheter has successfully passed through 360° of SC, its distal end will protrude from the opposite end of SC and can be delivered further until its tip is clear of DM and the two ends of the microcatheter will come to lie across each other. It is important that the AC is formed and pupil constricted. Placing interrupted 10/0 nylon deep scleral flap sutures at the apex and along the sides of the deep flap and tying them before executing the trabeculotomy maintains the AC with minimal need for viscoelastic. If, on the other hand, the surgeon prefers filling the AC with viscoelastic, this will also protect the AC from shallowing. The catheter exits between the tied sutures easily. The two ends of the catheter suture are then grasped with forceps, and as they are gently pulled apart, the purse-string effect tears through the TM producing a trabeculotomy, as seen in Fig. 5.5b. This movement should be continuous and smooth so that as the AC shallows the catheter does not become snagged on iris or too close to corneal endothelium. Just before completion of the trabeculotomy, the free end of the catheter is released so that it passes through the AC under the area of the intact Descemet-trabecular tissue as the other end is pulled out of the eye (i.e., the small section of the trabeculum and SC under the wound is left intact and contributes to watertight wound closure).

The incisions are closed as described for the double-flap technique above. If the majority of deep flap 10/0 nylon sutures have been pre-placed before removing the microcatheter, only one or two more may be required before addressing the superficial flap and conjunctiva. The immediate postoperative subconjunctival injections, drops, patch, and shield are also as above.

Problem-Solving

Finding SC. The comments made for finding SC in the probe section above also hold for the microcatheter approach. As it is so delicate, there are occasions when even in the presence of convincing blood reflux from presumed SC openings, the catheter tip cannot be introduced into SC. In these cases a tiny ragged tissue filament may be catching the tip; making a fresh deep scleral flap incision just adjacent and parallel to the original incision may create cleaner edges to the SC openings and allow the microcatheter tip to pass smoothly.

Obstruction. If the microcatheter encounters an obstruction in SC, the first maneuver is to withdraw the catheter a small distance and then dilate the area by injecting viscoelastic (a single "click" of the attached hub, Ellex). Often, withdrawing the microcatheter and cannulating SC from the opposite opening overcome the obstruction. Changing the AC dynamics by either softening the eye a little, or filling it with BSS or viscoelastic, may also change the dynamics of the canal and allow the catheter to pass. If unable to pass the microcatheter 360°, it may be worth making a second scleral ab externo cutdown over the arrested illuminated tip, to execute a partial sectoral trabeculotomy along the section of SC cannulated.

Misdirection. If the illuminated tip deviates away from the peri-limbal area, it is either in a collector channel or the suprachoroidal space. If a collector channel deviation is suspected, try viscodilation as above combined with applying the flat end of a forcep over the suspected collector duct connection to encourage the catheter to remain in SC. If the iris twitches with advancement of the microcatheter, it has perforated into the AC. In this case further careful searching for the opening to SC is required, though once there is a DM perforation, the catheter may preferentially adopt that course. Trying cannulation from the opposite side may avoid the DM perforation and be more successful.

Blunted Suture (Ab Externo)

Operation (Video 5.3)

Surgical Technique. A corneal traction suture is placed and the globe rotated away from the surgeon to achieve adequate exposure of the surgical site. A 4–5 mm fornix-based conjunctival flap is dissected from the limbus posteriorly with an inferior radial relaxing incision. Conjunctiva and Tenon capsule should be dissected completely off the underlying sclera to allow clean scleral incisions. Cleaning episcleral tissue off the globe with strokes of a curved blade (e.g., Beaver blade) and gentle cautery also help prepare the surgical site.

A half-thickness, 3–4 mm × 3–4 mm scleral flap is fashioned starting approximately 4 mm behind the limbus and carried anteriorly to the limbal area. SC is identified either using a deep radial scleral incision over the suspected location of SC or a deep scleral flap as in the double-flap technique described above.

A fishhook-shaped fragment of 6-0 polypropylene suture is cut with sufficient length to be approximately 50% larger than circumference of the cornea (65–80 mm). The tip of the curved end of the suture is blunted by bringing high-temperature disposable cautery close (but not touching) to melt it into a mushroom cap shape. A small smooth rounded end is required for smooth passage through SC.

The blunted end of the prepared suture is introduced into the opening of SC and fed further for about 5–10 mm as shown in Fig. 5.6. It should pass easily without significant resistance. Its position in the canal should be verified by gonioscopy which should allow the bright blue suture and mushroom cap to be detected, even in the presence of corneal edema. Having verified its initial location, the suture is progressively fed into SC, with periodic gonioscopy. Once the suture has successfully passed through 360° of SC, its distal end will protrude from the opposite end of SC and can be delivered further or grasped using jewelers or other fine-tipped forceps. Great care should be taken not to perforate DM with the tips of the forceps. It should be noted that sometimes the blunted advancing end of the suture will pass through the "far end" of SC and make a second circumferential course, so that it needs to be lifted from the SC at its cut end to retrieve it.

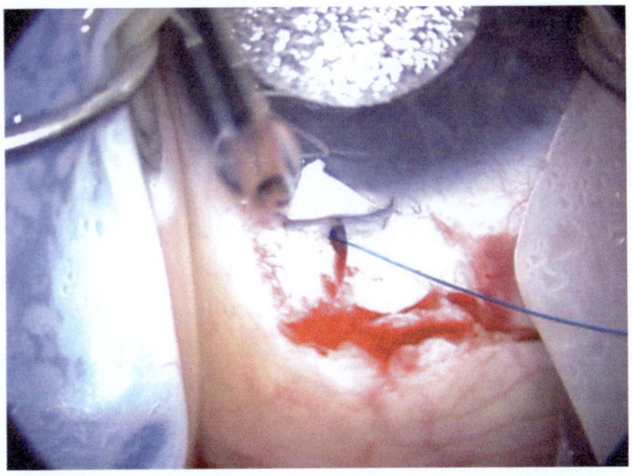

Fig. 5.6 Circumferential trabeculotomy with blunted suture filament. (Courtesy of Allen D. Beck, MD)

A small paracentesis is made, and an intracameral miotic agent such as acetylcholine chloride is injected followed by viscoelastic. The two ends of the blunted suture are grasped with needle holders and gently pulled in opposite directions "cheese-wiring" into the AC through SC and TM.

The incisions are closed as above. The immediate postoperative subconjunctival injections, drops, patch, and shield are also applied as for other angle surgeries.

Problem-Solving

Finding SC. Similar maneuvers to those described above for the metal probe and illuminated microcatheter technique are appropriate for blunted suture approaches.

"Lost" Polypropylene Suture. If the suture position in SC cannot be verified gonioscopically, one should not continue to feed it into the eye. The options are to try passing it in the opposite direction from the opposite SC opening, or to switch to an illuminated microcatheter if available, or to perform a conventional metal trabeculotomy or goniotomy.

Obstruction. If an obstruction is encountered, a first maneuver is to make a paracentesis, fill the AC with viscoelastic, and attempt moving the suture past the obstruction. Alternatively a second 6/0 polypropylene suture can be fashioned in the same way as the first, and threaded into SC from the opposite direction, leaving the original suture as a stent in SC. Other options are to switch to an illuminated microcatheter approach or to perform a conventional metal trabeculotomy or goniotomy.

Inadvertent AC Entry. If the AC is inadvertently entered, i.e., there is a full-thickness perforation, the AC should be maintained with BSS and/or viscoelastic. As it is more challenging to perform a paracentesis on a soft eye, some surgeons prefer to perform a small long oblique paracentesis prior to starting SC dissection and thus have more control should inadvertent perforation occur. SC dissection and cannulation can still be performed in the presence of a small perforation providing the eye is not dangerously soft.

Post-op Management

The postoperative management of the various forms of trabeculotomy (conventional or circumferential) and goniotomy is very similar.

Drops. A small amount of anti-inflammatory medication (usually prednisone drops) and antibiotic are used. A miotic is usually prescribed to keep tension on the iris and its insertion both to avoid peripheral anterior synechiae (PAS) formation and theoretically to help keep the freshly incised lips of trabeculotomy apart. A typical regimen would be:

1. Topical corticosteroid 4 × day tapering by one drop daily over 5-day intervals, or starting 2 hourly during waking hours, with a rapid taper
2. Miotic (pilocarpine 1% or 2%) 3–4 × day for 1 month; in newborns, pilocarpine 1% 1–2 × day for 1 month
3. Topical antibiotic 4 × day for 5–7 days

In newborns or medically fragile babies, great care should be taken with dosage of eye drops as adverse effects may be less easily identified and more profound than in older children (e.g., pyloric spasm from pilocarpine). In these children, lower concentrations and less frequent drop instillation should be considered and medications stopped if side effects develop.

Assessment. The child is reviewed on the first postoperative day. Cooperation is usually limited, but there are clues as to how the child is faring. The eye should be comfortable once the trauma of removing the patch has receded. Mild photosensitivity is possible. The AC should be formed, with an air bubble visible (if used) and the pupil round. The globe tension should be physiological to palpation (if unable to perform tonometry). Providing there is a general impression that the eye is in a satisfactory condition, there is no need to subject the child to a distressing examination. If there is any question of posterior segment complication, a B scan is helpful. If the chamber is flat, the pupil is distorted (suggestive of iris incarceration or prolapse through the wound), or the eye is excessively firm, return to the operating room, or initiate other therapeutic measures. If the wounds have been well sutured and the surgery itself uncomplicated, it is unusual for the chamber to be anything other than slightly shallowed. A small hyphema may be present but usually resolves quickly (within days) and is often far milder than anticipated given bleeding witnessed during surgery. A large hyphema should be cause for concern and closer monitoring and scrutiny.

Frequency of Evaluation. Providing there are no concerns about complications, a typical schedule of review is a visit to clinic on postoperative day 1, week 1, and week 2 and then possibly for an examination under anesthesia (EUA) a month after surgery. Follow-up thereafter is dictated by the response to surgery and whether the second eye requires treatment as well. As confidence grows that the glaucoma is stable, the intervals can be extended so that usually, at about 3 months postoperatively, three monthly evaluations (which may require EUA in the very young and uncooperative) are sufficient.

Interventions. Further surgical interventions would be required if there were serious complications. If nylon sutures have been used, these are removed at the first postoperative EUA.

Complications

Trabeculotomy is subject to all the general risks of any intraocular surgery. Failure to appropriately identify SC before inserting the trabeculotome, suture, or catheter can lead to trauma of the angle structures, cornea, iris, or lens. Ensuring there is a good view of the angle (internal approach) before and during surgery, and familiarity with the anatomy, especially in the buphthalmic eye, can help limit these complications.

Some hyphema is common as blood refluxes from SC (as in Fig. 5.3), but this is usually inconsequential and resolves within the first couple of days of surgery. More significant hyphemas are more likely if there is intraoperative trauma of the ciliary body or iris root and may be persistent [28, 31]. Occasional profound hypotony has been reported [32] and is most likely due to inadvertent or unrecognized cyclodialysis cleft or inadvertent full-thickness drainage. There have also been occasional reports of subretinal blunted suture misdirection [4, 33, 34] or vitreous loss after posterior extension of the deep radial scleral incision [14].

Hyphema

Intraoperative hyphema may compromise the gonioscopic view of the angle. Increasing the IOP can help tamponade this (e.g., injecting viscoelastic into the AC) though the blood can become suspended in the viscoelastic and thus continue to compromise the view. Irrigating the AC and promptly reforming it with viscoelastic may help, though there can be recurrent bleeding as the eye is decompressed. Some but not all surgeons believe it is important to remove all viscoelastic at the end of the case, to avoid IOP spikes and possible splits in DM. There is no harm in leaving some blood in the AC – it is remarkable how quickly it clears postoperatively. It is important to suture all wounds tightly to avoid hypotony which could encourage further hemorrhage. If it is not possible to view the angle for safe introduction of the suture or microcatheter, the eye should be closed and an external approach adopted.

A postoperative hyphema that is persistent (potentially amblyogenic), or accompanied by raised IOP that does not respond to medical measures, will require washout of the AC.

Perforation

A full-thickness perforation of the trabecular-Descemet area results in aqueous egress and a less well-supported ocular wall and angle structures. Intraoperatively this can be somewhat remedied by injecting viscoelastic to keep the AC formed. Prior to dissecting SC, performing a small tangential paracentesis and injecting acetylcholine chloride and a small amount of viscoelastic so as not to overinflate the eye help avoid perforation as slightly decompressing the globe prior to working in this delicate area reduces the tension on exposed trabecular-Descemet membrane. Using moistened sponge tips at this point can also prevent inadvertent perforation from a sharp edge. However it is important to remove all viscoelastic at the conclusion of surgery as the globe should be watertight and viscoelastic is not cleared as quickly as in an eye with an external filter (such as trabeculectomy or tube). Furthermore, presence of viscoelastic in the AC may mask leaking or oozing from wounds, which are critical to detect to avoid postoperative hypotony or inadvertent blebs.

Hypotony

Chronic hypotony is unusual following successful trabeculotomy as IOP lowering is achieved by internal drainage into SC and beyond in a closed system with downstream resistance. At most, the AC shallows slightly and recovers within a day or two. If hypotony is anticipated from the course of the operation and all measures have been taken to close the incisions as securely as possible, a depot of viscoelastic left in the AC may stabilize the IOP for a couple of days to allow early wound healing to occur.

If hypotony is persistent or severe enough to produce iridocorneal touch, the child should be taken back to surgery and the cause of hypotony identified and addressed.

Descemet Trauma

Most complications in trabeculotomy are related to handling of the probe. If the metal probe is turned into the AC with the tip too close to the corneal endothelium, a Descemet tear or detachment may result. If small, the detachment is harmless, but larger detachments may result in overlying corneal decompensation. If detected early, the Descemet scroll can be repositioned and tamponaded with an air bubble or a suture passed through the cornea to tack it down.

Iridodialysis and Cyclodialysis Cleft

These complications are due to incorrect positioning of the trabeculotome, blunted polypropylene suture, or microcatheter posterior to the scleral spur. This should be suspected if the catheter appears to be threading too freely into the eye, the blue suture tip is not identifiable by gonioscopy, and/or the illuminated microcatheter tip courses away from the limbus. This can damage iris root and lead to cyclodialysis if the trabeculotomy is completed. The management is dictated by the consequences which can be benign or include hypotony, hemorrhage, and the potential for later acute IOP elevation if a cleft closes spontaneously. If hypotony is profound or persistent, cleft repair may be required. There are several approaches described in the adult literature, such as cautery, sulcus tension ring, and various suturing techniques.

Scleral Flap Casualties

The sclera in buphthalmic eyes may be very thin, especially at the limbus. Therefore, dissection of the superficial and the deep scleral flaps must be performed with great caution. Button holes, flap tears, leaking suture tracks, and gapes may all lead to overfiltration. If these cannot be addressed with suturing, they can be sealed by covering with a scleral or corneal patch graft.

Disinsertion of the scleral flap hinge can be repaired by one or several U-shaped 10/0 nylon sutures (round needle) passed from the limbal base through the corresponding disinserted flap edge and then back through the limbus with the knot tied on the corneal side. This will pull the disinserted flap back to its limbal base and provide a watertight closure.

Leak or Inadvertent Bleb

Any leak in a buphthalmic eye is likely to cause hypotony and therefore should be addressed without delay. For most children this would require a return to the OR for resuturing. In buphthalmic eyes, spatulated needles may leave tracks that leak, especially when sutures are tied under tension, and so lamellar passes (rather than full thickness) and round-bodied needles can be helpful (e.g., 10/0 nylon on a round-bodied needle). An inadvertent bleb may "convert" the surgery to a form of trabeculectomy or "filtering trabeculotomy" which, provided the bleb is healthy and the IOP not too low, can be managed as for trabeculectomy.

Outcomes

The success rates and outcomes of conventional trabeculotomy are comparable to those of goniotomy in similar patient groups as they result in similar alteration to the angle anatomy. In such patient cohorts, success rates of up to approximately 90% have been reported for trabeculotomy [2–5, 35–41]. Those studies which report longer follow-up durations show a gradual reduction in success over time [38, 39, 41].

In general, the angle surgeries are most successful in primary congenital glaucoma [36]. Presentation at an age of less than 3 months [3, 4] or greater than a year [36] or with advanced buphthalmos (axial length greater than 24 mm [3] or corneal diameter > 14 mm [36]) is a poor prognostic factor. Other risk factors may also be at play to explain the variability in outcomes reported from different parts of the world [2–5, 35–41]. This has led to varying approaches to the management of pediatric glaucoma, which was well reflected in the survey of pediatric glaucoma surgeons conducted for the WGA Consensus Series on Childhood Glaucoma [42].

Circumferential trabeculotomy results have also been favorable in PCG, especially in the low-risk PCG group in which both IOP reduction and visual acuity were superior in the 360 trabeculotomy group compared to historical controls for both conventional (metal probe) trabeculotomy [31, 43, 44] and goniotomy [44, 45]. This has been corroborated by prospective randomized controlled trials in which circumferential trabeculotomy enjoyed favorable outcomes and lower reoperation rates compared to conventional trabeculotomy controls [46, 47]. In populations considered to experience more severe disease, circumferential trabeculotomy alone may be as successful as CTT with MMC [48].

Many studies include a mixed population of open-angle glaucomas making comparison of outcomes between these groups difficult to distinguish. While some surgeons will reserve the angle approach for cases with an immature angle typical of PCG, others regard trabeculotomy as the primary angle procedure of choice for aniridic glaucoma [42]. As experience with circumferential trabeculotomy grows, this is also being advocated for JOAG and glaucoma following cataract surgery [49, 50].

There have been no cost-effectiveness studies comparing these different forms of trabeculotomy. Arguments in favor of the circumferential approach are that it requires fewer EUAs and fewer surgeries in those eyes that would have required more than one procedure. However not all eyes require more than one angle procedure. A blunted polypropylene suture is much less costly than the illuminated microcatheter approach but then may be more complex and time-consuming when cannulation is tricky. When using an ab externo approach, circumferential trabeculotomy is time-consuming and takes longer than goniotomy or conventional trabeculotomy.

There has also been little reported on the impact of primary surgery on subsequent surgeries in a given child. A primary trabeculotomy could impact the performance of other intraocular surgeries in which there are periods of hypotony – theoretically intra- or postoperative blood reflux from the episcleral venous circulation could complicate surgeries such as cataract extraction, vitrectomy, corneal surgery, etc. Primary trabeculotomy may also affect the performance and success of future glaucoma surgeries depending on their relative location on the globe: alterations to globe anatomy and cellular wound healing pathways by surgical trauma may affect the integrity of future surgeries such as trabeculectomy, glaucoma drainage device (GDD), or cyclophotocoagulation.

Options After Failed Trabeculotomy

Surgery may be considered a failure either because it fails to lower IOP sufficiently or because it has caused complications that result in loss of vision. Determining the underlying cause for surgical failure or complication is important as it will contribute to decision-making for the subsequent management of the child.

In the case of conventional trabeculotomy in which only a section of the angle was treated, there may be benefit in further angle surgery to increase the extent of the circumference treated; this is dictated by the response to previous angle surgery and ease of access to the angle. Either a conventional or a microcatheter approach can be used [29]. There are also reports of successful circumferential trabeculotomy after prior goniotomy [28], though the predictability of such surgeries is uncertain and likely to be limited by scarring of SC.

If the angle is to be abandoned, the surgeries most commonly favored are trabeculectomy or GDD [42]. It is well known that trabeculectomy surgery fares best when performed on surgically naïve eyes in which there is no conjunctival or scleral scarring. For this reason, many glaucoma surgeons prefer trabeculotomy to be sited temporally or inferiorly, sparing the superior globe for future trabeculectomy, should it be required. If the superior location has already been used for an ab externo trabeculotomy, FTO, or CTT, it may be possible to convert the surgery into a functioning trabeculectomy if the flap architecture allows. Sclera that has previously been incised and healed tends to be friable, and fashioning a new flap that is robust enough for a safe trabeculectomy can be difficult. The deeper flap incision and opening into SC of a trabeculotomy is also a little more posterior than the ideal sclerostomy location for trabeculectomy and therefore more prone to hemorrhage [51]. In such eyes, many surgeons would prefer a GDD. In certain circumstances, transscleral cyclophotocoagulation may also be the preferred option.

Trabeculotomy Combined With External Filtration

Filtering Trabeculotomy (FTO)

This technique combines conventional metal probe trabeculotomy with elements of deep sclerectomy. Aqueous drains from the AC via the trabeculotomy openings into a scleral lake created beneath a superficial scleral flap and thence into a bleb as for trabeculectomy [24].

Operation (Video 5.4)

Surgical Technique. The preparation for FTO is similar to that for conventional trabeculotomy using a double-flap technique, as shown in Fig. 5.4. The conjunctival incision can be either at the limbus or in the fornix. A well-dissected clean superficial flap is important to achieve good closure; thin flaps are more likely to leak along suture tracks and at the margins.

Once the superficial scleral flap has been fashioned, a deep scleral flap is created within its margins extending anteriorly into SC. The deep flap is then resected at its base at the limbus to create a space, a scleral lake, to collect aqueous draining from the cut ends of SC. If needed, the openings to SC can be probed to confirm their location. The trabeculotome is then introduced into SC and a conventional trabeculotomy completed on each side. These steps are shown in Fig. 5.7a–d. The trabecular-Descemet membrane in the central area beneath the scleral flap is left intact which helps prevent bulk aqueous outflow (as occurs with trabeculectomy) and overfiltration. A depot of hyaluronic acid is placed in the scleral lake to maintain the space by avoiding contact and adhesion of the superficial scleral flap with the bed of the lake.

The superficial scleral flap is sutured with interrupted 10/0 nylon akin to trabeculectomy closure with a view to creating a healthy low bleb (see Fig. 5.7d). The conjunctiva is then closed.

Combined Trabeculectomy-Trabeculotomy (CTT)

In this procedure a conventional metal probe trabeculotomy is combined with a trabeculectomy. The intent is to provide a dual approach: the trabeculotomy addresses the developmentally abnormal angle structures, and the trabeculectomy provides an additional external filtration mechanism to lower IOP. The trabeculotomy is performed first and the trabeculectomy developed from the deep scleral dissection.

Operation (Video 5.5)

Surgical Technique. The eye is prepared for a superior surgery with a traction suture and topical epinephrine to blanche blood vessels. The conjunctiva and superficial scleral flaps are dissected as for conventional trabeculectomy. If MMC is to be used, it is best applied prior to opening the eye to avoid inadvertent seepage into the eye. There are also theoretical concerns that compared to adults, the soft collagen of the eyes of young babies, as well as the smaller body weight per unit of MMC, may result in greater systemic absorption of MMC than in adults though we are not aware of any reports of any systemic adverse effects from topically applied MMC in either adults or children. When considering the use of MMC, these concerns must be balanced with the risk of surgical failure in the individual situation. This is more fully addressed in the trabeculectomy section.

Figure 5.8a–h shows the main steps of this procedure. The superficial scleral flap is reflected and a deep radial incision dissected beneath it in the limbal area until SC is opened, as for conventional trabeculotomy. The trabeculotomy portion of the surgery is then performed. The SC incision is then extended anteriorly and a block of tissue excised to complete the sclerostomy portion of the trabeculectomy. This can be fashioned by blade, scissors, trephine, or punch and should be sized so as to be well covered by the superficial flap (e.g., a single bite of a pediatric-sized punch). A surgical iridectomy is then performed. The scleral flap is then sutured with interrupted 10/0 nylon. The outflow resistance can be tested by injecting fluid through a paracentesis or by adjusting flow through an AC maintainer. The conjunctiva is then closed meticulously to prevent any leak, with sutures buried to provide a comfortable eye.

Potential Modifications

Double Scleral Flap Technique. When a double scleral flap approach is used (as in Figs. 5.4 and 5.7), the deep flap can be excised at its base, akin to a deep sclerectomy or canaloplasty, which may make identifying SC easier [52].

AC Maintainer and Pre-placed Apical Scleral Flap Sutures. An AC maintainer and apical scleral flap sutures inserted before performing

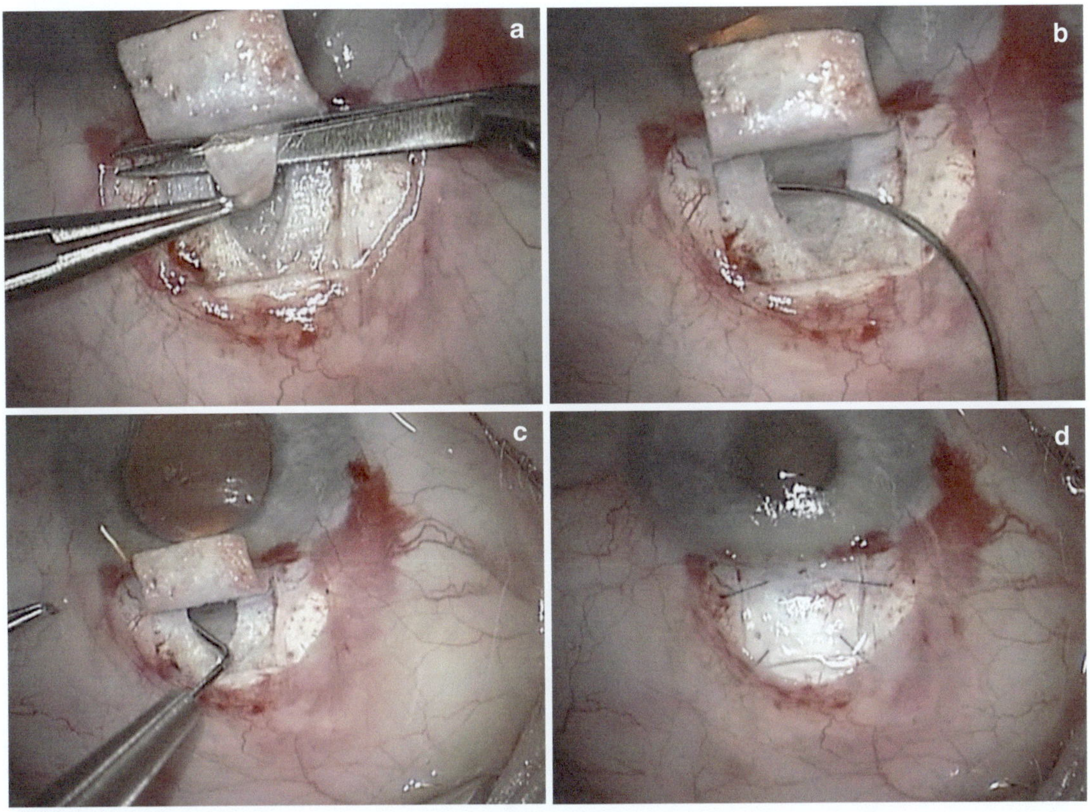

Fig. 5.7 Filtering trabeculotomy. (**a**) Removing deep flap to create scleral lake. (**b**) Probing opening of Schlemm canal. (**c**) Rotating probe into AC. (**d**) Superficial scleral flap closure. (Courtesy of Franz Grehn, MD, PhD)

the sclerostomy (an example of pre-placed scleral flap sutures can be seen in Fig. 5.8) reduce the duration of hypotony once the eye is open. Furthermore, an AC maintainer provides a more realistic assessment of flap fluid dynamics and closure, than when relying on viscoelastic to maintain the chamber.

Site of Sclerostomy. In conventional trabeculectomy, the sclerostomy is typically performed more anteriorly than in CTT where the deep scleral incision of the trabeculotomy is developed into a full-thickness sclerostomy. As this area is closer to CB and iris root, there is a greater risk of iris incarceration and hemorrhage. A modification to the technique is therefore to dissect the base of the superficial scleral flap further anteriorly, where a sclerostomy can then be made independent of the trabeculotomy incision.

Scleral Flap Suturing in Young and Buphthalmic Eyes. In very small children and buphthalmic eyes, it may be advantageous at times to use nylon sutures mounted on a round-bodied instead of a spatulated needle and pass the needle through the scleral lamella rather than full thickness. The tracks left by a cutting needle may leak, especially if there is tension causing the track to gape, and tight sutures may cut through the soft collagen of young eyes. Multiple sutures may be required to achieve adequate closure, and if there is leakage from their tracks, these should be replaced.

Post-op Management

As the goal of these surgeries is maintenance of a functioning bleb, concomitant with a greater risk of hypotony than for trabeculotomy alone, closer postoperative surveillance is necessary.

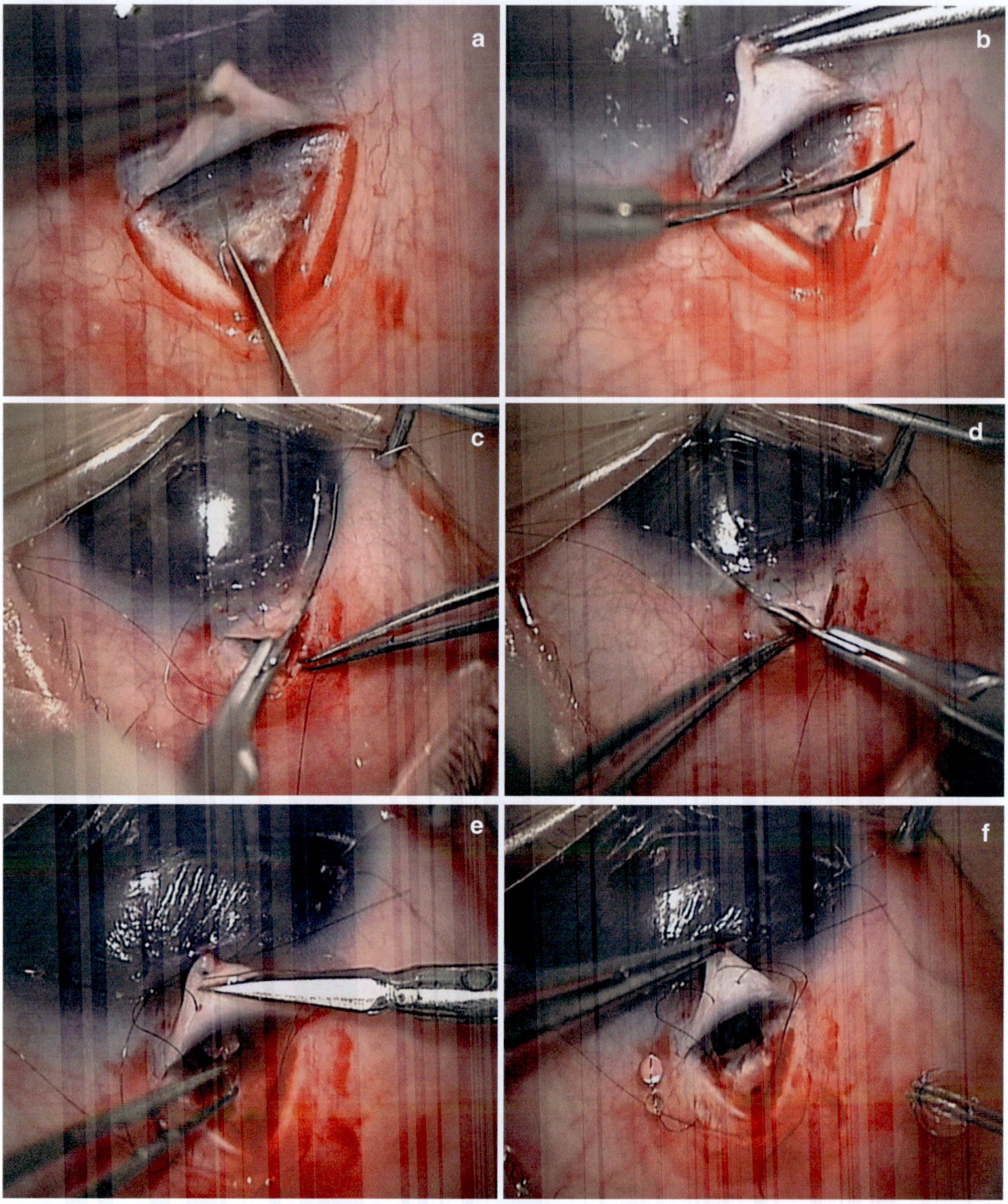

Fig. 5.8 Combined trabeculotomy-trabeculectomy. (**a**) Deep scleral radial incision into Schlemm canal. (**b**) Inserting trabeculotome into Schlemm canal. (**c**) Rotating probe into AC (right trabeculotomy portion). (**d**) Inserting and rotating probe into AC in opposite direction (left trabeculotomy portion). (**e**) Dissecting full-thickness deep scleral block. (**f**) Scleral block excised to create sclerostomy (trabeculectomy portion). (**g**) Peripheral iridectomy. (**h**) Scleral flap closure. (Courtesy of Professor Nader Bayoumi, Alexandria University, Egypt)

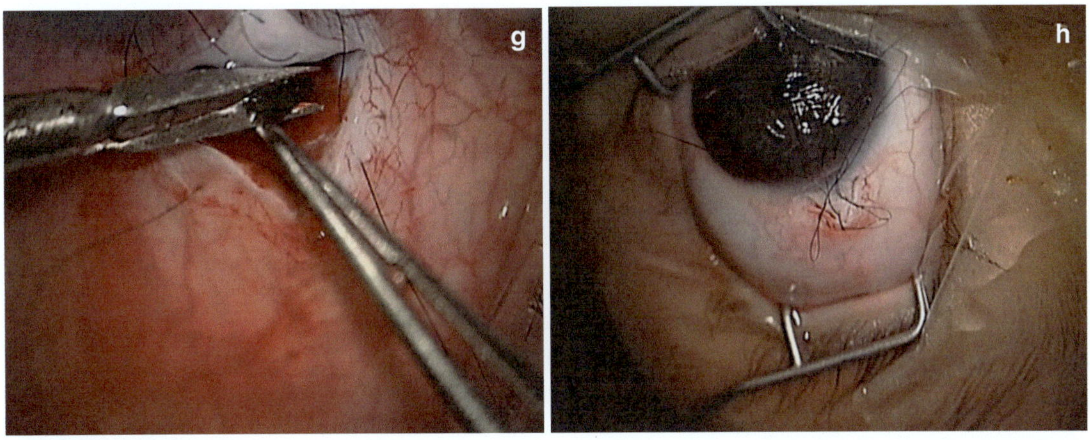

Fig. 5.8 (continued)

Complications

The complications of the combined procedure are the same as for each component alone. These may be compounded by greater surgical time and tissue manipulation inherent in a more extensive procedure.

Outcomes

Although debated [53, 54], CTT has been reported to perform better when compared, albeit retrospectively or with convenience controls, to either surgery performed alone. For example, studies from India [55] and China [16] report greater success rates for CTT than conventional (metal probe) trabeculotomy alone, while those from the Middle East [12, 14, 15, 20] and Africa [56] show greater success rates for CTT than trabeculectomy alone. It has been suggested that in these populations, it is the severity of disease, rather than choice of surgery, that accounts for the combined procedure performing better than its components performed separately. In other populations, single-surgeon series report good results on par with the other angle surgeries [57]. It has only been recently that the combined versus single surgery approaches have been tested against each other using a prospective randomized study design. Two studies, one comparing metal probe trabeculotomy to CTT [58] and the other circumferential trabeculotomy to CTT [48], found angle surgery alone as effective as CTT, at least in the short term. Longer-term studies report some "drift" over time with reduction in success rates with each year postoperatively [16, 39, 55, 59].

The majority of studies describing the outcomes of trabeculotomy remain single-surgeon series, retrospective in design and vulnerable to multiple sources of bias [60]. Most studies address PCG though some cohorts include other childhood glaucomas such as JOAG, glaucoma associated with aniridia, Sturge-Weber syndrome, and glaucoma following cataract extraction. In general, for both trabeculotomy alone or when combined with trabeculectomy, outcomes are better in PCG than in the secondary glaucomas.

Options After Failed FTO and CCT

Manipulations of the trabeculectomy flap by needling or adjustment of flap sutures can resuscitate a failing or failed CTT as in trabeculectomy alone. Needling can also be used to convert a FTO into a full-thickness procedure by carefully advancing the needle through the trabecular-Descemet membrane into the AC [24]. Alternatively, converting a FTO to a trabeculectomy can more formally be performed by re-opening conjunctiva, elevating the superficial scleral flap, advancing the scleral flap dissection anteriorly into the limbal area, and performing a sclerostomy and peripheral iridectomy as described for CTT above. A failed primary CTT can also be followed with a second trabeculectomy with MMC at a separate site [61], if there is adequate quality tissue and space beneath the upper lid. MMC can also be used when converting FTO to trabeculectomy. Further alternatives for failed FTO and CCT include GDD or cyclophotocoagulation.

Future Developments

This is a rapidly changing field and an exciting time in pediatric glaucoma surgery. New technologies developed for adult glaucoma may in turn bring greater safety and surgical success in childhood glaucoma. Well-conducted studies using standardized disease classifications, outcome measures, and pooled data resources will help improve the development and delivery of safe effective surgery in one of the most challenging specialties of medicine.

References

1. Barkan O. Operation for congenital glaucoma. Am J Ophthalmol. 1942;25(5):552–68.
2. SD MP Jr, McFarland D. External trabeculectomy for developmental glaucoma. Ophthalmology. 1980;87(4):302–5.
3. Dietlein TS, Jacobi PC, Krieglstein GK. Prognosis of primary ab externo surgery for primary congenital glaucoma. Br J Ophthalmol. 1999;83(3):317–22.
4. Akimoto M, Tanihara H, Negi A, Nagata M. Surgical results of trabeculectomy ab externo for developmental glaucoma. Arch Ophthalmol. 1994;112(12):1540–4.
5. Luntz MH, Livingston DG. Trabeculotomy ab externo and trabeculectomy in congenital and adult-onset glaucoma. Am J Ophthalmol. 1977;83(2):174–9.
6. Beck AD, Lynch MG. 360 degrees trabeculotomy for primary congenital glaucoma. Arch Ophthalmol. 1995;113(9):1200–2.
7. Sarkisian SR Jr. An illuminated microcatheter for 360-degree trabeculotomy [corrected] in congenital glaucoma: a retrospective case series. J AAPOS. 2010;14(5):412–6.
8. Grover DS, Godfrey DG, Smith O, Feuer WJ, Montes de Oca I, Fellman RL. Gonioscopy-assisted transluminal trabeculotomy, ab interno trabeculotomy: technique report and preliminary results. Ophthalmology. 2014;121(4):855–61.
9. Maul E, Strozzi L, Munoz C, Reyes C. The outflow pathway in congenital glaucoma. Am J Ophthalmol. 1980;89(5):667–73.
10. Sampaolesi R. Congenital glaucoma: long-term results of surgery. Dev Ophthalmol. 1987;14:166–76.
11. Mandal AK, Naduvilath TJ, Jayagandan A. Surgical results of combined trabeculotomy-trabeculectomy for developmental glaucoma. Ophthalmology. 1998;105(6):974–82.
12. Biedner BZ, Rothkoff L. Combined trabeculotomy-trabeculectomy compared with primary trabeculotomy for congenital glaucoma. J Pediatr Ophthalmol Strabismus. 1998;35(1):49–50.
13. Mandal AK, Prasad K, Naduvilath TJ. Surgical results and complications of mitomycin C augmented trabeculectomy in refractory developmental glaucoma. Ophthalmic Surg Lasers. 1999;30(6):473–80.
14. Mullaney PB, Selleck C, Al-Awad A. Combined trabeculotomy and trabeculectomy as an initial procedure in uncomplicated congenital glaucoma. Arch Ophthalmol. 1999;117(4):457–560.
15. al-Hazmi A, Awad A, Zwaan J. Correlation between surgical success rate and severity of congenital glaucoma. Br J Ophthalmol. 2005;89(4):449–53.
16. Zhang X, Du S, Fan Q, Peng S, Yu M, Ge J. Long-term surgical outcomes of primary congenital glaucoma in China. Clinics (Sao Paulo, Brazil). 2009;64(6):543–51.
17. Jalil A, Au L, Khan I, Ashworth J, Lloyd IC, Biswas S. Combined trabeculotomy–trabeculectomy augmented with 5-fluorouracil in paediatric glaucoma. Clin Exp Ophthalmol. 2011;39(3):207–14.
18. Dubey S, Agrawal A, Chauhan L, Mukherjee S, Douglas G. Combined trabeculotomy-trabeculectomy with antimetabolite and releasable suture: outcome with primary congenital glaucoma in a north Indian population. Nepal J Ophthalmol. 2015;7(1):16–25.
19. Harms H, Dannheim R. Epicritical consideration of 300 cases of trabeculotomy 'ab externo'. Trans Ophthalmol Soc U K. 1969;89:491–9.
20. Elder MJ. Combined trabeculotomy-trabeculectomy compared with primary trabeculectomy for congenital glaucoma. Br J Ophthalmol. 1994;78(10):745–8.
21. Mandal AK, Matalia JH, Nutheti R, Krishnaiah S. Combined trabeculotomy and trabeculectomy in advanced primary developmental glaucoma with corneal diameter of 14 mm or more. Eye (Lond). 2006;20(2):135–43.
22. al-Hazmi A, Zwaan J, Awad A. Effectiveness and complications of mitomycin C use during pediatric glaucoma surgery. Ophthalmology. 1998;105(10):1915–20.
23. Jalil A, Au L, Khan I, Ashworth J, Lloyd IC, Biswas S. Combined trabeculotomy-trabeculectomy

augmented with 5-fluorouracil in paediatric glaucoma. Clin Exp Ophthalmol. 2011;39(3):207–14.
24. Matlach J, Hipp M, Wagner M, Heuschmann PU, Klink T, Grehn F. A comparative study of a modified filtering trabeculotomy and conventional trabeculectomy. Clin Ophthalmol. 2015;9:483–92.
25. ElSheikha OZ, Abdelhakim MA, Elhilali HM, Kassem RR. Is viscotrabeculotomy superior to conventional trabeculotomy in the management of Egyptian infants with congenital glaucoma? Acta Ophthalmol. 2015;93(5):e366–71.
26. Tamcelik N, Ozkiris A, Sarici AM. Long-term results of combined viscotrabeculotomy-trabeculectomy in refractory developmental glaucoma. Eye (Lond). 2010;24(4):613–8.
27. Mandal AK. Primary combined trabeculotomy-trabeculectomy for early-onset glaucoma in Sturge-Weber syndrome. Ophthalmology. 1999;106(8):1621–7.
28. Beck AD, Lynch MJ, Crandall J, Mobin-Uddin O. Surgical outcomes with 360-degree suture trabeculotomy in poor-prognosis primary congenital glaucoma and glaucoma associated with congenital anomalies or cataract surgery. J AAPOS. 2011;15:54–8.
29. Shi Y, Wang H, Yin J, Zhang X, Li M, Xin C, et al. Outcomes of microcatheter-assisted trabeculotomy following failed angle surgeries in primary congenital glaucoma. Eye (Lond). 2017;31(1):132–9.
30. Alward WL. Chapter 11, Primary congenital glaucoma. Version 1.0. 28 Sep 2015. Iowa Glaucoma Curriculum. http://curriculum.iowaglaucoma.org/chapter/11. Accessed 12 Mar 2018.
31. Lim ME, Neely DE, Wang J. Comparison of 360 degree with traditional trabeculotomy in pediatric glaucoma. J AAPOS. 2015;19(2):145–9.
32. Gloor BR. Gefahren der 360 degrees-Fadentrabekulotomie [Risks of 360 degree suture trabeculotomy]. Ophthalmologe. 1998;95(2):100–3. [Article in German]
33. Neely DE. False passage: a complication of 360 degrees suture trabeculotomy. J AAPOS. 2005;9(4):396–7.
34. Wise J, Toygar O, Correa ZM, Miller DM, Sisk RA. Subretinal cannulation as a complication of suture trabeculotomy surgery in a pediatric patient. Retin Cases Brief Rep. 2017;11(1):79–82.
35. Luntz MH. Congenital, infantile, and juvenile glaucoma. Ophthalmology. 1979;86(5):793–802.
36. Quigley HA. Childhood glaucoma: results with trabeculotomy and study of reversible cupping. Ophthalmology. 1982;89(3):219–26.
37. Debnath SC, Teichmann KD, Salamah K. Trabeculectomy versus trabeculotomy in congenital glaucoma. Br J Ophthalmol. 1989;73:608–11.
38. Elder MJ. Congenital glaucoma in the West Bank and Gaza Strip. Br J Ophthalmol. 1993;77(7):413–6.
39. Meyer G, Schwenn O, Pfeiffer N, Grehn F. Trabeculotomy in congenital glaucoma. Graefes Arch Clin Exp Ophthalmol. 2000;238(3):207–13.
40. Tamcelik N, Ozkiris A. Long-term results of viscotrabeculotomy in congenital glaucoma: comparison to classical trabeculotomy. Br J Ophthalmol. 2008;92:36–9.
41. Yalvac IS, Satana B, Suveren A, Eksioglu U, Duman S. Success of trabeculotomy in patients with congenital glaucoma operated on within 3 months of birth. Eye (Lond). 2007;21(4):459–64.
42. Papadopoulos M, Edmunds B, Chiang M, Mandal A, Grajewski AL, Khaw PT. Glaucoma surgery in children. In: Weinreb RN, Grajewski A, Papadopoulos M, Grigg J, Freedman S, editors. Childhood glaucoma, WGA consensus series 9. Amsterdam: Kugler Publications; 2013. p. 95–134.
43. Shi Y, Wang H, Yin J, Li M, Zhang X, Xin C, et al. Microcatheter-assisted trabeculotomy versus rigid probe trabeculotomy in childhood glaucoma. Br J Ophthalmol. 2016;100(9):1257–62.
44. Neustein RF, Beck AD. Circumferential trabeculotomy versus conventional angle surgery: comparing long-term surgical success and clinical outcomes in children with primary congenital glaucoma. Am J Ophthalmol. 2017;183:17–24.
45. Girkin CA, Rhodes L, McGwin G. Goniotomy versus circumferential trabeculotomy with an illuminated microcatheter in congenital glaucoma. J AAPOS. 2012;16(5):424–7.
46. El Sayed Y, Gawdat G. Two-year results of microcatheter-assisted trabeculotomy in paediatric glaucoma: a randomized controlled study. Acta Ophthalmol. 2017;95(8):e713–9.
47. Shakrawal J, Bali S, Sidhu T, Verma S, Sihota R, Dada T. Randomized trial on illuminated-microcatheter circumferential trabeculotomy versus conventional trabeculotomy in congenital glaucoma. Am J Ophthalmol. 2017;180:158–64.
48. Temkar S, Gupta S, Sihota R. Illuminated microcatheter circumferential trabeculotomy versus combined trabeculotomy-trabeculectomy for primary congenital glaucoma: a randomized controlled trial. Am J Ophthalmol. 2015;159(3):490–7.
49. Dao JB, Sarkisian SR Jr, Freedman SF. Illuminated microcatheter-facilitated 360-degree trabeculotomy for refractory aphakic and juvenile open-angle glaucoma. J Glaucoma. 2014;23(7):449–54.
50. Lim ME, Dao JB, Freedman SF. 360-Degree trabeculotomy for medically refractory glaucoma following cataract surgery and juvenile open-angle glaucoma. Am J Ophthalmol. 2017;175:1–7.
51. Konstas AG, Jay JL. Modification of trabeculectomy to avoid postoperative hyphaema. The 'guarded anterior fistula' operation. Br J Ophthalmol. 1992;76(6):353–7.
52. Bayoumi NH. Deep sclerectomy in pediatric glaucoma filtering surgery. Eye (Lond). 2012;26(12):1548–53.
53. Khan AO. Trabeculotomy versus trabeculotomy-trabeculectomy for congenital glaucoma. Br J Ophthalmol. 2006;90(1):125.

54. Chang TC, Cavuoto KM. Surgical management in primary congenital glaucoma: four debates. J Ophthalmol. 2013;2013:612708.
55. Mandal AK, Gothwal VK, Nutheti R. Surgical outcome of primary developmental glaucoma: a single surgeon's long-term experience from a tertiary eye care centre in India. Eye (Lond). 2007;21(6):764–74.
56. Essuman VA, Braimah IZ, Ndanu TA, Ntim-Amponsah CT. Combined trabeculotomy and trabeculectomy: outcome for primary congenital glaucoma in a West Africa population. Eye (Lond). 2011;25(1):77–83.
57. Campos-Mollo E, Moral-Cazalla R, Belmonte-Martinez J. Combined trabeculotomy-trabeculectomy as the initial surgical procedure of primary developmental glaucoma. Arch Soc Esp Oftalmol. 2008;83(8):479–85. [Article in Spanish]
58. Khalil DH, Abdelhakim MA. Primary trabeculotomy compared to combined trabeculectomy-trabeculotomy in congenital glaucoma: 3-year study. Acta Ophthalmol. 2016;94(7):e550–e4.
59. Alsheikheh A, Klink J, Klink T, Steffen H, Grehn F. Long-term results of surgery in childhood glaucoma. Graefes Arch Clin Exp Ophthalmol. 2007;245(2):195–203.
60. Ghate D, Wang X. Surgical interventions for primary congenital glaucoma. Cochrane Database Syst Rev. 2015;1:CD008213.
61. Mandal AK, Walton DS, John T, Jayagandan A. Mitomycin C-augmented trabeculectomy in refractory congenital glaucoma. Ophthalmology. 1997;104(6):996–1003.

6 Pediatric Trabeculectomy

Maria Papadopoulos and Peng Tee Khaw

History

Trabeculectomy was first described by Cairns in 1968 in an attempt to replace full-thickness sclerostomy with a safer "guarded sclerostomy" associated with fewer complications [1]. With time trabeculectomy was to become, and still remains, the reference standard for filtering surgery worldwide. Following its introduction in adult glaucoma surgery, it was also adopted for use in children. Conventional techniques at the time such as Elliot trephining, iridencleisis, and cyclodialysis were associated with poor outcomes for refractory cases and significant complications in buphthalmic eyes, fuelling the search for alternative operations with better and safer outcomes [2, 3]. Furthermore, it gradually became evident that angle surgery even after multiple attempts was not always successful in primary congenital glaucoma (PCG), especially in older children [4], and even less so in secondary childhood glaucoma [5, 6].

Beauchamp and Park were the first in 1979 to publish trabeculectomy outcomes in children with advanced or refractory glaucoma. Most children in the series had previous surgery before trabeculectomy, and around 30% of eyes were aphakic at the time of surgery. Successful outcomes were low and complication rates high for which the authors cited numerous reasons, including "more rapid healing processes" [7]. Despite subsequent more encouraging reports of trabeculectomy in children without previous surgery (primary trabeculectomy) [8–10], excessive scarring in the region of the scleral flap remained a barrier to success in many cases. In the adult glaucoma literature, evidence was mounting that adjunctive therapy such as topical steroids [11] and 5-fluorouracil (5FU) [12] could improve outcomes by limiting the wound healing response and reducing fibrous tissue formation. However, the association of 5FU with complications such as corneal toxicity and the need for frequent postoperative subconjunctival injections made its use in children impractical. In 1991, Miller and Rice demonstrated the use of intraoperative beta radiation (750 cGy) to the surgical site improved trabeculectomy outcomes in children and was associated with diffuse elevated blebs with no increase in complications [13]. However, despite the simplicity of application, it never gained widespread use probably because of limited

Electronic Supplementary Material The online version of this chapter (https://doi.org/10.1007/978-3-319-54003-0_6) contains supplementary material, which is available to authorized users.

M. Papadopoulos (✉)
Glaucoma Service, Moorfields Eye Hospital, London, UK
e-mail: maria.papadopoulos@moorfields.nhs.uk

P. T. Khaw
National Institute for Health Research Biomedical Research Centre, Moorfields Eye Hospital and University College London Institute of Ophthalmology, London, UK

A. L. Grajewski et al. (eds.), *Surgical Management of Childhood Glaucoma*,
https://doi.org/10.1007/978-3-319-54003-0_6

access to the strontium[90] probes. The introduction in the late 1990s of mitomycin C (MMC), a potent inhibitor of fibroblast function, which could be applied at varying potencies and required only intraoperative exposure, offered major advantages over 5FU as an adjunct to trabeculectomy surgery in children. Although MMC was generally thought to improve trabeculectomy success, its association with significant, potentially blinding complications such as bleb-related infection led over the years to trabeculectomy falling out of favor in children and to alternative techniques to replace it, such as glaucoma drainage devices (GDD) [14–16].

However, the limited surgical armamentarium for childhood glaucoma and the fact that trabeculectomy was able to achieve lower mean intraocular pressure (IOP) and be less dependent on medication for IOP control than GDDs, led to a reevaluation of the technique in the late 1990s [17]. The resulting simple modifications to the surgical and antiscarring application technique have shown trabeculectomy in the twenty-first century to be associated with satisfactory outcomes in appropriate cases in children of all ages and with reduced complications [18, 19]. This is of particular relevance and importance to the developing world, where often the need is great but access to GDDs limited.

Indications and Contraindications

In PCG, the most common indication for trabeculectomy is failed angle surgery [20]. However, it can be considered as first-line surgery by surgeons unfamiliar with angle surgery, if angle surgery is not possible, or if the patient is unlikely to respond sufficiently to angle surgery (e.g., very early or late presentations). A further indication may be cases where very low target pressures are required (advanced optic disc damage or to improve corneal clarity) as the IOP can be potentially titrated. In juvenile open-angle glaucoma (JOAG), trabeculectomy is usually the procedure of choice [21], although 360° trabeculotomy may be effective in selected cases. For most phakic secondary glaucomas, trabeculectomy can be considered first-line due to the lower success rates of angle surgery compared to PCG. Possible exceptions include uveitic glaucoma [22], congenital rubella [5], and infantile presentations of Sturge-Weber syndrome (SWS) [23] when angle surgery may be attempted first.

Trabeculectomy is contraindicated in glaucoma secondary to malignant intraocular tumors to prevent the risk of tumor seeding. Relative contraindications to trabeculectomy surgery include aphakia or pseudophakia following congenital cataract surgery due to poor outcomes and Peters anomaly (moderate to severe forms) as it is our impression it's associated with an increased risk of trabeculectomy failure. The presence of a cataract requiring imminent surgery or corneal pathology that may require transplantation in the near future is also a relative contraindication because of the high risk of failure after pediatric anterior segment surgery. And, the inability to regularly review children in the postoperative period to assess bleb function and inflammation may compromise success.

Risk Factors for Failure

There are numerous risk factors for failure of trabeculectomy in children, which include age, severity of disease, previous surgery involving the conjunctiva, absence of a natural lens, and lack of cooperation with examination and with the administration of drops in the postoperative period.

Children have lower trabeculectomy success rates compared to adults [24]. It has been suggested that a thicker Tenon capsule in children acting as an impediment to filtration and as a large reservoir of fibroblasts results in an enhanced inflammatory and healing response in pediatric eyes [7, 25]. Infancy, especially less than the age of 1 year [26–29], has often been cited as a risk factor for failure; however, contemporary trabeculectomy results in infants suggest satisfactory long-term outcomes [19].

Conjunctival scarring [13, 24, 29–31], a legacy of previous surgeries, increases the risk of failure as does aphakia or pseudophakia following congenital cataract surgery [28, 32–34] and long-term drop use particularly when associated with conjunctival redness and inflammation [13].

Glaucoma filtering surgery, such as trabeculectomy, is unique in that the actual technique contributes only partially to success, with bleb management in the postoperative period being just as important. Failure tends to occur early in children, and so frequent postoperative examinations to assess the bleb and the ability to perform postoperative manipulations, such as suture removal, are crucial to trabeculectomy success. Regular and sometimes intensive steroid topical therapy is also often required to avoid failure from excessive inflammation. However, both these factors can be challenging for clinicians and parents due to difficulties with cooperation in infants and young children. Examinations under anesthesia (EUA) may be required possibly on a repeated basis to adequately monitor IOP and bleb progress. Although there are concerns related to multiple general anesthetics in children affecting development, they should be considered within the context of the high risk of blindness from glaucoma inadequately assessed or managed surgically.

Advantages and Disadvantages

For advantages and disadvantages of trabeculectomy with MMC, refer to Table 6.1 [20].

Table 6.1 Advantages and disadvantages of trabeculectomy with mitomycin C

Advantages	• Titration of postoperative IOP possible with corneal buried releasable sutures • Lower IOP achievable compared to GDD and therefore indicated if low IOP required, e.g., to clear hazy cornea • Less medication for IOP control compared to GDD • Fewer postoperative surgical revisions compared to GDD • No tube-related complications, e.g., corneal decompensation or tube retraction/exposure • May significantly clear cloudy corneas and avoid potential corneal surgery • Many surgeons worldwide have experience performing trabeculectomy
Disadvantages	• More invasive and higher complications than angle surgery • Need regular postoperative follow-up which may include examinations under anesthesia • Less likely to be successful if previous superior conjunctival surgery • Poor results in aphakic and pseudophakic patients even with MMC • Significant lifetime risk of endophthalmitis with thin, avascular bleb (more likely with small treatment areas of MMC and a limbal-based conjunctival flap)

Adapted from Papadopoulos et al. [20] with permission
IOP intraocular pressure, *GDD* glaucoma drainage device, *MMC* mitomycin C

Preoperative Considerations and Preparation

Once the decision is made that trabeculectomy is the best surgical option, it is vital to discuss the details of the surgery with the parents including likely success, the need for regular follow-up, and intensive postoperative drops along with the possibility of unplanned surgery should there be a complication. A "quiet eye" is necessary to maximize the chances of success, for example, in children with uveitic glaucoma who may need additional topical and/or systemic immunosuppression preoperatively.

Preoperatively it is important to also give consideration to the MMC dose, which depends on multiple factors such as the type of glaucoma, age, race, inflammatory state of the eye, previous surgical history, corneal clarity, severity of optic nerve damage, and the state of the fellow eye. For example, you are more likely to use a higher concentration of MMC if a combination of high-risk factors exists or if a low IOP is required to maximize corneal clarity or to preserve a very damaged optic nerve's function in advanced glaucoma.

The surgical instruments required are as per trabeculectomy for adult glaucoma surgery.

Table 6.2 Suggested instruments, suture, and consumables for pediatric trabeculectomy surgery

Instruments and knives
Eye speculum (e.g., Khaw pediatric or standard glaucoma speculum)
Needle holder
Fine, notched/grooved forceps
Tying forceps
Westcott scissors
Tooke knife
Calipers
15° Feather® blade
Angled crescent blade
Descemet membrane punch (e.g., Khaw small Descemet membrane punch 0.5 mm)
Vannas scissors (straight or curved)
Sutures and consumables
7/0 Mersilk for corneal traction suture
10–0 Nylon on a spatulated needle
23G needle on 3 ml syringe
Anterior chamber maintainer (e.g., Lewicky)
Bipolar diathermy
Mitomycin C
Merocel corneal shields
Balanced salt solution
20 ml syringe with 20G Rycroft cannula
Sterile air
Apraclonidine 0.5% (for hemostasis)
± Tear film strip
± Viscoelastic (e.g., Provisc or similar)

A small but adequate 500 μm sclerostomy can be created quickly with a Khaw Descemet membrane punch 7–101 (Duckworth & Kent, UK) and can be considered. An anterior chamber (AC) maintainer is mandatory for all cases. For MMC treatment, Merocel corneal shields (Beaver Visitec, UK) or pieces of a wick sponge can be used. In infants, consideration should be given to treating the undersurface of the scleral flap with a tear film strip (Clement Clarke, UK) soaked in MMC (Table 6.2).

Operation

Intraoperative Preparation

Following general anesthesia induction, a sterile field is prepared.

Surgical Technique

The aim of trabeculectomy surgery is to create a pathway for external drainage of aqueous from the AC to the subconjunctival space. Although there are many ways to successfully perform trabeculectomy surgery in children, contemporary trabeculectomy techniques have evolved with the aim of encouraging posterior aqueous flow and the development of diffuse drainage blebs to minimize complications while achieving satisfactory outcomes (Fig. 6.1). One such technique is the Moorfields Safer Surgery System [35], which emphasizes posterior aqueous flow through a fornix-based conjunctival flap, a large area of treatment with antiscarring agents, and short scleral flap radial incisions which discourage direct flow near the limbus (Fig. 6.2). Titration of postoperative IOP is possible with releasable or adjustable sutures. Buphthalmic eyes are especially prone to hypotony, flat anterior chambers, choroidal effusions, and suprachoroidal hemorrhage due to low scleral rigidity if aqueous flow is not well controlled. The potential for these complications should never be underestimated. Measures to minimize hypotony are essential in trabeculectomy surgery especially in cases such as aniridia and (SWS). In cases of SWS, some surgeons have suggested prophylactic measures such as sclerotomies with glaucoma surgery [36] to prevent suprachoroidal

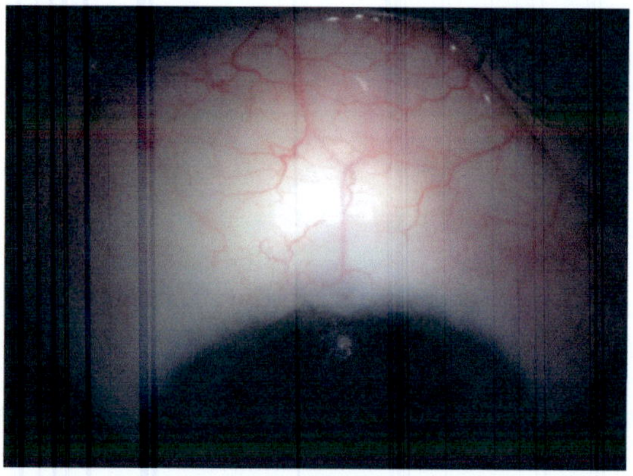

Fig. 6.1 Diffuse, elevated bleb using contemporary trabeculectomy surgery. (Courtesy of Maria Papadopoulos, MBBS, FRCOphth)

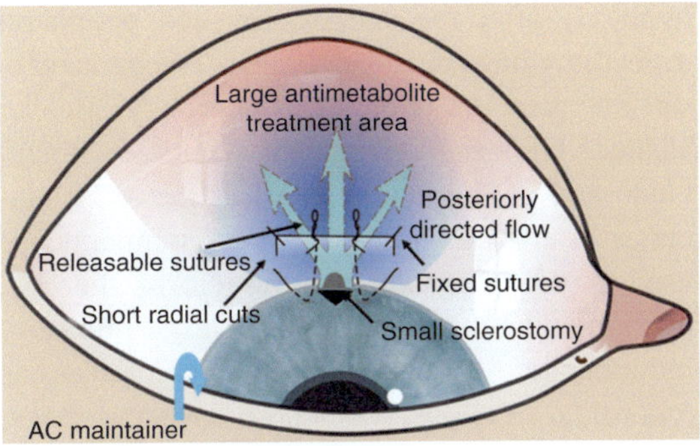

Fig. 6.2 Moorfields Safer Surgery System: a contemporary pediatric trabeculectomy technique for infants and children. (Courtesy of Peng Tee Khaw, PhD, FRCP, FRCS, FRCOphth, FRCPath, CBiol and Maria Papadopoulos, MBBS, FRCOphth)

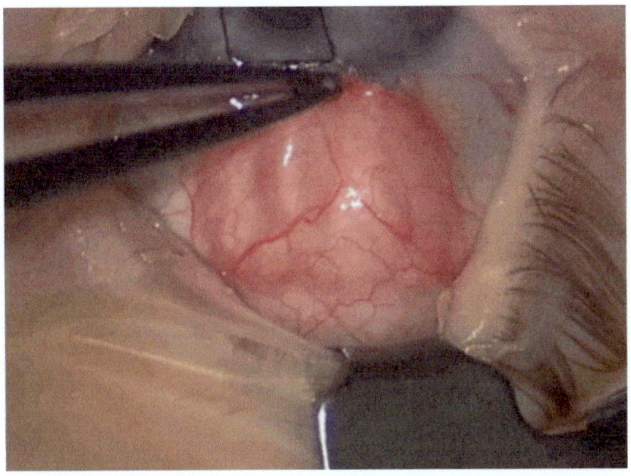

Fig. 6.3 Large treatment area with mitomycin C-soaked Merocel corneal shields. (Courtesy of Maria Papadopoulos, MBBS, FRCOphth)

effusion and hemorrhage, but others have questioned the need [37]. We feel that the use of an AC maintainer and secure closure techniques significantly reduce the rate of choroidal effusions and the need for prophylactic sclerotomies in these cases.

Moorfields Safer Surgery System

Adequate exposure of the superior fornix is necessary and can be achieved with a 7/0 Mersilk (Ethicon, US) corneal traction suture (see Table 6.2). Apraclonidine 0.5% drops are applied to the superior conjunctiva before the conjunctival incision to minimize intraoperative bleeding from the conjunctiva. We prefer this to adrenaline as it produces better blanching and less pupil dilatation. A superior fornix-based conjunctival flap is created by incising the conjunctiva and accessing the Tenon layer at the limbus with fine, notched forceps and Westcott scissors. The peritomy is extended to allow adequate access to the superior sclera to fashion the scleral flap. This is followed by posterior blunt dissection of the subconjunctival space, around 8 mm from the limbus, to create a space for antiscarring treatment. Any bleeding vessels are cauterized before a wide area of approximately 3 clock hours is treated with MMC-soaked Merocel corneal shields (Beaver Visitec, UK) (Fig. 6.3). In infants MMC treatment occurs after the scleral flap is fashioned so that the undersurface of the scleral flap can also be treated with a tear film strip (Clement Clarke, UK) cut to size and soaked in MMC. MMC is applied at concentrations varying between 0.2 and 0.5 mg/ml for 3 min before irrigation with 20 ml of balanced salt solution.

Diathermy is applied to blanch the area of incision, and loose episcleral tissue is cleared with a Tooke knife. At the 12 o'clock position, a 15° Feather® blade (PFM Medical, UK) is used to create a 5 mm partial thickness tangential incision which forms the posterior edge of the flap about 4 mm from the limbus. A rectangular (5 mm × 4 mm), lamellar scleral tunnel is then fashioned with an angled crescent blade beginning at the posterior incision and advancing anteriorly to the superficial limbus for the width of the initial incision with care not to enter the AC (Fig. 6.4). In infants with buphthalmic eyes, the wide limbus mandates the correct positioning of the scleral flap. The posterior edge of the flap should not be at the edge of the limbus but within more robust sclera to minimize cheesewiring of sutures. The sides of the scleral tunnel are then opened toward the limbus with the Feather® blade to create the scleral flap. Due to the elastic nature of sclera in children, these radial cuts should be short to enable tight closure without the need to suture the radial edge of the flap and to also encourage posterior aqueous flow and a diffuse bleb (Fig. 6.5).

A 10-0 nylon (Alcon, UK) is used to preplace intralamellar scleral sutures, with a fixed suture at each corner and two releasable sutures at the posterior edge of the scleral flap (Fig. 6.6). We avoid passing the needle full thickness through the sclera to avoid aqueous seepage around the needle track. Releasable sutures are preferable as they can be loosened or removed while under EUA in infants and young children and on the slit lamp in older children. The releasable loop is buried in a corneal slit parallel to the limbus, so it can be left indefinitely without the risk of infection. Preplacement of the sutures with a formed globe is easier than after the sclerostomy, and it also reduces the duration of intraoperative hypotony after the sclerostomy and peripheral iridectomy have been performed. The paracentesis for the AC maintainer (Lewicky, Beaver Visitec, UK) is then created with a Feather® blade and 21G green needle and the AC maintainer inserted in the AC. An AC maintainer is used in all cases to rapidly reform the AC, maintain the IOP intraoperatively, minimize intraoperative hypotony-related complications (choroidal effusions, suprachoroidal hemorrhage, vitreous prolapse with peripheral iridectomy), and facilitate the accurate judgment of flow through the scleral flap to ensure adequate flap closure.

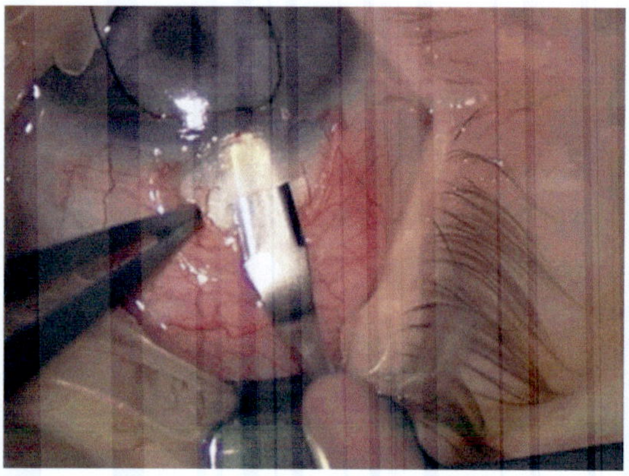

Fig. 6.4 Lamellar scleral tunnel fashioned with an angled crescent blade. (Courtesy of Maria Papadopoulos, MBBS, FRCOphth)

The AC is entered at the anterior edge of the scleral bed, and a 500 μm sclerostomy is created with a Khaw Descemet membrane punch 7-101 (Duckworth & Kent, UK) followed by a surgical iridectomy. The scleral flap is then sutured closed by tying the preplaced releasables first (four throws), followed by the fixed sutures in infants and children. The AC maintainer must be temporally turned off to soften the eye when tightening the sutures to prevent them from tearing the scleral flap. Further sutures are placed in the scleral flap as required with the aim of achieving minimal or slow aqueous flow through the flap at the end of procedure, e.g., gradual hydration of a sponge swab. A tenonectomy is not performed to minimize the theoretical risk of a thin bleb developing. The removal of the AC maintainer

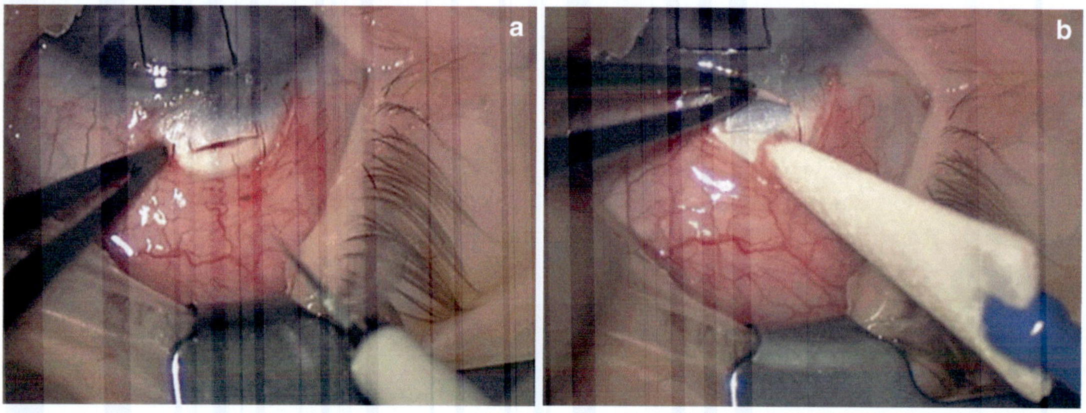

Fig. 6.5 Short radial cuts to encourage posterior aqueous flow and a diffuse bleb. (Courtesy of Maria Papadopoulos, MBBS, FRCOphth)

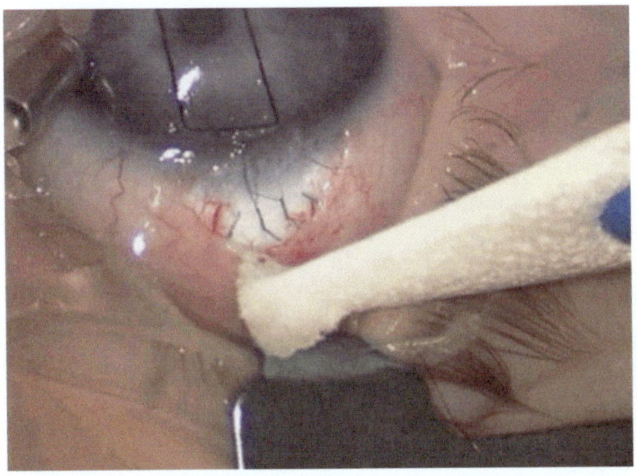

Fig. 6.6 Two fixed 10-0 nylon sutures at the edge of flap and two releasables with four throws at posterior edge of flap allowing minimal flow. (Courtesy of Maria Papadopoulos, MBBS, FRCOphth)

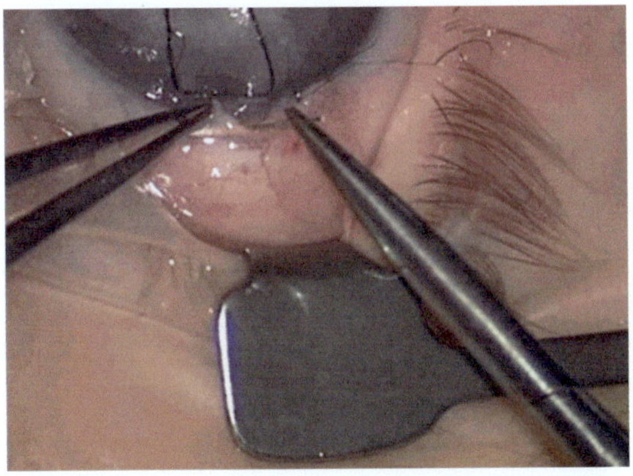

Fig. 6.7 Horizontal mattress suture for conjunctival closure. (Courtesy of Maria Papadopoulos, MBBS, FRCOphth)

with suturing of the paracentesis (required in buphthalmic eyes, unlike adults) is followed by conjunctival closure with 10-0 nylon sutures, all the while intermittently judging the depth of the AC and IOP. Purse-string sutures are used at the edges of the peritomy with either horizontal mattress sutures along the limbus (Fig. 6.7) or corneal buried, conjunctival sutures. Nylon suture ends are trimmed short to disappear in the corneal slit with corneal conjunctival closure, or cut short and covered well by a conjunctival frill with horizontal mattress suture closure along the limbus. This is to avoid discomfort and excessive eye rubbing which may lead to conjunctival wound dehiscence.

Viscoelastic (usually Provisc®, Alcon, UK) and air are occasionally left in the AC if the scleral flap cannot be secured by multiple sutures. Subconjunctival injections of steroid (betamethasone), antibiotic (cefuroxime), and often local anesthetic (Marcaine) to minimize postoperative pain and possibly reduce scarring by suppression of fibroblast activity are given at the end of the case. All eyes are patched overnight (Table 6.3) [20] (Video 6.1).

Antiscarring Agents

The main cause of filtration ceasing and trabeculectomy failure is fibrous tissue formation in the region of the scleral flap, which necessitates the use of an antiscarring agent in children. This is usually MMC due to its greater antiproliferative potency than 5FU and the need for only intraoperative exposure. In a small prospective series of 12 eyes of primary and secondary childhood glaucoma comparing the use of MMC (0.2 mg/ml, 88%) and perioperative 5FU to perioperative 5FU alone (maximum 6 injections), 7/8 eyes of the MMC and 5FU group were controlled off medications as opposed to 0/4 eyes in the 5FU group alone [38].

The greatest advance in MMC therapy has been the understanding that a wider application of MMC treatment is more likely to be associated with a diffuse elevated bleb as opposed to a focal avascular bleb and therefore associated with a significantly reduced risk of complications such as bleb-related infection [18, 19, 39] (Fig. 6.8). However, we suggest adjunctive MMC for those experienced in its use. The most appropriate MMC application method (i.e., whether to also treat under the scleral flap), concentration, and duration of exposure for children are unclear from the literature. The MMC dose is usually determined by the number of risk factors for scarring and the surgeon's familiarity with specific concentrations, but most surgeons use between 0.2 and 0.5 mg/ml. The duration of MMC exposure is best kept constant, and only the dose varied to establish consistency of use, with our preference being for 3 min [40]. An

Table 6.3 Pediatric trabeculectomy technique aimed at encouraging posterior flow and formation of diffuse bleb: important surgical points

Surgical steps	Surgical points/rationale
Corneal traction suture (7/0 Mersilk)	Allows adequate exposure Avoids hemorrhage from superior rectus muscle suture
Fornix-based conjunctival flap	Less likely to form a scar limiting posterior flow Allows better visualization of limbal anatomy
Wet field cautery	Hemostasis Avoids scleral shrinkage (important in thin sclera)
Antiscarring agents	Diffuse, large treatment to minimize risk of a focal, avascular bleb
Scleral flap	Consider fashioning scleral flap first before antiscarring treatment in infants to enable treatment under scleral flap Large scleral flap (4 × 5 mm) and as thick as possible Sutures less likely to cheesewire Greater resistance to aqueous outflow Posterior edge must be well beyond limbus to prevent cheesewiring of flap Dissection forward into cornea avoids iris, ciliary body, and vitreous incarceration Short radial cuts enough to allow reflection of scleral flap for the sclerostomy Greater the scleral elasticity (incision gap) the shorter the radial cuts Directs aqueous flow posteriorly to prevent cystic blebs
Preplaced scleral flap sutures before sclerostomy	Easier to place with formed globe Reduces duration of intraoperative hypotony after sclerostomy and PI performed Releasable sutures through posterior edge of scleral flap and fixed sutures at corners if scleral flap gapes, e.g., in infants Releasable loop buried in cornea so suture can be left indefinitely without risk of infection Can be adjusted or removed under anesthetic or slit lamp without laser
Paracentesis for anterior chamber (AC) maintainer	Oblique, peripheral, long tunnel with a 21G needle minimizes risk of inadvertent lens damage, avoids wound leak, and stabilizes infusion cannula Allows maintenance of intraoperative IOP preventing hypotony and potential choroidal effusions, suprachoroidal hemorrhage, and vitreous prolapse with PI Allows AC reformation Must turn off temporarily when tying scleral flap sutures tight to prevent cheesewiring Used to gauge flow through sclera flap and ensure adequate flap closure
Sclerostomy	Small sclerostomy punch (500 μm diameter) allows increased control of aqueous outflow both intra- and postoperatively and is quick to perform As anterior as possible prevents iris, ciliary body, and vitreous incarceration
Scleral flap closure	Tight closure vital with antiscarring agent use Add additional sutures as required to reduce flow
Fornix-based conjunctival closure	10–0 Nylon retains tension longer than dissolvable sutures with minimal inflammation Purse-string sutures at peritomy edges Corneal buried, conjunctival suture closure, or limbal horizontal mattress sutures
Prevention of postop hypotony	Appropriate concentration of MMC Short radial cuts direct flow posteriorly and minimizes anterior flow from scleral flap sides Tight scleral flap sutures with option to adjust or release at later stage Watertight conjunctival closure Suture paracentesis May leave viscoelastic in AC if high flow rate through scleral flap despite maximal suturing or if ciliary body shut down anticipated (uveitic cases)

Adapted from Papadopoulos et al. [20], with permission
IOP intraocular pressure, *AC* anterior chamber, *PI* peripheral iridotomy, *MMC* mitomycin C

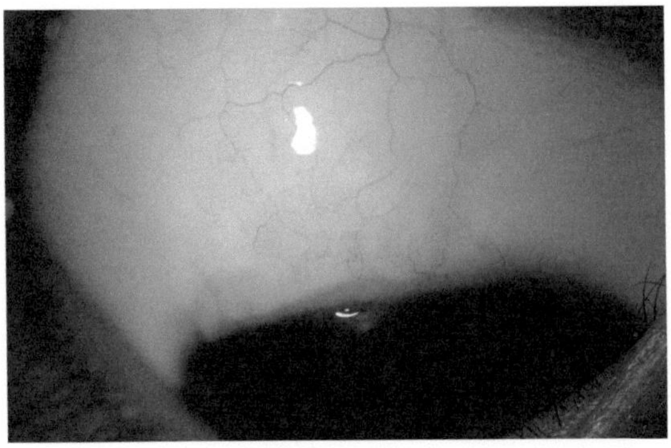

Fig. 6.8 Elevated, diffuse bleb following Moorfields Safer Surgery System trabeculectomy with a large treatment area of mitomycin C

approach when using MMC in infants following failed angle surgery is to use a low dose, e.g., 0.2 mg/ml, at the time of surgery which minimizes the risk and duration of early complications such as hypotony but then to "top up" with subconjunctival 5FU injections at the time of postoperative EUA, as indicated [19].

Potential Modifications

Trabeculectomy can be combined with trabeculotomy to theoretically provide two major outflow pathways and potentially better results than either operation performed alone, but there are no prospective comparisons of all three operations. Combined trabeculotomy-trabeculectomy (CTT) is advocated in some ethnic populations due to its higher incidence of successful IOP control retrospectively compared to these operations performed separately, for example, from the Middle East [41–43]. However, Dietlein et al. in a retrospective study comparing trabeculotomy, trabeculectomy, and CTT without antiscarring agents in PCG patients (Caucasian 71%, Turkish and Arabian 29%) demonstrated no statistical difference in success between the three operations after a median follow-up of 3 years [31]. The authors argued that success was determined more by the severity of the disease rather than the procedure. Conversely, Lawrence and Netland in a retrospective review of trabeculectomy versus CTT both with MMC (0.25 mg/ml, same average exposure time) in 40 eyes (mostly Caucasian and African-American) reported a lower success rate in the trabeculectomy group (70.6% versus 91.3%) at the last follow-up. Mean IOP was the same for both groups. Success was defined as IOP control (6–21 mm Hg) with or without glaucoma medications and without further glaucoma surgery or loss of light perception. However, there were significant differences between the two groups with regard to age (trabeculectomy group was older, 100 months versus 19 months), lens status (more aphakic/pseudophakic children in the trabeculectomy group), number of preoperative medications (higher in the trabeculectomy group), casemix (more PCG and anterior segment dysgenesis in the CTT group), and follow-up (longer for CTT group). Chronic hypotony was the cause of three of the five failures in the trabeculectomy group and one of the two in the CTT group [44].

With regard to CTT technique, once the trabeculotomy is performed, a block of sclera is removed at the limbus by scissors or punch by extending the initial Schlemm canal incision. As a result the sclerostomy is placed more posteriorly than is usual for trabeculectomy, which increases the likelihood of the iris incarceration. This can be avoided by making a separate more anterior incision under the hinge of the scleral flap for the sclerostomy. CTT is described in more detail in Chapter 5, Angle Surgery: Trabeculotomy.

Postoperative Management

Postoperatively, children receive intensive steroid drops (dexamethasone 0.1%) every 2–3 h and ointment at night (e.g., betamethasone ointment). Topical steroids are gradually weaned over 3–4 months or sooner as dictated by the degree of conjunctival inflammation and the IOP. Antibiotic drops (e.g., chloramphenicol) four times a day are usually stopped once exposed sutures are removed. Cycloplegics are not routinely administered but necessary when the AC is significantly shallow and/or choroidal effusions are present. A plastic shield over the operated eye at night time for the first month after surgery is advised.

An important consideration in the planning of a trabeculectomy in children concerns postoperative management. Failure tends to occur early in children, and so frequent monitoring in the early postoperative period is vital. Children should be examined the first postoperative day followed in cooperative older children and teenagers by weekly monitoring for the first month, as with adults, to examine for the presence of a bleb and the degree of bleb inflammation. Subsequent outpatient visits occur at greater intervals depending on bleb appearance and IOP control (Fig. 6.9). In infants, at least one EUA is often needed within the first month after surgery, preferably within the first 2 weeks. Jayaram et al. reported close postoperative monitoring of infants with EUAs at 1 week, 3 weeks, and 6 weeks following trabeculectomy surgery and average duration of postoperative topical steroids of around 3 months achieved satisfactory long-term outcomes off medications [19]. While under anesthesia, sutures can be loosened or removed, and subconjunctival 5FU (0.2–.3 ml of 5FU 50 mg/ml), steroids such as betamethasone, and local anesthetic can be injected adjacent to the bleb depending on the characteristics of the bleb and the degree of bleb inflammation. Monitoring for complications in the postoperative period is also important, and B-scan can be useful in uncooperative children to exclude choroidal effusions.

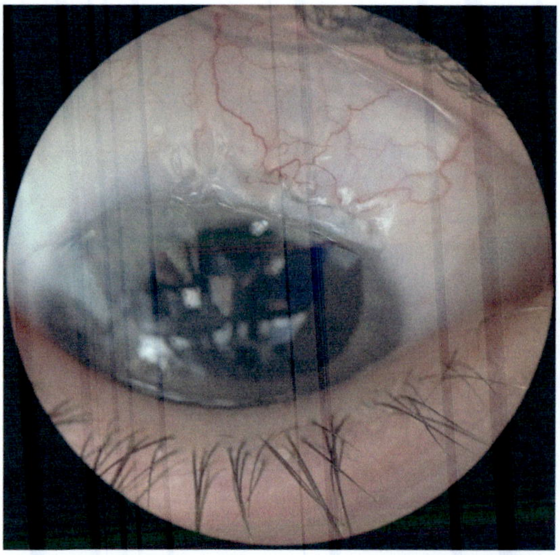

Fig. 6.9 A diffuse bleb with minimal inflammation 2 months post-trabeculectomy surgery. (Courtesy of Maria Papadopoulos, MBBS, FRCOphth)

Complications

There are a many challenges to successful trabeculectomy surgery. These relate not only to surgical technique but also to anatomical factors of a buphthalmic eye, which must be respected to minimize complications. The potential for complications in children after trabeculectomy, especially with MMC, cannot be overstated. Trabeculectomy surgery in young children has been associated with significant surgical complications including early hypotony, flat anterior chambers, choroidal effusions, and suprachoroidal hemorrhage along with retinal detachments and phthisis [14, 26, 32]. Thin avascular, cystic blebs, which use to be common [26, 28], predispose to late complications of bleb-related infection such as endophthalmitis and chronic bleb leaks [14, 28, 32]. However, with contemporary pediatric trabeculectomy techniques, most of these are now avoidable and have significantly decreased [18, 19, 45]. The most common complications associated with trabeculectomy are discussed, along with management and prevention. It is worth emphasizing the point that the best way to manage complications is to avoid them.

Hypotony

Hypotony is a potentially major sight-threatening complication of surgery due to the risk of suprachoroidal hemorrhage in buphthalmic eyes which can occur intra- or postoperatively. The risk is significantly higher in buphthalmic versus normal adult eyes, so careful attention to surgical technique is critical to avoid this potentially devastating complication. In addition to hemorrhage, hypotony can also result in a shallow or flat AC, which in phakic patients may precipitate or hasten cataract formation. Furthermore, lens-endothelial corneal touch can lead to endothelial decompensation and ultimately to corneal failure. Hypotony maculopathy and choroidal effusions can also develop.

Children with glaucoma are at high risk of hypotony with trabeculectomy surgery for many anatomical reasons. The thin sclera of buphthalmic eyes and the reduced scleral rigidity of pediatric eyes result in a tendency for the eye to collapse at low pressures. A sufficiently thick scleral flap is vital for the adequate closure of the flap to avoid hypotony and to prevent sutures cheesewiring the flap causing full-thickness holes and leaks. However, it is made challenging by the scleral thinness of buphthalmic eyes. Elastic sclera tends to gape when incised requiring increased suture tension to close the incision. Furthermore, if the sclera is very thin, other modalities such as GDD surgery might be more appropriate.

Children with SWS who have choroidal hemangiomas are especially prone to large serous choroidal effusions, even at relatively normal IOP, and also to suprachoroidal hemorrhage in the early postoperative period. In light of this, it could be argued that an alternative operation to trabeculectomy such as GDD (with the use of an AC maintainer, a tight tunnel with a 25 gauge needle, both an extraluminal ligature (6-0 Vicryl) and an intraluminal stent (3-0 Supramid) to restrict flow with a Baerveldt implant) should be considered in SWS patients with choroidal hemangiomas. Postoperative hypotony with this technique may be less likely compared to trabeculectomy in which early postoperative IOP may be less predictable despite efforts to avoid low IOP. Uveitic patients also carry an increased risk of hypotony and its consequences thought to be due to ciliary body shutdown from surgically induced inflammation, so inflammation must be suppressed pre- and postoperatively with topical and if necessary systemic immunosuppression. Children with aniridia are particularly vulnerable to lens-endothelial touch due to an absent iris to separate an anteriorly displaced lens and the cornea, and so hypotony should be avoided at all costs.

Early hypotony following trabeculectomy is potentially common and has been reported in almost 50% of cases [28]. However, more recent literature suggests a lower incidence of around 10% [19]. Choroidal effusions and flat anterior chambers associated with early hypotony following trabeculectomy surgery have been reported at a rate of 22% [32] and 10% [26], respectively, in the past. With recent modifications to the trabeculectomy technique, these complications have been significantly reduced to a choroidal effusion rate of 10% and no cases of flat anterior chambers [19]. Chronic hypotony associated with trabeculectomy can also occur but is much less common and has been reported at a rate of 0–8% [14, 15, 19].

The management of hypotony depends on the degree of hypotony and is targeted toward its cause. Buphthalmic eyes with significant hypotony should not be managed conservatively by observation for very long due to the real risk of suprachoroidal hemorrhage. Following trabeculectomy, early hypotony is often due to overfiltration rather than a limbal bleb leak with fornix-based conjunctival flaps, which is uncommon due to the new closure techniques. If the IOP is low but the AC is reasonably formed and there are no choroidal effusions, the patient can be observed with the frequency of topical steroids reduced to encourage healing and a cycloplegic, e.g., atropine, added. However, if the AC is very shallow or flat and/or there are significant choroidal effusions, it is appropriate to consider injecting viscoelastic into the AC with a reduction in the frequency of topical steroids, or further surgery if the cause is excessive filtration through the scleral flap which can be resolved with the addition of further sutures. Dealing with the consequences of hypotony alone such as drainage of choroidal effusions should be avoided as these resolve once the cause of hypotony is addressed and the IOP rises.

To prevent hypotony and suprachoroidal hemorrhage during surgery, the use of an AC maintainer is advised. Furthermore, incisions such as paracentesis should be adequately sutured as they may not remain watertight with stromal hydration as they do in adults, due to reduced pediatric corneal rigidity. Postoperative hypotony following trabeculectomy can be minimized by using an appropriate concentration of MMC at the time of surgery to minimize prolonged early hypotony, fashioning as thick a scleral flap as possible with short radial cuts to minimize leakage through the scleral flap sides, tight scleral flap lamellar sutures to avoid cheesewiring and watertight conjunctival closure. Occasionally the use of a small amount of cohesive viscoelastic can help maintain the AC and the IOP in the first 24–48 h after surgery if the flap allows slightly too much flow despite maximal suturing.

Bleb-Related Infection

Infection can develop in a bleb usually as a late complication of trabeculectomy surgery and is very serious as it is potentially rapidly blinding. Bleb-related infection (BRI) refers to a spectrum of disease severity ranging from infection limited to the bleb (blebitis) to fulminant endophthalmitis (bleb-related endophthalmitis). Blebitis is generally regarded as an isolated bleb infection without clinically apparent vitreous involvement, whereas bleb-related endophthalmitis (BRE) is generally regarded as extension of the infection into the eye (in which case a vitreous biopsy and intraocular antibiotics are indicated) [46]. BRI can occur following any filtration surgery in which there is a bleb such as trabeculectomy and combined trabeculotomy-trabeculectomy. Studies from the adult literature report a more virulent spectrum of organisms responsible for BRI such as *Streptococcus* species, *Haemophilus influenzae*, and *Pseudomonas aeruginosa* [46, 47] than those causing acute post-cataract surgical endophthalmitis which are usually gram-positive organisms introduced at the time of surgery. In the pediatric literature, the pathogens are often not reported. When they are reported, the organisms are consistent with those found in adults [28]. Generally, visual acuity outcomes in BRE are worse than in acute onset endophthalmitis after cataract surgery, but most cases of blebitis achieve vision back to or within one line of preinfection visual acuity [14, 47].

Numerous risk factors for BRI exist but by far the most important relates to bleb morphology, that is, an avascular, thin-walled, cystic bleb which results in compromised physical and immunological defenses against organisms (Fig. 6.10). The use of MMC has long been thought to cause thin avascular blebs, and although it may play a role, these types of blebs have been associated with glaucoma surgery well before the introduction of antiscarring agents [48]. Recent publications suggest that the development of these blebs is more likely related to application and surgical technique rather than the use of MMC per se [18, 19, 39]. Other risk factors for infection include chronic bleb leak [14, 49], interpalpebral or inferior placement of the trabeculectomy [50], contact lens use [51, 52], and bacterial conjunctivitis [52, 53].

BRI is believed to occur more frequently in children compared to adults due to poor hygiene [54] with rates varying from none up to 17% in a study with a mean follow-up period of 28 months [14, 32]. Bleb-related endophthalmitis has been reported in up to 9% of pediatric MMC trabeculectomies [14, 32].

BRI is usually symptomatic and may present with foreign body sensation, photophobia, blurred vision, pain, conjunctival inflammation, or purulent discharge. A prodrome of a few days

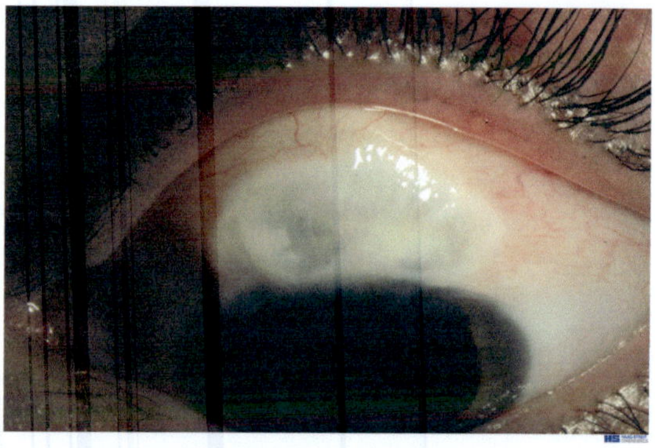

Fig. 6.10 An "at-risk" bleb: thin, avascular, cystic bleb at risk of infection. (Courtesy of Maria Papadopoulos, MBBS, FRCOphth)

is characteristic of blebitis, whereas sudden onset and rapid progression suggests endophthalmitis. Children who present with a short prodrome of 24–48 h should be closely observed for progression of signs. In early blebitis there is intense conjunctival inflammation limited to the area immediately around the bleb, which helps distinguish it from generalized conjunctivitis, and this relative disparity alerts the clinician to the bleb as the source of the symptoms. The thin, cystic, avascular bleb is white against the hyperemic surrounding conjunctiva and is known as the "white-on-red" appearance (Fig. 6.11). This can progress to a mucopurulent infiltrate of the bleb and a purulent discharge. A thin slit lamp beam through the bleb may show a hypopyon within it. There may be an associated bleb leak. AC activity is variable and vitritis may be present indicating endophthalmitis. A B-scan is indicated if the presence of vitritis cannot be clinically assessed. Typically ultrasound shows low- to medium-density vitreal echoes with endophthalmitis. Conjunctival and eyelid cultures from BRE have been found to correlate poorly with intraocular cultures [47, 52].

BRI should be treated early and aggressively to maximize visual function as long-term visual prognosis depends on the extent of the infection, the virulence of the organism, and the timing of therapy. Blebitis, being a precursor of endophthalmitis, is more effectively treated at an earlier stage resulting in a better prognosis [46, 53]. Acute management is determined by the stage of disease, whether it is blebitis or endophthalmitis. There are no randomized, controlled trials which have established the optimum antibiotic regimen for the treatment of BRI. However, topical and systemic broad-spectrum antibiotics are indicated to cover the diverse spectrum of pathogens which may be responsible. The quinolones have a good broad-spectrum cover for gram-positive and gram-negative organisms. The 4th-generation quinolones (e.g., moxifloxacin, gatifloxacin, and besifloxacin) have better gram-positive coverage including significant activity against *Strep. pneumoniae* and *Staphylococcus* species resistant to 2nd- and 3rd-generation quinolones. Systemic moxifloxacin is usually avoided in children because of the theoretical risk of arthropathy in weight-bearing joints, but ciprofloxacin and amoxicillin/clavulanic acid can be considered instead. Consideration should be given to the addition of polymyxin B for multidrug-resistant bacteria and gram-negative bacteria and vancomycin for methicillin-resistant *Staphylococcus aureus* (MRSA). Later the antibiotic regimen can be refined according to the child's response to treatment and to the culture and sensitivity results. Children with BRI require frequent topical antibiotics (e.g., moxifloxacin hourly day and night). Cases of blebitis should be reevaluated within 4–6 h to check for signs of progression such as increasing symptoms, deterioration of vision, and/or cellular activity in the aqueous or vitreous. Hospital admission should be considered for clinical or social reasons when there are concerns that adequate treatment cannot be administered at home. BRE must also be treated with intravitreal antibiotics once aqueous and vitreous samples have been taken.

The value of intravitreal steroids in the treatment of BRE has also not been established although it may be associated with better visual outcomes [55]. The rationale is that the inflammatory response compounds the tissue destruction caused by the inciting infection. Topical steroids are recommended (e.g., dexamethasone 0.1%).

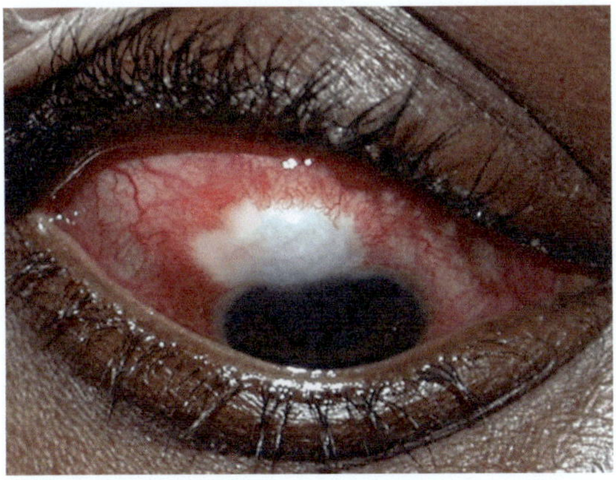

Fig. 6.11 "White-on-red" bleb appearance associated with bleb-related infection. (Courtesy of Maria Papadopoulos, MBBS, FRCOphth)

Clear guidelines for the role of vitrectomy versus vitreous tap and intravitreal antibiotics alone in BRE are lacking. In theory, vitrectomy decreases the bacterial load and associated toxins, helping to preserve retinal function. It is advisable to consider a vitrectomy if there is significant vitreous involvement or in culture-positive patients showing no improvement after vitreous tap and injection. Furthermore, in children, vitrectomy may be the best way to obtain a satisfactory sample for culture and diagnostic purposes.

Late management of an episode of BRI usually involves a decision about whether surgical intervention is indicated to minimize the risk of further infection. Bleb filtration function is usually maintained after infection and often not an issue [14, 32]. Multiple factors must be considered such as a bleb which extends into the interpalpebral fissure, poor contralateral vision, poor hygiene, persistent bleb leak, ability of the patient to follow advice and act on the symptoms or signs of infection, and the accessibility to ophthalmic care. This last factor would definitely lower the threshold for surgical intervention. Bleb revision involving bleb excision and conjunctival advancement is the most definitive treatment. However, this alone will not prevent recurrence of a thin avascular bleb if scleral thinning or a full-thickness sclerostomy is evident at the time of the revision and is not also addressed with a simultaneous patch graft. Revising the bleb may lead to loss of IOP control. Bleb revision should be delayed until the infection has completely resolved which may be several weeks or months after the acute episode.

With regard to the prevention of infection of an "at-risk" bleb, the role of prophylactic antibiotics is controversial and has not been proven to decrease the incidence of infection. However, it may be appropriate in children with "at-risk" blebs who may be unable to reach an ophthalmologist urgently for assessment and treatment (e.g., while on vacation) to be given a broad-spectrum antibiotic to use if symptoms develop, until they can reach an ophthalmologist. If an avascular cystic bleb develops after surgery, parents should be informed about the risk and seriousness of bleb-related infection. They should be advised to report immediately to an ophthalmologist should symptoms or signs of bleb-related infection occur such as localized conjunctival injection, increasing pain, or an AC hypopyon. Children with filtering blebs, especially those which are "at risk," experiencing bacterial conjunctivitis should be treated with a topical bactericidal antibiotic and closely observed during and after treatment for the development of intraocular inflammation. Furthermore, a history of prior bleb infection should prompt even greater vigilance as this has been calculated to increase the risk of developing endophthalmitis approximately 12-fold [52].

The prevention of a "bleb at risk" is vital as it puts the child at a lifetime risk of infection and potential blindness. Wells et al., in a retrospective comparative study undertaken in children and young adults, demonstrated a significant reduction in the incidence of a thin avascular bleb and serious bleb-related complications with modifications such as a large area of antiscarring treatment, fornix-based conjunctival flap, and fashioning a scleral flap which encourages posterior flow [18]. Furthermore, antiscarring agents should be cautiously and appropriately selected according to the patient's risk factors for failure. Inferiorly placed blebs should be avoided, as should blebs with nasal and temporal extensions within the interpalpebral fissure. Releasable sutures should always be buried and antibiotics used when sutures are exposed.

Chronic Bleb Leak

Chronic bleb leaks tend to occur late in thin, avascular blebs which are fragile and easily traumatized especially by children, and may be intermittent. A leak should always be excluded in such blebs with fluorescein 2%. Reported rates of late bleb leaks from older pediatric trabeculectomy literature range from 3 to 23% [14, 28, 32]. However, in recent studies using contemporary surgical techniques when performing MMC trabeculectomies in children, there were no early or late bleb leaks [19, 45].

Chronic, late leaks are usually refractory to conservative measures such as a bandage contact lens due to poor tissue integrity. Often surgical revision is necessary with excision of the unhealthy conjunctival tissue and advancement of healthy conjunctiva with well-vascularized edges. To prevent the recurrence of a thin, avascular, cystic bleb, any scleral defects must be addressed with a patch graft. Repairing the bleb leak may lead to loss of IOP control.

The prevention of chronic bleb leaks is best achieved with contemporary pediatric trabeculectomy techniques which minimize the risk of a thin, avascular bleb developing as discussed above (see Fig. 6.2).

Outcomes

Criteria for success in published papers on trabeculectomy are largely based on IOP control either with (qualified success) or without (complete success) topical medications along with the absence of serious complications. Published studies of trabeculectomy for childhood glaucoma are all retrospective which makes comparison difficult as success is influenced potentially by a number of factors such as definition of success, patient's age and race, previous surgery, surgical technique, dose and duration of MMC, use of 5FU postoperatively, casemix (primary and secondary glaucomas), inclusion of non-phakic patients, and duration of follow-up. This makes the answering of questions regarding who are the best candidates for trabeculectomy and which is the most appropriate MMC dose or duration difficult to answer.

Early results of unenhanced trabeculectomy by Beauchamp and Parks in 25 eyes (44% PCG, 32% aphakic) were poor with only 50% success after a mean overall follow-up of 18 months and with a 20% complication rate. However, only 3 of the 25 eyes had a primary trabeculectomy (i.e., first operation on a virgin eye) [7]. Subsequent authors reported even lower success rates of 35% for trabeculectomy in childhood glaucoma after longer follow-up of around 3–5 years [24, 29]. These poor results were speculated to be due to multiple previous ocular surgery and age. In light of these findings, surgeons considered performing primary trabeculectomy. Fulcher et al. reported their findings in 20 Caucasian eyes (65% PCG) with primary, unenhanced trabeculectomy with a success rate (IOP of ≤ 18 mm Hg and clinical stability) of 92% in children with PCG and 86% in children with secondary childhood glaucoma (all phakic) and no serious complications, after a mean follow-up of almost 8 years [10]. These improved results likely reflected the fact that all patients were Caucasian and phakic and had no previous surgery. However, success of trabeculectomy as a primary procedure in certain populations was found to be lower at 54–72% [42, 56]. Elder reported results of unenhanced primary trabeculectomy in 44 eyes of Palestinian Arab children with PCG of 72% cumulative success (IOP of ≤ 21 mm Hg and no medication) with few complications, after a mean follow-up of only 2 years [42].

Despite encouraging reports of primary trabeculectomy in some groups, excessive scarring remained a barrier to success for many cases especially those cases refractory to previous glaucoma surgery. The introduction of MMC was thought to improve success in such cases [57]. Overall, the success of MMC trabeculectomy in children has been reported to be 59–95% with short follow-up of 2 years or less [14, 26, 27, 32, 57], reducing to 55–60% after 6–7 years mean follow-up [19, 58]. Publications suggest that the dose of MMC does not affect success or complication rates [27, 59]. Al Hazmi et al., in a large retrospective series of 150 PCG eyes undergoing trabeculectomy with variable MMC concentrations (0.2 or 0.4 mg/ml) and times of exposure (2–5 min), showed no significant difference in outcomes and complications [27].

Infancy (less than 2 years of age) has been reported to be a significant risk factor for MMC trabeculectomy failure. Outcomes in infants less than 1 year of age vary between 15 and 43% [26–28, 32] after less than 2 years of follow-up with the lower rates in series with aphakic patients [28, 32]. Beck et al. reported that being aged less than 1 year at the time of surgery was associated with almost a sixfold risk of failure [32]. For infants less than 2 years of age, Al Hazmi et al. described a success rate of 39% (IOP < 21 mmHg without topical medications) in 66 eyes (unreported follow-up) in a study population of PCG patients from the Middle East [27]. In a smaller series of 24 eyes with both primary and secondary childhood glaucoma (17% aphakic), Beck et al. reported a cumulative success rate of only 19% (IOP < 23 mmHg with topical medication) at 6 years in infants less than 2 years of age [15]. More recently, in a similar aged series of 40 eyes of phakic patients with primary and secondary childhood glaucoma, Jayaram et al. reported a cumulative probability of success of 60% at 7 years [19]. Almost all successful cases were not using topical IOP-lowering medications at final follow-up. For infants less than 1 year of age, 70% were successful at the end of follow-up.

A consistently reported risk factor for trabeculectomy failure, even with MMC, is glaucoma following congenital cataract surgery [28, 32–34]. In a study by Freedman et al. with a series of 21 eyes treated with MMC trabeculectomy (0.4 mg/ml, 3–5 min) and postoperative 5FU, the qualified success rates for phakic versus aphakic eyes (n = 7) were 64% to 29%, respectively, after 23 months [28]. Azuara-Blanco et al. further highlighted this point in a series of 21 eyes treated with MMC trabeculectomy (0.4 mg/ml, 1–5 min) who found 0% complete success after 18 months in aphakic eyes (n = 8) [33]. Beck et al. reported aphakia to carry an almost threefold risk of failure [32].

As the Tenon capsule is thought to be implicated in the higher failure rate of children, a recent 24-month prospective study by Awadein and El Sayed compared MMC trabeculectomy alone (0.4 mg/ml, 3 min) and MMC trabeculectomy with partial tenonectomy in 64 eyes of children with glaucoma [60]. A tenonectomy of about 8 mm in diameter to include the area over the scleral flap and expected bleb was performed from a fornix-based conjunctival flap leaving behind the "thinnest conjunctiva possible." There was no significant difference between the two groups with regard to age, lens status, diagnosis, and prior glaucoma surgeries. The mean postoperative IOP was significantly lower in the group who underwent tenonectomy throughout follow-up as were the number of medications from the third postoperative month. Complete success (IOP 5–21 mm Hg without medications and signs of glaucoma progression) and qualified success (with medications) were the same in both groups. More failures (uncontrolled IOP despite maximum tolerated medical treatment, further glaucoma surgery, or devastating complication) occurred in the non-tenonectomy group (30%) compared to the tenonectomy group (55%), but this was not significant. After multivariate analysis, only the number of prior glaucoma surgeries was a predictor of failure. With regard to bleb morphology, the authors report that the tenonectomy group had blebs with "thinner walls" and that encapsulation occurred significantly less frequently in the tenonectomy group (3% versus 25%). There was only one case of endophthalmitis that occurred in a child who did not have a tenonectomy, and there were no cases of chronic bleb leak. Furthermore, less needling and 5FU injections were necessary in the tenonectomy group (3% versus 25%). Although this paper suggests a possible role for tenonectomy in pediatric trabeculectomy, the potential for the development of thin blebs at risk of infection and leaks in the longer term is a concern.

Another approach to improve trabeculectomy success was attempted by Mahdy et al., through the use of intraoperative subconjunctival bevacizumab (Avastin), a recombinant humanized monoclonal vascular endothelial growth factor (VEGF) antibody to modulate the wound healing effects of VEGF. In a prospective paired-eye study design, they compared MMC (0.4 mg/ml, 3 min) trabeculectomy alone in one eye and MMC trabeculectomy with bevacizumab (2.5 mg in 0.2 mls) in the fellow eye of 12 children with refractory glaucoma [61]. Following limbal-based conjunctival flap closure, bevacizumab was injected subconjunctivally over the scleral flap area. Sham injections were performed in the fellow MMC trabeculectomy alone group. There were no significant differences between the two groups with regard to preoperative IOP, lens status, and diagnosis. The mean postoperative IOP was significantly lower in the group who had subconjunctival bevacizumab at 1-year follow-up. Complete success (IOP 5–21 mm Hg without medications and no further glaucoma surgery or visually devastating complications) and qualified success (with medication) were significantly better in the subconjunctival bevacizumab group (complete success 75% versus 58% and qualified success 92% versus 75%, respectively). Shallow AC was the most common complication in each group (17%). One case in MMC trabeculectomy group alone developed late bleb-related endophthalmitis after 3 months and resulted in phthisis bulbi (8.33%). Although off-label use of drugs is common in pediatric ophthalmology and bevacizumab as an adjunct may improve MMC trabeculectomy results, further study of anti-VEGF agents to assess the safety and efficacy of these drugs in this population is needed [62].

Despite the fact that the aim of surgery is to preserve vision in children, visual outcomes are rarely reported in the literature. In Beauchamp and Park's paper, visual acuity was assessed in 18 of the 26 eyes, and the best acuity was 20/200. Where trabeculectomy visual outcomes in children are described, the majority of eyes maintain visual acuity within two Snellen lines; however, in a study by Beck et al. from 1998, 11% of eyes were reported to have lost more than 2 lines of vision or progressed to no light perception attributable to devastating surgical complications [32]. More recently, Jayaram et al. reported final overall visual acuity outcomes of 34.2% seeing 20/40 or better, 89.5% seeing 20/200 or better, and no cases of loss of light perception [19]. Hopefully future studies will evaluate success not only in terms of IOP control and visual acuity but also with regard to functional vision and quality of life measures.

Comparison to Other Techniques

The accepted alternative to trabeculectomy following failed angle surgery is the insertion of a glaucoma drainage device (GDD). Success rates or success probabilities at last follow-up vary from 31 to 97% with variable follow-up from 1 to 7 years [63]. In infants, success of GDD at 1 year is reported at 74–87% [15, 64] with 53% survival at 6 years after surgery [15], comparable to the trabeculectomy outcomes of Jayaram et al. [19]. MMC trabeculectomy compared to GDDs may achieve lower mean IOP [32] and of significance be less dependent on medication for IOP control [19, 32, 63]. In one study, only 14% of infants undergoing GDD surgery achieved IOP control without topical medications [64] compared to 62.5% (25/40) trabeculectomy cases [19]. However a major difference between trabeculectomy and GDD surgery is the significant burden of associated complications in the latter group often requiring surgical revision. Beck et al. reported 46% of eyes with a GDD required one or more operations due to a complication related to the implant (most commonly tube corneal touch and exposure), in contrast to 12.5% of eyes in trabeculectomy group [15]. Tube malposition, erosion, and endophthalmitis are consistently reported with greater frequency in the pediatric compared to adult population [63]. Tube malposition requiring further surgery has been reported in 26–35% of cases [15, 64]. Of concern is particularly the rate of corneal decompensation in the longer term for these children following GDD surgery.

Trabeculectomy has also been compared to deep sclerectomy both with MMC (0.2 mg/ml, 1 min) in a small series of children with uveitis as primary procedures and found to be more successful with regard to IOP control off medications (88% versus 50%) with all failed cases of deep sclerectomy requiring further glaucoma surgery [65].

Options After Failed Surgery

When trabeculectomy fails to control IOP, a popular option is to consider bleb needling with an antiscarring agent such as 5FU or MMC if the sclerostomy is patent. The MMC is best injected subconjunctivally posterior to the bleb and before needling while the intraocular pressure is still high, to prevent inadvertent intraocular entry after needling. Repeated needling may be necessary with early failure. Other options after failed trabeculectomy include repeating the trabeculectomy at an adjacent site with a higher dose of MMC or a GDD [20].

References

1. Cairns JE. Trabeculectomy. Preliminary report of a new method. Am J Ophthalmol. 1968;66(4):673–9.
2. Scheie HG. Results of peripheral iridectomy with scleral cautery in congenital and juvenile glaucoma. Trans Am Ophthalmol Soc. 1962;60:116–39.
3. Gregersen E, Kessing SV. Congenital glaucoma before and after the introduction of microsurgery. Results of “macrosurgery” 1943–1963 and of microsurgery (trabeculotomy/ectomy) 1970–1974. Acta Ophthalmol (Copenh). 1977;55(3):422–30.
4. Lister A. The prognosis in congenital glaucoma. Trans Ophthalmol Soc U K. 1966;86:5–18.
5. Rice NS. The surgical management of congenital glaucoma. Aust J Ophthalmol. 1977;5:174–9.
6. Luntz MH. Congenital, infantile, and juvenile glaucoma. Ophthalmology. 1979;86(5):793–802.
7. Beauchamp GR, Parks MM. Filtering surgery in children: barriers to success. Ophthalmology. 1979;86(i):170–80.
8. Burke JP, Bowell R. Primary trabeculectomy in congenital glaucoma. Br J Ophthalmol. 1989;73(3):186–90.
9. Turacli ME, Aktan SG, Sayli BS, Akarsu N. Therapeutical and genetical aspects of congenital glaucomas. Int Ophthalmol. 1992;16(4–5):359–62.
10. Fulcher T, Chan J, Lanigan B, Bowell R, O'Keefe M. Long-term follow up of primary trabeculectomy for infantile glaucoma. Br J Ophthalmol. 1996;80(6):499–502.
11. Starita RJ, Fellman RL, Spaeth GL, Poryzees EM, Greenidge KC, Traverso CE. Short- and long-term effects of postoperative corticosteroids on trabeculectomy. Ophthalmology. 1985;92(7):938–46.
12. The Fluorouracil Filtering Surgery Study Group. Fluorouracil filtering surgery study one year follow-up. Am J Ophthalmol. 1989;108(6):625–35.
13. Miller MH, Rice NS. Trabeculectomy combined with beta irradiation for congenital glaucoma. Br J Ophthalmol. 1991;75(10):584–90.
14. Sidoti PA, Belmonte SJ, Liebmann JM, Ritch R. Trabeculectomy with mitomycin-C in the treatment of pediatric glaucomas. Ophthalmology. 2000;107(3):422–9.
15. Beck AD, Freedman S, Kammer J, Jin J. Aqueous shunt devices compared to trabeculectomy with mitomycin C for children in the first two years of life. Am J Ophthalmol. 2003;136(6):994–1000.
16. Tanimoto SA, Brandt JD. Options in pediatric glaucoma after angle surgery has failed. Curr Opin Ophthalmol. 2006;17(2):132–7.
17. Khaw PT, Wilkins MR, Shah P. Glaucoma surgery. In: Easty DL, Sparrow JM, editors. Oxford textbook of ophthalmology. New York: Oxford University Press; 1999.
18. Wells AP, Cordeiro MF, Bunce C, Khaw PT. Cystic bleb formation and related complications in limbus-versus fornix-based conjunctival flaps in pediatric and young adult trabeculectomy with mitomycin C. Ophthalmology. 2003;110(11):2192–7.
19. Jayaram H, Scawn R, Pooley F, Chiang M, Bunce C, Strouthidis NG, et al. Long-term outcomes of trabeculectomy augmented with mitomycin-C undertaken within the first two years of life. Ophthalmology. 2015;122(11):2216–22.
20. Papadopoulos M, Edmunds B, Chiang M, Mandal A, Grajewski AL, Khaw PT. Glaucoma surgery in children. In: Weinreb RN, Grajewski A, Papadopoulos M, Grigg J, Freedman S, editors. Childhood glaucoma, WGA Consensus series 9. Amsterdam: Kugler Publications; 2013. p. 95–134.
21. Chang TC, Brookes J, Cavuoto K, Bitrian E, Grajewski AL. Primary congenital glaucoma and juvenile open-angle glaucoma. In: Weinreb RN, Grajewski A, Papadopoulos M, Grigg J, Freedman S, editors. Childhood glaucoma, WGA Consensus series 9. Amsterdam: Kugler Publications; 2013. p. 137–53.
22. Bohnsack BL, Freedman SF. Surgical outcomes in childhood uveitic glaucoma. Am J Ophthalmol. 2013;155(1):134–42.
23. Olsen KE, Huang AS, Wright MM. The efficacy of goniotomy/trabeculotomy in early-onset glaucoma associated with the Sturge-Weber syndrome. J AAPOS. 1998;2(6):365–8.
24. Gressel MG, Heuer DK, Parrish RK 2nd. Trabeculectomy in young patients. Ophthalmology. 1984;91(10):1242–6.
25. Skuta GL, Parrish RK. Wound healing in glaucoma filtering surgery. Surv Ophthalmol. 1987;32(3):149–70. Review
26. Susanna R Jr, Oltrogge EW, Carani JC, Nicolela MT. Mitomycin as adjunct chemotherapy with trabeculectomy in congenital and developmental glaucomas. J Glaucoma. 1995;4(3):151–7.
27. al-Hazmi A, Zwaan J, Awad A, al-Mesfer S, Mullaney PB, Wheeler DT. Effectiveness and complications of mitomycin C use during pediatric glaucoma surgery. Ophthalmology. 1998;105(10):1915–20.
28. Freedman SF, McCormick K, Cox TA. Mitomycin C-augmented trabeculectomy with postoperative wound modulation in pediatric glaucoma. J AAPOS. 1999;3(2):117–24.
29. Inaba Z. Long-term results of trabeculectomy in the Japanese: an analysis by life-table method. Jpn J Ophthalmol. 1982;26(4):361–73.
30. Broadway DC, Grierson I, Hitchings RA. Local effects of previous conjunctival incisional surgery and the subsequent outcome of filtration surgery. Am J Ophthalmol. 1998;125(6):805–18.

31. Dietlein TS, Jacobi PC, Krieglstein GK. Prognosis of primary ab externo surgery for primary congenital glaucoma. Br J Ophthalmol. 1999;83(3):317–22.
32. Beck AD, Wilson WR, Lynch MG, Lynn MJ, Noe R. Trabeculectomy with adjunctive mitomycin C in pediatric glaucoma. Am J Ophthalmol. 1998;126(5):648–57.
33. Azuara-Blanco A, Wilson RP, Spaeth GL, Schmidt CM, Augsburger JJ. Filtration procedures supplemented with mitomycin C in the management of childhood glaucoma. Br J Ophthalmol. 1999;83(2):151–6.
34. Mandal AK, Bagga H, Nutheti R, Gothwal VK, Nanda AK. Trabeculectomy with or without mitomycin-C for paediatric glaucoma in aphakia and pseudophakia following congenital cataract surgery. Eye (Lond). 2003;17(1):53–62.
35. Khaw PT, Chiang M, Shah P, Sii F, Lockwood A, Khalili A. Enhanced trabeculectomy: the Moorfields Safer Surgery System. Dev Ophthalmol. 2012;50:1–28.
36. Budenz DL, Sakamoto D, Eliezer R, Varma R, Heuer DK. Two-staged Baerveldt glaucoma implant for childhood glaucoma associated with Sturge-Weber syndrome. Ophthalmology. 2000;107(11):2105–10.
37. Eibschitz-Tsimhoni M, Lichter PR, Del Monte MA, Archer SM, Musch DC, Rm S, Moroi SE. Assessing the need for posterior sclerotomy at the time of filtering surgery in patients with Sturge-Weber syndrome. Ophthalmology. 2003;110(7):1361–3.
38. Snir M, Lusky M, Shalev B, Gaton D, Weinberger D. Mitomycin C and 5-fluorouracil antimetabolite therapy for pediatric glaucoma filtration surgery. Ophthalmic Surg Lasers. 2000;31(1):31–7.
39. Cordeiro MF, Constable PH, Alexander RA, Bhattacharya SS, Phaw PT. Effect of varying the mitomycin-C treatment area in glaucoma filtration surgery in the rabbit. Invest Ophth Vis Sci. 1997;38(8):1639–46.
40. Wilkins M, Occleston A, Kotecha A, et al. Sponge delivery variables and tissue levels of 5-fluorouracil. Br J Ophthalmol. 2000;84(1):92–7.
41. Elder MJ. Congenital glaucoma in the West Bank and Gaza Strip. Br J Ophthalmol. 1993;77(7):413–6.
42. Elder MJ. Combined trabeculotomy-trabeculectomy compared with primary trabeculectomy for congenital glaucoma. Br J Ophthalmol. 1994;78(10):745–8.
43. Al-Hazmi A, Awad A, Zwaan J, Al-Mesfer SA, Al-Jadaan I, Al-Mohammed A. Correlation between surgical success rate and severity of congenital glaucoma. Br J Ophthalmol. 2005;89(4):449–53.
44. Lawrence SD, Netland PA. Trabeculectomy versus combined trabeculotomy-trabeculectomy in pediatric glaucoma. J Pediatr Ophthalmol Strabismus. 2012;49(6):359–65.
45. Low S, Hamada S, Nischal KK. Antimetabolite and releasable suture augmented filtration surgery in refractory pediatric glaucomas. J AAPOS. 2008;12(2):166–72.
46. Brown RH, Yang LH, Walker SD, Lynch MG, Martinez LA, Wilson LA. Treatment of bleb infection after glaucoma surgery. Arch Ophthalmol. 1994;112(1):57–61.
47. Ciulla TA, Beck AD, Topping TM, Baker AS. Blebitis, early endophthalmitis, and late endophthalmitis after glaucoma-filtering surgery. Ophthalmology. 1997;104(6):986–95.
48. Sugar HS. Complications, repair and reoperation of antiglaucoma filtering blebs. Am J Ophthalmol. 1967;63(4):825–33.
49. Soltau JB, Rothman RF, Budenz DL, Greenfield DS, Feuer W, Liebmann JM, Ritch R. Risk factors for glaucoma filtering bleb infections. Arch Ophthalmol. 2000;118(3):338–42.
50. Caronia RM, Liebmann JM, Friedman R, Cohen H, Ritch R. Trabeculectomy at the inferior limbus. Arch Ophthalmol. 1996;114(4):387–91.
51. Bellows AR, McCulley JP. Endophthalmitis in aphakic patients with unplanned filtering blebs wearing contact lenses. Ophthalmology. 1981;88(8):839–43.
52. Mandelbaum S, Forster RK, Gelender H, Culbertson W. Late onset endophthalmitis associated with filtering blebs. Ophthalmology. 1985;92(7):964–72.
53. Waheed S, Liebmann JM, Greenfield DS, Ritterband DC, Seedor JA, Shah M, Ritch R. Recurrent bleb infections. Br J Ophthalmol. 1998;82(8):926–9.
54. Golde KT, Gardiner MF. Bacterial conjunctivitis in children: a current review of pathogens and treatment. Int Ophthalmol Clin. 2011;51(4):85–92.
55. Kangas TA, Greenfield DS, Flynn HW Jr, Parrish RK 2nd, Palmberg P. Delayed-onset endophthalmitis associated with conjunctival filtering blebs. Ophthalmology. 1997;104(5):746–52.
56. Debnath SC, Teichmann KD, Salamah K. Trabeculectomy versus trabeculotomy in congenital glaucoma. Br J Ophthalmol. 1989;73(8):608–11.
57. Mandal AK, Walton DS, John T, Jayagandan A. Mitomycin C-augmented trabeculectomy in refractory congenital glaucoma. Ophthalmology. 1997;104(6):996–1001.
58. Giampani J Jr, Borges-Giampani AS, Carani JC, Oltrogge EW, Susanna R Jr. Efficacy and safety of trabeculectomy with mitomycin C for childhood glaucoma: a study of results with long-term follow-up. Clinics (Sao Paulo). 2008;63(4):421–6.
59. Ozkiris A, Tamcelik N. Long-term results of trabeculectomy with different concentrations of mitomycin C in refractory developmental glaucoma. J Pediatr Ophthalmol Strabismus. 2005;42(2):97–102.
60. Awadein A, El Sayed YM. Excision of tenon capsule in pediatric trabeculectomy: a controlled study. J Glaucoma. 2016;25(1):39–44.
61. Mahdy RA, Al-Mosallamy SM, Al-Sawad MA, Bor'i A, Wm E-H. Evaluation the adjunctive use of combined bevacizumab and mitomycin C to trabeculectomy in the management of recurrent pediatric glaucoma. Eye (Lond). 2016;30(1):53–8.
62. Averyn RL. Extrapolating anti-vascular endothelial growth factor therapy into pediatric ophthalmology: promise and concern. J AAPOS. 2009;13(4):329–31.

63. Chen TC, Chen PP, Francis BA, Junk AK, Smithy SD, Singh K, Lin SC. Pediatric glaucoma surgery: a report by the American Academy of Ophthalmology. Opthalmology. 2014;121(11):2107–15.
64. Almobarak F, Khan AO. Complications and 2-year valve survival following Ahmed valve implantation during the first 2 years of life. Br J Ophthalmol. 2009;93(6):795–8.
65. Heinz C, Koch J, Heiligenhaus A. Trabeculectomy or modified deep sclerectomy in juvenile uveitic glaucoma. J Ophthalmic Inflamm Infect. 2011;1(4):165–70.

Glaucoma Drainage Devices

7

James D. Brandt, Naama Hammel, Cecilia Fenerty, and Tanya Karaconji

Introduction

The treatment of primary congenital glaucoma (PCG) and the many secondary forms of glaucoma in childhood was revolutionized in the 1940s with the introduction of targeted surgery of the anterior chamber angle: goniotomy *ab-interno* [1] and trabeculotomy *ab-externo* [2, 3], both of which are discussed elsewhere in this book. Retrospective studies of both trabeculotomy and goniotomy in patients with PCG demonstrate success rates as high as 75–90%. However, even in the best of hands, some 20% or more of primary angle surgeries eventually fail, due to the underlying structural defect, the severity of the glaucoma at presentation, or the underlying diagnosis. Secondary glaucomas presenting in infancy such as aniridia, Axenfeld-Rieger anomaly, Peters anomaly, and glaucoma following cataract surgery (GFCS) often respond poorly if at all to primary angle surgery. When angle procedures like goniotomy or trabeculotomy fail, cannot be performed due to abnormal anatomy, or are felt unlikely to succeed based on the underlying presentation, surgeons are then confronted with choosing an alternative. One increasingly attractive option is the implantation of a glaucoma drainage device (GDD). This chapter will review the current status of GDDs in the management of childhood glaucoma including general principles of these devices, surgical techniques, and a review of the current pediatric GDD literature. We hope to provide useful guidance to surgeons confronting this clinical challenge.

All GDDs share a common design – they employ a biocompatible silicone tube placed in the anterior chamber (AC) or vitrectomized posterior chamber in order to shunt aqueous humor to the subconjunctival space [4]. This potential space between the sclera and the overlying Tenon capsule and conjunctiva is then maintained by an external biocompatible "plate" made of silicone or acrylic which varies in surface area. Once healing has occurred, the IOP-lowering effect of a GDD is roughly proportional to the inner surface area of the capsule surrounding the plate [5, 6].

History

The first purpose-designed GDD was that of Molteno [7], introduced in the early 1970s. In the first iteration of his procedure, the circular acrylic

Electronic Supplementary Material The online version of this chapter (https://doi.org/10.1007/978-3-319-54003-0_7) contains supplementary material, which is available to authorized users.

J. D. Brandt (✉) · N. Hammel
Department of Ophthalmology and Vision Science, University of California, Davis, Sacramento, CA, USA
e-mail: jdbrandt@ucdavis.edu

C. Fenerty · T. Karaconji
Manchester Royal Eye Hospital, University of Manchester, Manchester, UK

A. L. Grajewski et al. (eds.), *Surgical Management of Childhood Glaucoma*, https://doi.org/10.1007/978-3-319-54003-0_7

plate was sutured to the equatorial sclera and the tube tucked out of the way for subsequent retrieval (Stage 1). Some weeks later, after a fibrous capsule had formed around the plate, the tube was then retrieved (without violating the plate capsule) and inserted into the eye to drain aqueous humor (Stage 2). Molteno subsequently described the use of a Vicryl® (polyglactin) (Ethicon Somerville NJ, USA) tie to temporarily occlude the tube long enough for a capsule to develop around the equatorial implant [8], thus avoiding a two-stage procedure. In either case, glaucoma medications are used to lower intraocular pressure (IOP) until the device is fully functioning some 6 to 8 weeks later.

Currently available GDDs are listed in Table 7.1 and can broadly be categorized based by whether they are valved (e.g., Ahmed glaucoma valve) or non-valved designs (e.g., Molteno™, Baerveldt®, and Aurolab aqueous drainage implant devices) and then further categorized by plate surface area. Non-valved implants must be temporarily occluded to prevent early hypotony until sufficient fibrosis has developed around the plate to prevent hypotony; valved devices allow flow immediately after surgical implantation.

Considerations for Surgeons Experienced with GDD Surgery in Adults

It's often stated that children are not simply little adults, and certainly their eyes don't behave like little adult eyes. Glaucoma surgeons experienced in placing GDD in adult eyes must modify their usual surgical technique for the pediatric eye. Covered in more detail in this chapter, the following is a partial listing of things to note when tackling these cases:

- *Consider ocular size when choosing a glaucoma implant.* An adult-sized implant can usually be placed in a buphthalmic eye, but in nanophthalmic or microphthalmic eyes, a shorter implant must be chosen to avoid impinging on the optic nerve.
- *The sclera of buphthalmic eyes is very thin.* Suture passes can easily perforate the sclera leading to a retinal detachment. A longer, shallow pass may be necessary to adequately secure the implant in place.
- *Ocular growth must be accounted for in selecting tube position and length.* Around 3 millimeters of tube length must remain in the AC to accommodate for progressive buphthalmos or normal ocular growth in young children. Tube retraction in the growing eye is a late complication that can generally be avoided.
- *Forward tube movement is common.* In the pediatric eye, tubes tend to straighten out over time and will erode through overlying sclera and peripheral cornea. It is generally best to position AC tube entry as posterior as possible away from the cornea (sometimes through a surgical iridectomy) to avoid late corneal complications.
- *Pars plana placement may be considered in aphakic and pseudophakic eyes.* In children, placement in the pars plana must be accompanied by a meticulous and thorough vitrectomy. Late occlusion with vitreous remnants and retinal detachment are common (~ 20%) [9].

Specific Glaucoma Drainage Devices

Molteno™ Glaucoma Drainage Devices

The Molteno drainage implant was the pioneering GDD first described in 1969 [7]. It provided the foundation on which all of the currently available GDDs are based. The Molteno™ implant is a non-valved device con-

Table 7.1 Currently marketed glaucoma drainage devices

Name	Type	Model	Materials	Valve/drainage mechanism	Plate surface area (mm^2)	Manufacturer	FDA/CE approval status	Website
Ahmed glaucoma valve	Valved	FP7 (flexible plate)	Medical-grade silicone	Elastomer membrane	184	New World Medical	FDA and CE	http://www.newworldmedical.com/product-fp7
		FP8 (flexible plate – pediatric)	Medical-grade silicone	Elastomer membrane	102	New World Medical	FDA and CE	http://www.newworldmedical.com/product-fp8
		S2	Medical-grade polypropylene	Elastomer membrane	184	New World Medical	FDA and CE	http://www.newworldmedical.com/product-s2
		S3 (pediatric)	Medical-grade polypropylene	Elastomer membrane	85	New World Medical	FDA and CE	http://www.newworldmedical.com/product-s3
Baerveldt® glaucoma implant	Non-valved	BG 103–250 glaucoma implant	Medical-grade silicone	Open tube	250	Johnson & Johnson Vision	FDA and CE	https://surgical.jnjvision.com/us/iols/other/baerveldt-glaucoma-implants
		BG 101–350 glaucoma implant	Medical-grade silicone	Open tube	350	Johnson & Johnson Vision	FDA and CE	
		Pars plana BG 102–350 glaucoma implant	Medical-grade silicone	Open tube with Hoffman elbow	350	Johnson & Johnson Vision	FDA and CE	
Molteno™	Non-valved	Molteno™ SS	Medical-grade acrylic	Open tube	185	Molteno Ophthalmic	FDA and CE	https://www.molteno.com/molteno-glaucoma-drainage-devices
		Molteno™ SL	Medical-grade acrylic	Open tube	245	Molteno Ophthalmic	FDA and CE	
		Pediatric/microphthalmic P1	Medical-grade acrylic	Open tube	80	Molteno Ophthalmic	FDA and CE	
Aurolab aqueous drainage implant (AADI)	Non-valved		Silicone	Open tube	350	Aurolab (a manufacturing division of Aravind Eye Institute, Madurai, India)	CE	http://www.aurolab.com/glaucoma-shunt.asp

FDA US Food and Drug Administration, *CE* European Commission

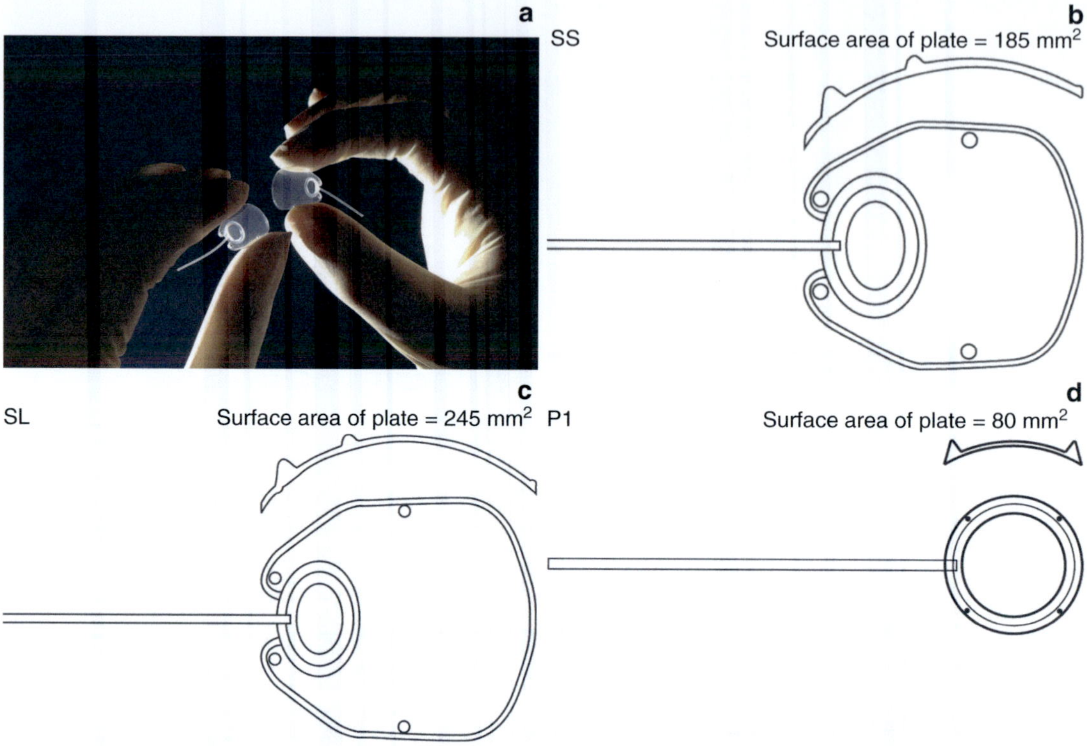

Fig. 7.1 (**a**) The Molteno3™ S-Series of glaucoma drainage devices; the model SS (right) has a surface area of 185 mm^2, the model SL (left) has a surface area of 245 mm^2; (**b**) diagram of model SS; (**c**) diagram of model SL; (**d**) diagram of model P1. Model P1 is designed for very small pediatric or nanophthalmic eyes and has a surface area of 80 mm^2. (Courtesy of Molteno Ophthalmic Ltd., Dunedin, New Zealand)

sisting of a silicone tube attached to an end plate placed 9–10 mm posterior to the limbus within the subconjunctival space. The plate is sutured to the sclera and covered by a thick flap of Tenon tissue and conjunctiva. A permeable fibrovascular bleb forms over the plate, the surface area of which contributes to the amount of aqueous drainage and the final level of IOP [10] along with the thickness of the bleb capsule.

The original Molteno™ implant consisted of a single 13 mm diameter plate molded from acrylic with a surface area of 135 mm^2. The single plate is inserted between two rectus muscles in the chosen quadrant. The double-plate Molteno™ implant was introduced in 1981 and consists of two plates, one of which is attached to the silicone tube in the AC, while a second tube connects the two plates forming a total surface area of 270 mm^2.

Currently marketed (Molteno Ophthalmic, Ltd., Dunedin, New Zealand) Molteno™ implants (Fig. 7.1) are the Molteno3™ S-Series, the SS (185 mm^2), and SL (245 mm^2) models, both designed for single-quadrant placement, and the Molteno™ P1 (80 mm^2) designed for implantation in eyes with axial lengths shorter than 17 mm.

Baerveldt® Glaucoma Drainage Devices

Introduced in 1990, the Baerveldt® glaucoma implant (BGI) is a non-valved device with a silicone tube attached to one of two sizes of external silicone plate (250 and 350 mm^2). The company (Johnson & Johnson Vision, Santa Ana CA, USA) also markets a 350 mm^2 version for implantation in the pars plana with the tube specially

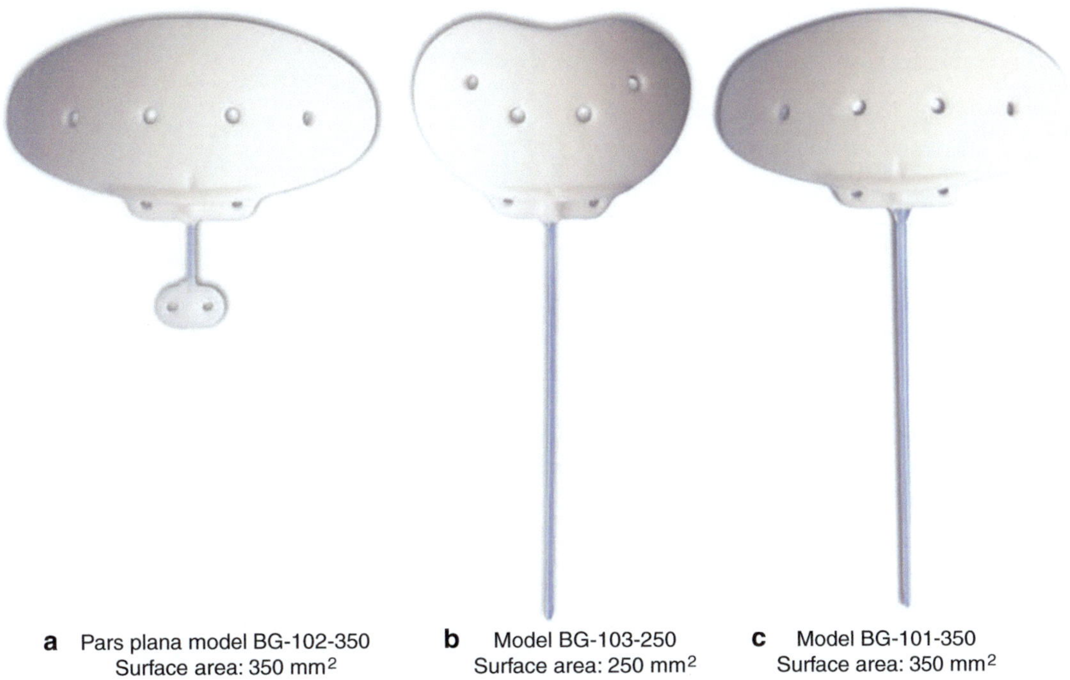

Fig. 7.2 The Baerveldt® glaucoma implant comes in three models: Model BG 101–350 (**a**) has a surface area of 350 mm^2; Model BT103–250 (**b**) has a surface area of 250 mm^2; Model 102–350 (**c**) has a surface area of 350 mm2 and is designed with a Hoffman Elbow for insertion into the pars plana. (Courtesy of Johnson & Johnson Vision, Santa Ana CA, USA)

modified with a Hoffman elbow for this purpose. All are designed for surgical implantation in a single quadrant (Fig. 7.2).

The "wings" of the plate are intended for placement under the adjacent rectus muscles. When positioned in this manner, the front edge of the implant rests approximately 8 mm posterior to the limbus. All BGIs are made of smooth, tumble-polished, pliable medical-grade silicone. Barium is incorporated into the silicone, which results in a white, radio-opaque device. The plates are designed with four holes to allow a tissue "bridge" to develop between the upper and lower surfaces of the eventual capsule to limit the size of the bleb and thus reduce the likelihood of restrictive strabismus and diplopia.

Ahmed Glaucoma Valves

The Ahmed glaucoma valve (AGV) received the US Food and Drug Administration (FDA) approval in November 1993. The implant consists of three parts: a plate made of medical-grade silicone, polypropylene, or porous polyethylene, depending on the model; a drainage tube fabricated of medical-grade silicone; and a valve mechanism (Fig. 7.3). The non-obstructive, self-regulating valve mechanism consists of thin silicone elastomer membranes 8 mm long by 7 mm wide enclosed within Venturi-shaped chamber. The membranes are pretensioned to open and close in response to IOP variations, in the range of 8–12 mmHg, and so reduce the rate of early postoperative hypotony [11, 12]. After implantation, aqueous humor flows into the trapezoidal chamber of the valve.

Aurolab Aqueous Drainage Implant (AADI)

The Aurolab aqueous drainage implant (AADI) was introduced in 2013 by Aurolab (a manufacturing

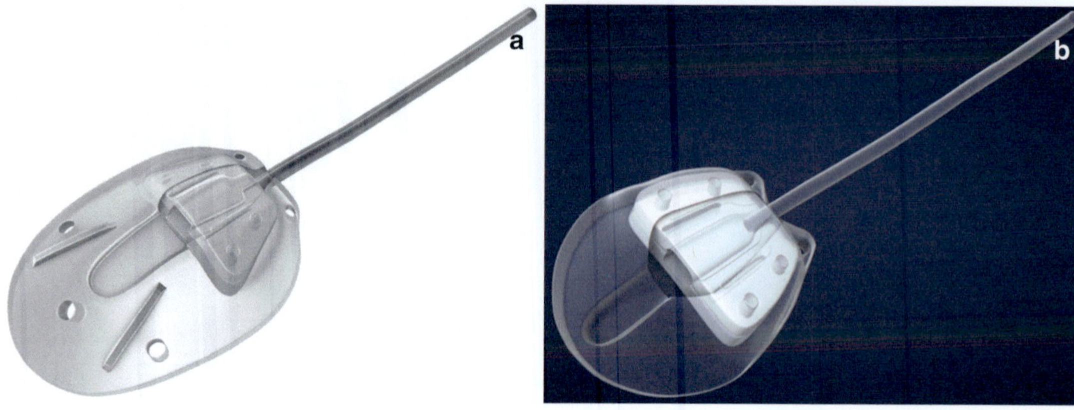

Fig. 7.3 Ahmed glaucoma valve FP7 (**a**) is a valved silicone glaucoma drainage device (GDD) implant with a surface area of 184 mm^2; the Ahmed glaucoma valve FP8 (**b**) is a GDD designed for small pediatric or nanophthalmic eyes, with a surface area of 102 mm^2. (Courtesy of New World Medical, Rancho Cucamonga CA, USA)

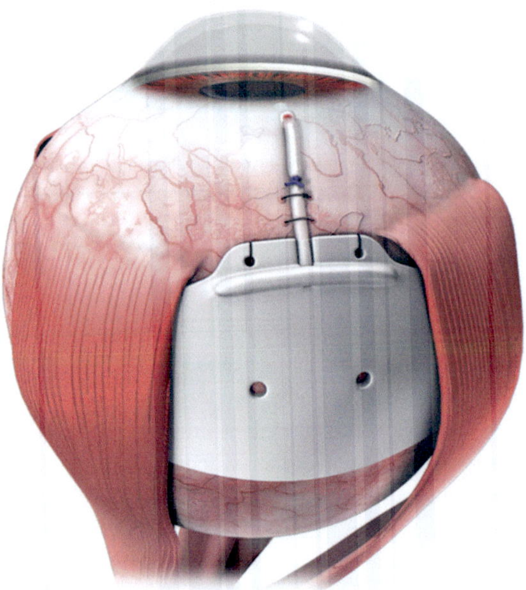

Fig. 7.4 Aurolab aqueous drainage implant (AADI) is a CE Mark approved, low-cost copy of the BG 101–350 Baerveldt® glaucoma implant (Fig. 7.2a above). (Courtesy of Aurolab, Madurai, India)

division of Aravind Eye Institute, Madurai, India). The AADI is a low-cost (~ US$50), non-valved GDD designed to replicate the BGI with a 350 mm^2 plate area (Fig. 7.4). Professor George Baerveldt authorized the use of his very successful design, and the device was manufactured in collaboration with the Bascom Palmer Eye Institute, Miami, Florida. Originally designed for use in India and other low-resourced countries, the device has received CE (European Commission) marking approval and is becoming broadly available in those countries that accept the CE mark for regulatory approval. It is not approved by the FDA and is therefore unavailable in the United States. Kaushik and colleagues [13] recently reported a prospective interventional study on 34 eyes of 31 children with refractory childhood glaucoma in which the AADI was implanted. Their results show an efficacy and safety profile that is comparable with published reports of the BGI and Ahmed glaucoma valve implants in children.

Indications and Contraindications

Glaucoma drainage devices are employed in childhood glaucoma when conventional angle surgery (goniotomy or trabeculotomy) has already failed or is believed unlikely to work. At such a point in clinical decision-making, most surgeons choose between a GDD and a trabeculectomy with anti-scarring agents. GDD surgery is also indicated when trabeculectomy is unlikely to work, e.g., in eyes with glaucoma following congenital cataract surgery or when trabeculectomy with anti-scarring agents has failed.

Advantages and Disadvantages

Table 7.2 broadly summarizes the pros and cons of GDD and trabeculectomy. There are no prospective randomized clinical trials comparing the two procedures in children. The Tube versus Trabeculectomy (TVT) study [14, 15] was a prospective randomized clinical trial comparing the Baerveldt® glaucoma implant to mitomycin C augmented trabeculectomy in adults greater than 18 years of age with prior failed trabeculectomy or prior cataract surgery. After 5 years of follow-up, the GDD group had a higher success rate than the trabeculectomy group with comparable complication rates, visual acuity outcomes, and medication burden. Although not directly applicable to the pediatric age group, GDDs are used most often in the eyes of older children with scarred conjunctiva, so the TVT provides at least some guidance to the surgeon considering a GDD or a trabeculectomy in such eyes.

Another consideration in balancing the decision between a trabeculectomy and a GDD is whether or not further surgical interventions are anticipated. The functioning of a well-established trabeculectomy will tend to diminish or even fail after further surgeries such as penetrating keratoplasty or even after uncomplicated cataract removal [16], e.g., in

Table 7.2 Pros and cons of glaucoma drainage devices compared to trabeculectomy in children

	Glaucoma drainage device		Trabeculectomy with MMC	
	Pros	Cons	Pros	Cons
Technique	Can be done with cloudy cornea	Violates conjunctiva Hardware in the eye	Can be performed with cloudy cornea No hardware left in the eye	Violates conjunctiva
Outcomes	Effective long-term IOP reduction, even after failed trabeculectomy Most likely to survive future intraocular surgery	Higher long-term IOP compared with trabeculectomy More likely to require supplemental medications Further surgery for complications more likely [73]	Lower long-term IOP Supplemental medications less likely	Poor results in glaucoma following cataract surgery even with MMC Less likely to survive future intraocular surgery
Complications	Lower risk of endophthalmitis	Risk of intra- and postoperative hypotony Risk of tube-related complications: corneal decompensation, cataract, tube erosion, migration, and obstruction Greater risk of postoperative motility disturbance	No tube-related complications	Risk of intra- and postoperative hypotony Lifelong risk of postoperative endophthalmitis if avascular bleb develops, especially if contact lenses are required
Quality of life	Contact lens wear possible (important for aphakic eyes with glaucoma) Post-op care involves fewer manipulations, reducing number of EUAs			Contact lens wear not recommended Post-op care requires frequent visits for close follow-up and possible suture adjustments/5FU injections which in turn might require more frequent EUAs

IOP intraocular pressure, *EUA* examination under anesthesia, *MMC* mitomycin C, *5FU* 5 Fluorouracil uveitic eyes. In eyes likely to need additional surgery after glaucoma surgery, a GDD is much more likely than trabeculectomy to continue functioning postoperatively. For this and other reasons, we firmly believe that a team approach to complex childhood glaucoma is key to successful outcomes, especially one that engages cornea, pediatric, and vitreoretinal specialists early on to develop a long-term plan of care that includes the proper sequencing of interventions.

Preoperative Considerations and Preparation

Preoperative examination and planning are essential for successful surgical outcomes. In infants and young children, a thorough examination sufficient to plan surgery may not be feasible in the clinic, and the decision on surgical approach may only be made in the operating room following an examination under anesthesia (EUA). The EUA for patients with childhood glaucoma is discussed in detail in Chapter 3.

Important Considerations for GDD

Axial Length Measurement of the axial length is important in the baseline assessment and ongoing monitoring of children with glaucoma. Progressive increases in the axial length of an eye in excess of normal growth may indicate poorly controlled IOP. In the context of planning for a GDD, axial length measurement may influence device selection (see below). In buphthalmic eyes that are adult size or larger, adult GDDs are commonly used.

Conjunctival mobility, which may constrain which quadrant is best for GDD implantation or preclude a trabeculectomy if the choice between procedures has not yet been made. It is often useful to inject balanced salt solution (BSS) into the subconjunctival space with a 30-gauge needle to help delineate episcleral scarring.

Gonioscopy, which will help visualize the presence of iris strands, membranes, or peripheral anterior synechiae (PAS) which might interfere with the insertion of the tube into the AC. If implantation is planned in a quadrant with broad PAS, a surgical peripheral iridectomy can be performed through a small corneal incision in the area of planned tube insertion to avoid having the tube end up under the iris.

Anterior chamber depth and lens status, visualized clinically by slit lamp, under the operating microscope, gonioscopy, or by ultrasound. This is done to determine if tube insertion into the AC can be safely performed both avoiding tube-corneal touch and damage to the crystalline lens. In pseudophakic or aphakic eyes, it may be preferable to place the tube in the ciliary sulcus or pars plana in combination with a pars plana vitrectomy or through a surgical peripheral iridectomy to keep the tube as far away from the corneal endothelium as possible.

Size of the palpebral aperture and motility of the globe are important in providing surgical access to insert a GDD. It may be necessary to perform a lateral canthotomy in some cases of small palpebral aperture to gain sufficient access for surgery. Ocular motility considerations include how to handle the GDD placement when strabismus is present before surgery, especially if the eye to be operated has had prior extraocular muscle surgery. An additional topic, and one which is beyond the scope of this chapter, includes how to handle strabismus induced or worsened by GDD placement.

Scleral Integrity The eyes which have had previous surgical procedures, trauma, or transscleral laser may have areas of scleral thinning which will influence the choice of quadrant used for GDD placement.

Choice of GDD Patch Although many surgeons will use commercially available patches (e.g., Tutoplast® pericardium, dura, or fascia lata) or donor grafts (e.g., sclera or cornea), some surgeons prefer to fashion a long scleral tunnel to cover the tube.

Choice of GDD

The decision of which implant to use in a specific case is based on a number of factors, including the underlying glaucoma diagnosis, level of IOP and ability to control IOP medically, ocular size, orbital anatomy, and finally surgeon preference.

Glaucoma Diagnosis GDDs lower IOP in all forms of childhood glaucoma, and there are no prospective randomized clinical trials comparing the different implants in children on which to base device choice. However, the specific form of disease may influence the choice of implant. In children with the potential for decreased aqueous production, e.g., eyes with uveitis or eyes that have already undergone cyclodestructive procedures, a valved or smaller surface area non-valved implant may be a better choice to avoid hypotony.

IOP Level The level of IOP and the ability to control the IOP with medications postoperatively can influence the choice between a valved or non-valved implant. The adult literature suggests that the non-valved 350 mm^2 Baerveldt® glaucoma implant may be superior to the Ahmed glaucoma valve in terms of long-term IOP-lowering and medication burden [17]. Hence, if the IOP in a child can be controlled with medications for 6 to 8 weeks while the non-valved implant is temporarily occluded, the surgeon may choose to use a Baerveldt implant in the hope of achieving slightly better long-term IOP control. In contrast, the Ahmed glaucoma valve lowers IOP immediately, which may be of prime importance especially if the child is in pain, has advanced glaucoma, and cannot tolerate medications or if corneal edema is causing amblyopia.

Ocular Size and Orbital Anatomy Often by the time pediatric eyes have already failed one procedure and require GDD surgery, the eyes have grown to adult size or larger. In such cases, adult-sized implants may usually be implanted without too much difficulty. As noted earlier, IOP-lowering is roughly proportional to plate size, so it is generally in the long-term interest of the child to implant an adult implant whenever possible. In contrast, when GDDs are used as primary surgery or in very young infants with small eyes (e.g., those with true microphthalmia), the physical size of adult implants comes into play.

GDDs are best implanted with the anterior edge of the plate at least 8 mm posterior to the surgical limbus. When an adult-sized GDD is placed in this position, the posterior edge of the implant plate may impinge on the optic nerve in young infants. Margeta and colleagues [18] measured the limbus to optic nerve distance in the superior temporal quadrant in 15 pediatric autopsy eyes. Figure 7.5 demonstrates that in a pediatric eye with axial length of 19 mm, an adult-sized Ahmed Model FP7 glaucoma valve, placed in the inferior nasal quadrant with the anterior edge sutured 7 mm from the limbus, overlaps the optic nerve to a significant degree. The Freedman-Margeta formula (http://people.duke.edu/~freed003/GDDCalculator/) offers a way to determine limbus to optic nerve distance in pediatric and small eyes in order to reduce the risk of optic nerve impingement by the posterior edge of the GDD plate. The Ahmed glaucoma valve is available in pediatric sizing (FP8 and S3 versions) as is the Molteno™ implant (P1 version); the posterior edge of the 350 mm^2 BGI and the AADI can be easily trimmed with a heavy surgical scissors to create a cutout to accommodate the optic nerve. The 250 mm^2 version of the BGI is designed with a posterior notch to avoid overriding the optic nerve.

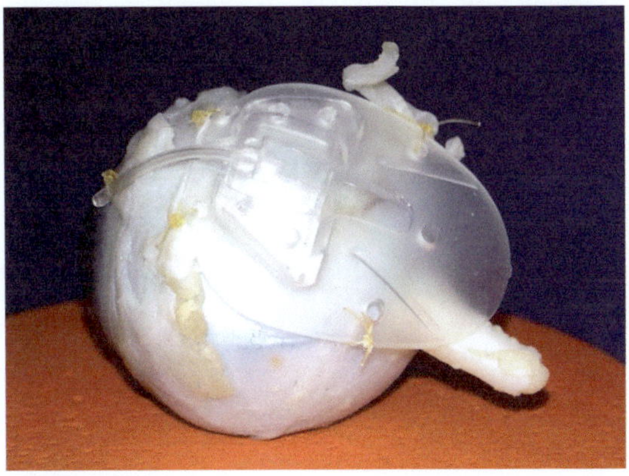

Fig. 7.5 Photograph of a pediatric autopsy eye (axial length 19 mm), showing an Ahmed Model FP7 glaucoma drainage device sutured in the superonasal quadrant. The anterior edge of the plate is located 7 mm from the limbus; note the extensive overlap of the posterior edge of the Ahmed device plate and the optic nerve. (Courtesy of Milica Margeta, MD, PhD and Sharon Freedman MD)

Operation

Intraoperative Preparation

The surgical field should be cleaned with sterile iodine or chlorhexidine-based preparation fluid, the area dried, and a surgical drape placed over the eye. Self-adhesive ophthalmic drapes with a transparent window and a pocket to collect irrigation fluid are desirable. This may be applied with the lids open and the lashes everted so that when the drape is cut open to apply a lid speculum, the lashes are retained underneath the sticky drape without straying into the surgical field.

With the lids held open by an ophthalmic speculum, a drop of 1:10,000 adrenalin or other topical ocular sympathomimetic drug may be instilled to promote vasoconstriction of the conjunctiva and episclera and minimize tissue bleeding.

The usual position for a GDD is in the superior temporal quadrant. The surgeon will generally be positioned superiorly or in the superior temporal position approximately 45° from the vertical; if the microscope permits, the assistant can be positioned superiorly.

Surgical Technique

A recommended set of instruments and suture materials for GDD surgery are listed in Table 7.3. Implantation of GDDs in pediatric patients requires special attention to the size of the eye and orbit, the thickness of the sclera, and the positioning of the tube in an eye that will continue to grow.

Traction Suture A corneal traction suture is placed in alignment with the intended quadrant to rotate the eye inferior-nasally to provide the best surgical exposure. This may be placed through partial-thickness cornea in the mid-periphery of the same quadrant or at the limbus on either or both side(s) of the planned entry site. The conjunctiva and surgical exposure are then evaluated for scarring, and sufficient room to place a GDD is confirmed.

Conjunctival Incision Most surgeons perform fornix-based conjunctival flaps (e.g., the incision is made at the limbus) for GDD implantation, but a limbus-based conjunctival flap (where the incision is placed approximately 6–8 mm posterior to the limbus) has several advantages in pediatric eyes. It facilitates placement of the sutures securing the plate to the sclera in the very tight pediatric orbit, and the incision can be closed confidently in a watertight manner that will not unravel if the child rubs the eye vigorously. And importantly in children with aphakia, contact lens use can often be resumed within days of surgery. In contrast, incisions at the limbus are more uncomfortable for children, and contact lenses cannot be resumed for several weeks in most cases. In a retrospective comparison of limbal-based to fornix-based incisions for GDDs in adults, Suhr et al. found no difference in IOP outcomes [19].

Another important consideration for incision type arises in children with aniridia. In these patients, limbal stem cell deficiency arises that leads to corneal conjunctivalization and opacity later in life. A limbal incision, cautery, and mitomycin C application are likely to be detrimental

Table 7.3 Recommended instruments and suture materials for glaucoma drainage devices implant surgery

Instruments and knives		Sutures and consumables	Device related
Eye speculum	Tenotomy scissors		GDD of choice
Caliper	Vannas scissors – straight, curved	7-0 Vicryl® or Mersilk for corneal traction suture	BSS on a 27- or 30-gauge cannula
Muscle hook	Mini-crescent blade	8-0 nylon on a spatulated needle	23- or 25-gauge needle
Conjunctival forceps	MVR blade/supersharp	8-0 or 9-0 Vicryl® for conjunctival closure	Patch graft material
Tying forceps	Conjunctival clamp	Viscoelastic	
Colibri forceps	Needle holder	Anterior chamber infusion	

GDD glaucoma drainage device, *BSS* balanced salt solution, *MVR* micro vitreoretinal to the limited reserve of stem cells in these patients. For patients with aniridia, a limbal-based (limbus sparing) conjunctival technique is recommended, and the use of MMC is avoided.

Device Preparation and Placement Once the conjunctival incision is made, dissection and elevation of Tenon capsule from the episclera are carried out, and the adjacent rectus muscles are identified with a muscle hook. Tenotomy scissors are used to clear all adhesions and check ligaments posterior to the incision to clear the potential space for the implant and to facilitate the easy implantation of the selected device. Alternatively, blunt dissection of the correct plane may be started with scissors and completed with two squint hooks inserted back-to-back in this pocket and pulled gently apart, as demonstrated in the Video 7.1.

Before implanting an AGV, it is imperative that the surgeon "prime" the device with BSS. The silicone leaflets of the valve device stick together during manufacture, and if they are not primed with BSS, the device will fail. A 27- or 30-gauge cannula on a syringe filled with BSS is inserted into the tip of the silicone tube. BSS is gently injected into the tube, and flow is observed through the valve leaflets under the microscope [20]. Once this is done, the device is "primed," and implantation in the selected quadrant may proceed.

A muscle hook may be used to engage the superior rectus muscle; the AGV device can be grasped gently with smooth forceps with care taken not to crush the portion of the device housing the valve mechanism. With forward traction on the muscle hook, the device is placed between the two rectus muscles and pushed posteriorly. When adequate preparation of the quadrant and clearance of adhesions or check ligaments has been done, the device will achieve a resting position with the anterior suture holes approximately 8 mm posterior to the limbus.

In the case of a BGI or AADI, the superior rectus muscle is engaged with a muscle hook and the implant plate grasped with large non-toothed forceps (e.g., Nugent or Moorfields forceps) and the appropriate wing of the implant placed under the muscle. A second non-toothed forceps is then used to grasp the opposite wing of the implant, and the muscle hook removed from under the superior rectus and repositioned under the lateral rectus muscle. The plates of these devices are quite flexible, so by grasping and bending the plate, the temporal wing can be easily placed under the lateral rectus muscle. The implant is then gently pulled forward to verify that it has achieved a good position between and under the two rectus muscles. It is not pulled tightly up under the muscle but rather should rest gently behind the muscle insertions with the suture holes positioned some 8–10 mm posterior to the limbus.

Because the BGI and AADI devices are not valved, the tube portion of the device must be temporarily occluded. In adults, this can be done with absorbable sutures, sutures that can be lasered or with a rip cord that is removed later at the slit lamp in older children and adults and in the operating room in young children. The absorbable suture technique is appropriate in young children and is described here along with the optional modification of an intraluminal stent to reduce the chance of hypotony. A suture of 6-0 or 7-0 polyglactin suture is tied around the silicone tube a few mm anterior to the plate. A 27- or 30-gauge cannula on a syringe filled with BSS is inserted into the tip of the silicone tube, and complete occlusion of the tube is confirmed. Ligation of the implant tube can be performed based on the surgeon's preference either on the back table of the operating room before implantation or under the operating microscope after the device is in place or sutured to the sclera. Any flow through the tube must be avoided in children as a flat chamber is likely to result that will necessitate an early return to the operating room.

In addition to the extraluminal absorbable tie, an intraluminal stent may be used to partially occlude the lumen. A nonabsorbable suture thread (e.g., 3-0 Prolene® or 3-0 Supramid®) is used with one end fed into the GDD tube at the plate and the distal end tracked beneath the conjunctiva, often into the inferior fornix. Following the absorption of the extraluminal tie at 6–8 weeks, the presence of this intraluminal stent mitigates the risk of hypotony. If, however, the IOP remains poorly controlled after the absorption of the Vicryl tie, the stent may be subsequently removed by making a small incision over its distal end in the lower fornix and the whole thread pulled out remotely from the device. The conjunctival incision is closed with a pre-placed Vicryl purse string suture.

Plate Suturing The next step in the procedure is to affix the plate to the sclera. A suture on a spatulated needle is used to make a deep partial-thickness pass just in front of the plate taking care not to penetrate the sclera, which can be quite thin in a buphthalmic eye. The suture is then passed through the fixation hole of the implant and tied down tightly to minimize plate movement. When possible, the knot should be rotated into the fixation holes to avoid the short lengths of suture eroding through to conjunctiva resulting in irritation or serious infection. Molteno described the use of 7-0 silk to secure the plate of his device to the sclera [7], and others advocate the use of nonabsorbable sutures, such as polyester (Mersilene®) or polypropylene (Prolene®). Current implants are designed with holes in the plate that allow tissue "rivets" to form between the sclera, through the hole, and to the capsule above. Once these tissue rivets are formed during the first few months of healing, the implant will not move.

Silk can cause significant local inflammation, and nonabsorbable sutures may cause the overlying conjunctiva to break down or erode, sometimes many years later. We recommend 8-0 Nylon to secure the implant in place on the sclera. Nylon has sufficient tensile strength to tie down the implant tightly; the material begins to degrade only after a year or so has passed, long after the tissue rivets have secured the implant in place. After several years, the nylon disintegrates, eliminating the risk of late conjunctival erosion.

Tube Implantation Insertion of the tube into the AC is the most challenging aspect of pediatric GDD surgery. The surgeon must account for an AC that may be shallow but also plan for the long-term growth of the eye.

An AC paracentesis is performed (e.g., using an MVR blade); if the child was dilated for an EUA or photography, a quick-acting miotic is first injected into the eye to constrict the pupil. A viscoelastic substance is injected, or an AC infusion inserted, to avoid intraoperative hypotony. The scleral surface anterior to the plate is cleared of adhesions, and gentle cautery is applied, if required, to dry the surface. When a limbus-based conjunctival flap has been created, the assistant can use a surgical conjunctival clamp (Khaw conjunctival clamp [Duckworth & Kent Ltd., Baldock, Hertfordshire, UK], Khaw/Shah 4 mm conjunctival clamp [Duckworth & Kent], or Lama cross-action 5 mm conjunctival forceps [Moria Inc., Doylestown PA, USA]) to grasp the flap and provide good surgical exposure (Fig. 7.6). The tube entry in children is usually created in an oblique direction so that the tube can be left long enough to accommodate growth without extending into the pupillary aperture. The tube is laid down on to the intended path of implantation and is trimmed to an appropriate

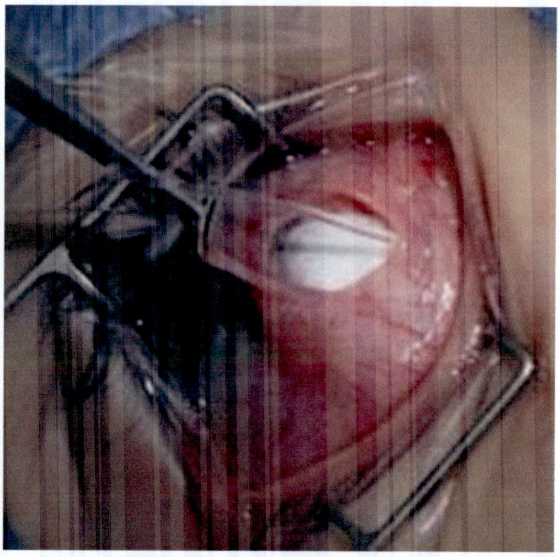

Fig. 7.6 Placement of an Ahmed glaucoma valve in the inferior nasal quadrant through a limbal-based conjunctival incision. The adult-sized plate (Model FP7) has already been sewn in place approximately 10 mm posterior to the limbus in this buphthalmic eye with a 25 mm axial length. Lama cross-action conjunctival forceps provide excellent exposure. (Courtesy of James D. Brandt, MD)

length creating an anteriorly oriented beveled tip. Before entering the eye with a needle to create a pathway for the tube, the AC is reassessed and the previously placed side-port incision used to deepen the chamber with viscoelastic as necessary. This side-port incision should be oriented in such a way that if the tube is misdirected in the eye, a Sinskey hook or iris spatula can be used to redirect the tube into the correct position. If the implant is positioned in such a way that the tube will enter the eye in an area of broad PAS or other obstructions, a surgical peripheral iridectomy can be created through a small corneal incision just inside the limbus. In this manner, the tube can be inserted more posteriorly and then rest in front of the iris but well back from the cornea. Any such corneal incision must be closed with a 10-0 suture of Nylon or Vicryl® as it will leak in a pediatric eye unless sutured.

In adults, a 23-gauge needle is often used to create the tube entry site; in children, the sclera is sufficiently flexible that a 25-gauge needle can be used and the tube can be inserted without too much difficulty. The use of a narrower gauge needle to fashion the tunnel also reduces the risk of leakage of aqueous around the tube and hypotony. Moving the tube entry site several millimeters back from the limbus avoiding a corneal track is important to avoid late erosions, but doing so can make it challenging to get the angle just right to avoid an anteriorly vaulted tube that touches the corneal endothelium. The beveled tip of the tube is then advanced into the needle tract and pushed forward with fine forceps. Alternatively, the tube may be inserted with the assistance of a fine blunt-tipped cannula by engaging the tip firmly onto the bevel of the trimmed tube and passing the cannula gently through the scleral tunnel taking the tube with it (Video 7.2). The surgeon should watch for the tube to enter the AC periphery where expected; if it does not, the tube may have migrated under the iris, in which case another pass can be tried or a surgical iridectomy created as noted above.

Once the tube has been inserted into the eye, the external portion should be secured to the sclera with a nonabsorbable suture (e.g., 9-0 Nylon) which helps to stabilize the tube. This both reduces the risk of migration out of the eye and also reduces outward bowing of the tube which may increase the susceptibility to erosion through the conjunctiva.

The tube must be covered to prevent its erosion through the overlying conjunctiva over time. The tube may be covered either with autologous tissue or with donor sclera or cornea obtained from an eye bank or dehydrated and preserved donor dura mater or pericardium [21]. This graft material is usually sutured into place with one or two sutures of fine (8-0 or 9-0) polyglactin; a permanent suture is not needed as graft materials rapidly incorporate into the surrounding Tenon capsule or conjunctiva.

Although autologous tissue may be obtained from fascia lata or temporalis fascia, many glaucoma surgeons now advocate using the patient's own sclera to support and cover the tube. This can be challenging in the thin sclera of a buphthalmic eye but can be done in a number of ways, the simplest of which is by creating a scleral flap. Alternatively, a long tunnel in the patient's native sclera may be created using a bent needle starting some 5 mm posterior to the limbus. Another method employs a small minicrescent blade (1.25 mm in width) (Video 7.3) that can be used to tunnel in the sclera up to about 2 mm posterior to the limbus, then completing the entry into the eye with a 25-gauge needle.

Once the tube has been inserted, any viscoelastic remaining in the eye is expressed through the side-port incision or washed out with irrigation. While some viscoelastic may be left in the eye safely when a valved implant is placed, it should be aggressively removed from the eye when a non-valved implant is used, as any retained viscoelastic will cause a dramatic rise in IOP. The AC is then refilled to a physiologic level with BSS to determine where the tube will end up in relation to the iris or cornea. If the tube is vaulted too far forward and risks touching the endothelium with eye rubbing, it is far better to revise the tube position and/or length at the initial surgery than returning to the operating room months or years later after endothelial loss has occurred.

Incision Closure Tenon layer and conjunctiva are securely sutured to ensure adequate coverage of the plate, tube, and patch graft/scleral flap, preferably with absorbable sutures to avoid returning to the operating room and further anesthetic exposure to deal with irritating sutures. A sub-Tenon injection of long-acting local anesthetic performed during closure can help with early postoperative pain relief.

The sclera is often thin in pediatric eyes and the tissues less rigid than adult eyes. It is therefore frequently necessary to suture the paracentesis used for the AC infusion or viscoelastic in order to avoid postoperative leaks; 10-0 monofilament Vicryl® is used when available for the same reason described above.

At the end of the operation, the eye should be inspected to ensure that the implant plate, patch graft, and intraocular portion of the tube are in a good position, that the AC is well formed, and that a clear red reflex can be seen. Fluorescein drops or strips can be used to inspect the conjunctiva and cornea of leaks, and instillation of a cycloplegic such as atropine will assist in deepening the AC. A subconjunctival injection of corticosteroid and antibiotic is commonly performed at the end of the procedure.

Modifications to Standard Technique

Some modifications to the technique of GDD surgery have already been mentioned and relate to surgeon preference and experience; however, modifications to the standard technique may be dictated by scarring and tissue distortion from previous surgery and trauma or by the underlying diagnosis.

Conjunctival Scarring Although superotemporal placement of the drainage device is often preferred, circumstances may dictate that a superonasal or inferior placement of the tube is required. Examples include eyes where previous glaucoma surgery has taken place in the superior temporal quadrant or where PAS preclude entry of the tube into the AC at that site.

The use of explants for the repair of retinal detachments is infrequent now; however, if a GDD is required in this circumstance, placement of the plate may need to be behind or even on top of the explant. Before placing a GDD in such eyes, it is essential to ensure that adequate and sufficiently mobile Tenon capsule and conjunctiva are available to cover the hardware before placing such a device.

Prior Strabismus Surgery If a rectus muscle has been resected in the quadrant planned for the GDD placement, one needs to prepare for additional scarring around the muscle insertion, but usually careful technique will allow the GDD surgery to proceed without major modification. By contrast, a previous rectus muscle recession (e.g., lateral rectus for a planned GDD in the superior temporal quadrant) may call for a modified GDD procedure, especially in the case of a planned Baerveldt GDD. Basically, for a Baerveldt to be placed in a quadrant where an adjacent rectus recession has previously occurred, the surgeon must identify the insertion of the recessed muscle and then may either trim the front of the respective wing to allow that wing to be placed behind the recessed rectus muscle (personal communication, SFF) or may trim the back of the respective wing, such that the wing is entirely in front of the rectus muscle. This latter technique may lead to making the anterior portion of the bleb in front of the muscle much more visible, which is often cosmetically problematic, and is therefore not recommended. It may be preferable in this case to place the plate in the superonasal quadrant, that is, in the quadrant with the resected rather than the recessed horizontal muscle. In the case of a preexisting strabismus, such as an exotropia, the surgeon may elect to recess the lateral rectus muscle concurrent with the GDD placement (especially in the case of a planned Baerveldt implant), because the muscle will be much harder to access after the GDD surgery. As described above, it is recommended that the anterior portion of the, respectively, Baerveldt wing be trimmed to allow the recessed rectus to remain anterior to the Baerveldt wing.

Glaucoma Following Cataract Surgery (GFCS) GDDs are frequently the preferred primary procedure in the management of glaucoma following cataract surgery, particularly in aphakic eyes where contact lens is planned. In this circumstance, a trabeculectomy is contraindicated due to increased risk of bleb-related endophthalmitis.

A success rate for controlling the IOP following cataract surgery has been reported of up to 90% at 1 year [22], and in addition, GDDs allow children to more easily wear contact lens refractive correction which assists with management of amblyopia. Tube insertion may be performed in the sulcus or the pars plana to avoid complications of corneal tube touch [23]. Doing so avoids leaving hardware at or near the limbus where aphakic contact lenses can lead to late-onset conjunctival breakdown over the tube; furthermore, pars plana insertion of the tube protects the corneal endothelium from tube-corneal touch. However, eyes which have undergone cataract surgery may be particularly susceptible to occlusion of the tube tip by capsular remnants, "Elschnig pearls" of residual cortical material, or vitreous. To mitigate this risk, it is essential to consider performing excision of lens pearls, and/or further vitrectomy if the eye is aphakic, and the tube should be positioned away from the iris and capsule.

Vitreous incarceration into the tube can happen shortly after surgery or many years later; in a retrospective review of Baerveldt® implants placed through the pars plana, Vinod et al. [9] reported vitreous tube obstruction in 19% of their series, occurring 3–112 months after implantation.

Any mobile vitreous will eventually find its way to the tube tip and occlude it. It is absolutely necessary to perform a meticulous pars plana vitrectomy prior to tube insertion in order to prevent this late complication. If corneal clarity prevents a good view, a surgical endoscope can be used to perform the vitrectomy [24]. The anterior core vitrectomy routinely performed at the time of pediatric lensectomy is insufficient; even in an aphakic eye that was vitrectomized at the time of cataract extraction, the vitreous base must be shaved down aggressively under direct visualization and an attempt made to cause a posterior vitreous detachment to elevate and remove the posterior hyaloid face. In young children in particular, the posterior hyaloid face is difficult to detach during vitrectomy, and it is this posterior shell of vitreous and hyaloid that can detach years later.

Care should be taken to ensure that the tube is trimmed to a length which allows direct visualization of the tip, particularly when it is inserted through the pars plana as this assists in diagnosing or excluding occlusion as a cause of GDD failure.

Sturge-Weber Syndrome Patients with Sturge-Weber syndrome may have associated choroidal hemangioma, and it is important to diagnose this prior to surgical intervention. Precipitous reduction in IOP or hypotony may result in a suprachoroidal hemorrhage, which can be sight threatening. Choroidal effusions are more common and may even occur undetected in the early postoperative period (Fig. 7.7). It is therefore essential to take measures to avoid both intraoperative and postoperative hypotony. The use of an AC infusion is helpful to maintain the IOP while the tube tunnel is fashioned and the tube inserted. Care should be taken to ensure that the tube tunnel is tight and that there is no peri-tube leak following insertion. The use of extraluminal tube restricting ligatures and intraluminal stents in non-valved devices is essential; great caution is recommended if a valved device is chosen and implanted without ligating the tubing, as choroidal effusions may be severe in the early postoperative period. Choroidal effusions may occur at higher-than-expected IOP in the presence of choroidal hemangioma, and it is advisable to omit glaucoma medications until review on the first postoperative day confirms the IOP. B-scan ultrasound examination is useful in monitoring for choroidal effusion.

Uveitis Surgical intervention in an eye with uveitis risks exacerbating inflammation which, in turn, may threaten the success of surgery. It is therefore desirable to optimize both systemic and

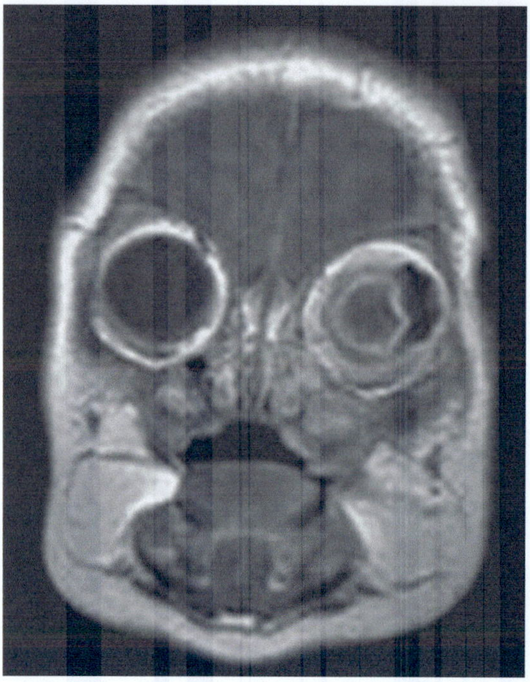

Fig. 7.7 Coronal reconstruction of an MRI performed on an infant with Sturge-Weber syndrome to evaluate central nervous system involvement in the disease. The scan was acquired 1 week after implantation of an Ahmed glaucoma valve in the superior temporal quadrant of the left eye. Note the lucent area representing the silicone implant, along with the annular choroidal effusion. The effusion had resolved by the next clinic visit and was never observed clinically. (Courtesy of James D. Brandt, MD)

topical immunosuppression before performing glaucoma surgery, and this may require collaboration with the pediatric rheumatologist. Complications of GDD surgery particularly related to poor control of intraocular inflammation include occlusion of the tube tip with fibrin, ciliary body shutdown, and hypotony. Hypotony is a risk in these eyes even in the absence of active inflammation as a consequence of poor ciliary function, and the risk is particularly high if the eye has previously undergone cyclodestructive procedures which are advised against in these eyes. Care should therefore be taken when performing GDD surgery to avoid over-drainage. For this reason, valved devices may be useful in these eyes, and if a non-valved device is preferred, the use of a restricting ligature and intraluminal stent is advisable. The choice of a small plate size in either a valved or non-valved device is also helpful.

Aniridia Aniridic eyes have limbal stem cell deficiency that leads to corneal conjunctivalization and opacity later in life. As previously mentioned, a limbal-based (limbus sparing) conjunctival technique is recommended, and the use of MMC is avoided in children with aniridia.

In addition, careful positioning of the tube in the AC is necessary to avoid it touching the lens, which is unprotected by the iris, as this results in cataract formation (Fig. 7.8). Tubes are commonly inserted into the eye in a radial or slightly oblique angle; however, a more aggressively tangential approach is used in cases of aniridia where it is desirable to avoid having the tube lying across the unprotected lens; a similar approach is sometimes taken in the setting of a corneal graft when it is desirable to have the tube lie beneath the host cornea rather than under the graft (Video 7.4).

The Role of Antimetabolites in GDD Surgery

Pediatric eyes frequently mount an exuberant healing response to the implantation of a foreign body such as a GDD; for this reason, some pediatric glaucoma surgeons advocate the use of antimetabolites at the time of surgery. Costa and colleagues performed a masked, randomized prospective clinical trial comparing the intraoperative use of MMC (0.5 mg/ml × 5 min] to BSS in adults older than 18 years of age undergoing AGV implantation (three of their subjects carried the diagnosis of "congenital glaucoma," but they were adults at the time of the study) [25]. They found no difference in short-term success at 1 year.

The role of antimetabolites in GDD success has yet to be established in the pediatric population. There are no prospective, randomized clinical trials comparing the intraoperative use of mitomycin C (MMC) in pediatric implants. Cui and colleagues performed a retrospective review of adjuvant treatment with antifibrotic agents during and after AGV implantation and reported

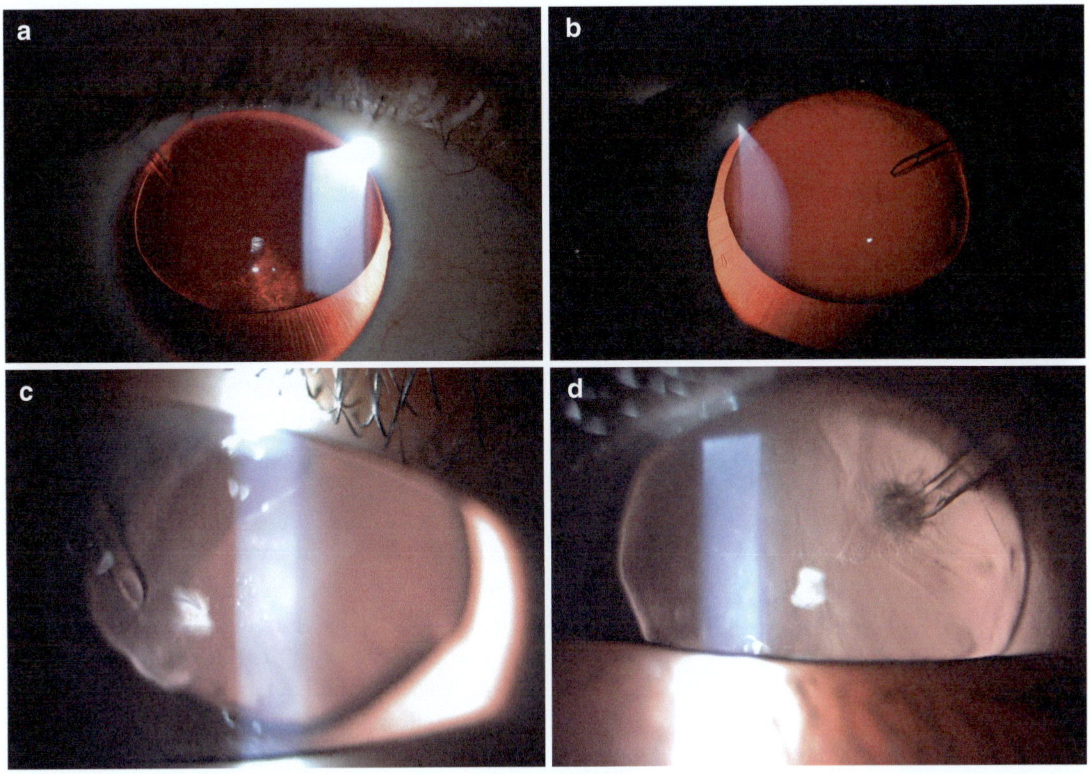

Fig. 7.8 (**a**, **b**) Bilateral glaucoma drainage devices placed at age 8 in a boy with glaucoma associated with aniridia. There is no tube-lens touch, but over the last 5 years, the lenses slowly dislocated upward, as shown, and developed early posterior subcapsular cataract with visual acuity in the 20/50 range bilaterally (patient does not have foveal agenesis). (**a**, **b** Courtesy of James D. Brandt, MD). (**c**) Tube of a Baerveldt glaucoma drainage device inserted at a tangent so that it lies near the equator of the lens (the thinnest portion of the lens) to avoid the tube touching the lens. (**d**) Tube of a Baerveldt glaucoma drainage device in an aniridic eye. The tube is inserted in a radial direction with the tip of the tube approaching the anterior pole of the lens (the thickest portion of the lens) resulting in the tube touching the lens and causing a localized opacity. (**c**, **d** Courtesy of Cecilia Fenerty, MD, FRCOphth)

decreased frequency of the hypertensive phase commonly observed with this device and improved surgical outcomes at 1 year [26]. A retrospective, nonrandomized study of AGV both with and without mitomycin C (MMC) in aphakic glaucoma showed no difference in IOP control between groups [27]. A larger retrospective study demonstrated worse outcomes after 2 years of follow-up in eyes receiving AGV plus MMC [28], though this may be due to differences in underlying diagnosis and previous number of surgical interventions between groups. A prospective randomized study looking at AGVs augmented with either Bevacizumab, MMC, or no MMC found higher success rate groups receiving both Bevacizumab and MMC at 1 year [29].

The bottom line is that the long-term safety and efficacy of the adjunctive use of antimetabolites in pediatric GDD surgery are not known. A surgical registry approach to capturing data on pediatric GDD surgery over many years may be the best way to determine the risk/benefit balance of antimetabolites in this population for whom long-term outcomes are so important.

Postoperative Management

Postoperative medication includes topical broad-spectrum antibiotic (e.g., chloramphenicol or fourth-generation fluoroquinolone), topical steroid (e.g., prednisolone acetate 1% or dexamethasone

0.1%), and often a topical cycloplegic (e.g., atropine 1% or cyclopentolate 1%). When a non-valved device has been implanted using an extraluminal tie and/or intraluminal stent, it may also be necessary to continue topical glaucoma medication until the extraluminal suture is absorbed and the tube opens. For those children with a valved tube, the device will function immediately, and often all the regular glaucoma medications can be stopped.

Pain relief is usually adequately managed with acetaminophen appropriately dosed by weight, with the addition of a systemic nonsteroidal anti-inflammatory drug if required.

Children are examined on the first postoperative day, and assessment should be directed to identify potential complications of surgery as detailed below. It is usually impossible to formally measure IOP in a young child on the first postoperative day, but if necessary the IOP may be estimated by gentle digital palpation over the closed lid. External examination will reveal any purulent discharge or bleeding, and ocular examination should aim to confirm the presence of a formed AC and clear red reflex. If necessary, a B-scan ultrasound examination can assist in assessment.

At 1 week after surgery, a more detailed exam is usually possible. In the presence of nonabsorbable sutures on the conjunctiva or cornea, antibiotic drops should be continued until they are removed. However, when absorbable sutures have been used for closure, antibiotics can be stopped within the first week or two postoperatively. The key issues during the first month or so after GDD surgery are infection surveillance, AC status, IOP, and tube positioning. If the IOP is very low, and the AC is very shallow or flat, reformation with viscoelastic in the operating room is urgently necessary to avoid corneal failure or cataract. B-scan ultrasound can help determine if choroidal effusions are present, and this can be done even in a crying infant in the clinic setting.

Topical cycloplegic, if used, may be stopped shortly after surgery if there is no hypotony and the AC remains deep. However, this medication may be temporarily reinstated around the time of opening of the extraluminal tie if there is a significant risk of hypotony. Topical steroid therapy should be tapered postoperatively according to the presence and grade of AC activity and external conjunctival hyperemia, usually over 1–2 months.

Management of valved versus non-valved GDDs diverges significantly in the postoperative period. In the case of a valved implant, preoperative glaucoma medications are usually discontinued to prevent hypotony. For those children who have had a non-valved device inserted utilizing an absorbable suture extraluminal tie, a critical time for review is around 6–7 weeks postoperatively when the tie usually spontaneously releases. In order to avoid hypotony at this time, it may be advisable to reduce or stop glaucoma medication a few days in advance. By this point, a fibrous capsule will have formed around the plate; this capsule offers resistance to outflow and thus avoids hypotony.

Further, EUA may be required to fully assess tube function and IOP control or for the removal of nonabsorbable sutures or the intraluminal stent. This should be planned at or beyond 6 weeks following surgery at which time any absorbable extraluminal tie will have spontaneously opened.

The "hypertensive phase" following GDD implantation is a widely recognized phenomenon, particularly with the Ahmed glaucoma valve [30], and is associated with high postoperative IOPs [31]. Approximately 4–6 weeks after implantation, the capsule forming around the AGV tends to thicken and offer more resistance to aqueous outflow. It is important to monitor for the onset of the hypertensive phase and if necessary reinstitute glaucoma medications at the earliest indication of a rise in IOP [32]. In a prospective study in adults, Pakravan and colleagues demonstrated that early aqueous suppression resulted in improved long-term IOP reduction and reduced the frequency of the hypertensive phase [33].

Complications

Although GDDs offer some benefits over other surgical procedures, they also carry the risk of significant complications. Complications which are particularly common or are unique to GDDs are described below.

Hypotony

Hypotony may be a serious and sight-threatening complication which may occur as an early, medium-term, or late complication of GDD surgery. It is often associated with a shallow or flat AC, maculopathy, choroidal effusion, serous retinal detachment, or suprachoroidal hemorrhage. Postoperative review should place an emphasis on assessing for the presence of hypotony and associated complications so that treatment can be initiated early. Further complications such as PAS, cataract, or phthisis may ensue if hypotony is not appropriately managed.

Buphthalmic eyes, which are large with little scleral rigidity, are particularly at risk of the complications of hypotony. Perioperatively, hypotony is avoided by the use of viscoelastic agents or AC infusion to maintain the AC. The use of appropriate-sized devices, small gauge needle entry, valved devices, and suture restriction of non-valved devices as described above reduces the risk of postoperative hypotony. In circumstances when hypotony occurs despite the above measures, assessment needs to be made as to whether this is due to over-drainage or under production of aqueous (ciliary body shutdown).

Over-drainage in the early postoperative period may occur due to:

- Leakage around the tube at the site of the scleral tunnel
- Failure of the valve mechanism in a valved device
- Lack of adequate restriction of a non-valved device
- Drainage via a different path, e.g., preexisting trabeculectomy exposed during GDD surgery, iatrogenic cyclodialysis cleft

Over-drainage may occur as a medium-term or late complication when a restricting ligature is released or an intraluminal stent removed in a non-valved device. Tube exposure (described below) may also result in leakage and over-drainage as a late complication. Management of clinically significant hypotony due to over-drainage will require surgical intervention to identify and remediate the underlying cause. The use of an AC infusion assists in identifying areas of aqueous leakage around the tube or through the tube when extraluminal restriction is not adequate. Suturing the tube tunnel on either side of the tube may stop leakage from this site; however, sometimes it is also helpful to use a small amount of Tenon capsule to plug the leak. Tubes which are draining because of inadequate restriction will require an additional tighter tie to be applied. In the extreme situation where these measures do not stop leakage, the tube is removed from the tunnel, which should be sutured closed. The surgeon should then decide whether to fashion a fresh tunnel or simply tuck the tube out of the way for later reinsertion, thus converting the surgery to the "two-stage" approach described at the beginning of the chapter.

Ciliary body shutdown as a primary cause of postoperative hypotony is most commonly encountered in eyes with glaucoma secondary to uveitis or in eyes that have previously undergone multiple ciliary ablations. Eyes which suffer a period of hypotony may additionally suffer ciliary body shutdown and aqueous hyposecretion as a consequence of ciliary body detachment with choroidal effusions. Primary ciliary body shutdown may require additional restriction or stenting of the tube to limit drainage while awaiting restoration of ciliary body function. In addition to aggressive management of any underlying inflammation, consideration should be given to artificially elevating the IOP by use of viscoelastic, BSS, gas (e.g., filtered air or 20% SF_6), or a combination of these into the AC.

Tube Occlusion

Tube occlusion may occur early or late in the postoperative period, and for this reason, it is important in siting the tube and trimming its length to ensure that the tip is directly visible. In eyes having undergone cataract surgery, occlusion may be related to capsular remnants, lens pearls, or vitreous as described elsewhere in this chapter. Fibrin may also occlude the tube from intraocular inflammation postoperatively or blood in the presence of a hyphema.

Rates of tube obstruction in different pediatric glaucomas with different drainage devices range from 6% to 20% [34–44]. Surgical removal of the obstruction is often required. The options depend on the underlying cause but may involve a combination of tube flushing, AC washout, vitrectomy, iridectomy, or removal of the valve mechanism in an AGV.

Patients with a late-onset vitreous incarceration present with sudden, marked IOP elevation after months or years of good IOP control. B-scan ultrasound reveals no bleb over the plate, indicating blockage of the tube. If the patient can cooperate, vitreous incarceration can be seen in the tube tip at the slit lamp or with a gonioscopy prism in a dilated eye. Vinod and colleagues [23) recommend a surgical approach in such patients. It is not sufficient to simply perform a vitrectomy; these tubes are usually blocked with a plug of condensed vitreous that must be removed with end-grasping retinal forceps (Fig. 7.9); if only a simple vitrectomy is performed, this now amputated plug will be free to travel up the tube and cause permanent failure. Once the vitreous plug and remaining mobile vitreous are cleared from the tube, full function of the GDD is usually restored, and IOP returns to pre-occlusion levels; B-scan ultrasound will reveal the presence of a filtering bleb over the equatorial plate, confirming flow through the system.

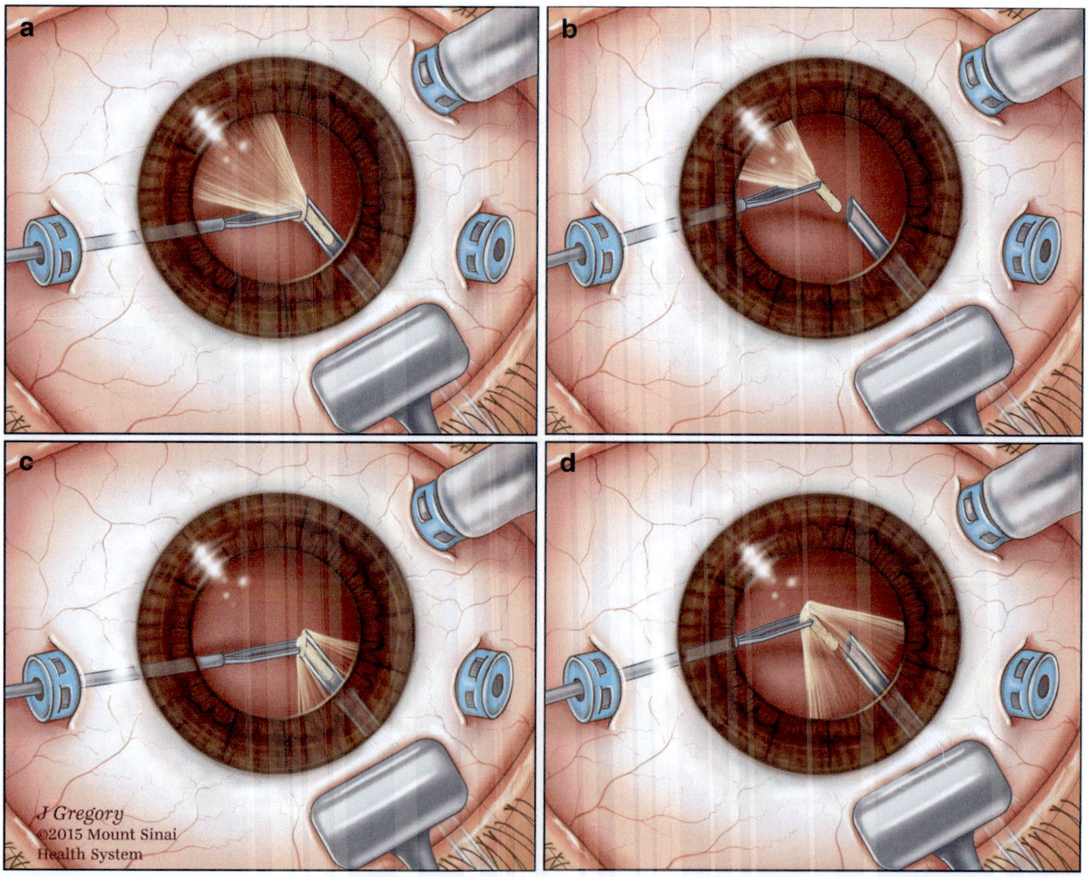

Fig. 7.9 Technique of pars plana vitrectomy to remove a vitreous plug occluding a tube as described by Vinod and colleagues. Note that a simple vitrectomy is insufficient – end-grasping forceps must be used to remove the condensed vitreous plug or the plug will be free to travel up the tube and cause permanent failure. (From Vinod et al. [30]. Illustration by Jill K. Gregory, CMI. Reprinted with permission from ©Mount Sinai Health System, New York NY, USA)

Tube Touch

Corneal touch and endothelial damage occurs when the tube is sited anteriorly in the AC and particularly if the intracameral portion of the tube is long. *Corneal opacification* occurs at the site of tube touch with endothelial damage resulting in *corneal edema* and *decompensation*. The tunnel for the tube should be constructed so that the tube enters the AC in front of and parallel to the iris. If the intracameral portion of the tube is too long, it may be observed at the slit lamp to sweep from side to side or forward and back when the patient blinks or when touching the eyelid on examination. In a young child, tube touch may be intermittent with eye rubbing, and a focal area of corneal edema near the tube tip seen at EUA may be the only clue that this is happening and may require shortening or repositioning of the tube.

Iris touch may occur if the tube is sited too far posteriorly in the AC. This may result in *chafing of the iris* with localized atrophy or *chronic uveitis*. This may also be associated with *corectopia,* particularly if the iris root is involved; corectopia on this basis is particularly common in eyes with Sturge-Weber syndrome (Fig. 7.10).

Lens touch results in cataract and may be a consequence of a tube which is too long, sited too far posteriorly, or in a radial rather than tangential direction.

The treatment of tube touch complications is ultimately surgical and is carried out by shortening and/or resiting the tube. In some cases of anterior segment tube-related complications, it is may be necessary to reposition the tube posteriorly through the pars plana [45].

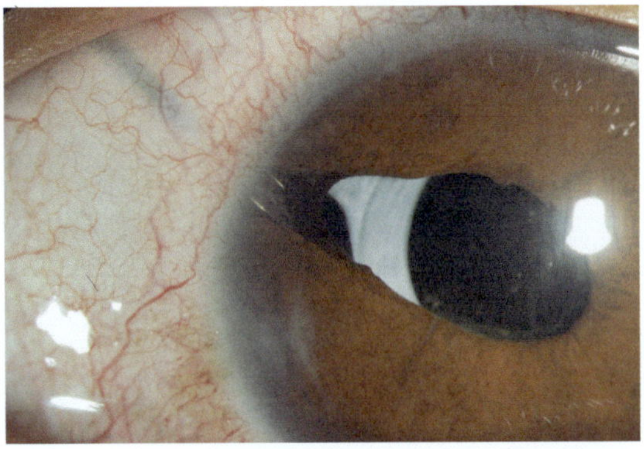

Fig. 7.10 Tube-related corectopia. Teenager with chronic uveitic glaucoma who underwent placement of an Ahmed Glaucoma Valve about 5 years earlier combined with phacoemulsification and injection of an Ozurdex™ dexamethasone implant (Allergan, Dublin, Ireland) who returns with maintained IOP control and good vision. Note the iris is dragged to the tube insertion. This may be avoided by performing a localized peripheral iridectomy and inserting the tube more posteriorly through the iridectomy so that the iris cannot adhere to the base of the tube. (Courtesy of James D. Brandt, MD)

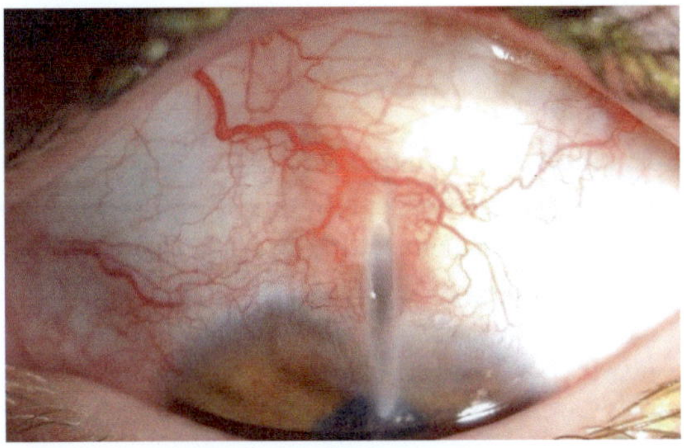

Fig. 7.11 Exposed tube. A teenage female with uveitis underwent Baerveldt tube surgery for secondary glaucoma. However, the tube tunnel was very superficial and anterior; note the long tunnel within the corneal stroma. Although the plate was sutured to the sclera, the tube was not sutured against the sclera (e.g., with a box suture) and as a consequence bowed anteriorly. Over time, the donor scleral patch graft overlying the tube melted away and the tube eroded through the conjunctiva, and the patient presented complaining of pain and discomfort. (Courtesy of Cecilia Fenerty MD, FRCOphth)

Erosion

Erosion of the GDD through the conjunctiva (Fig. 7.11) may result in infection *(endophthalmitis), leak, or hypotony*. Securing the plate and the tube with sutures as described above ensures the device does not sit raised over the underlying scleral plane with the overlying conjunctiva stretched over the device surface. The use of a patch graft cushions the conjunctiva from the ridge of the tube and the anterior plate and further reduces the risk of erosion. However, if the conjunctiva is under tension when replaced to cover the GDD (e.g., as a consequence of scarring from previous surgery or trauma), it is more likely to erode over the tube or plate.

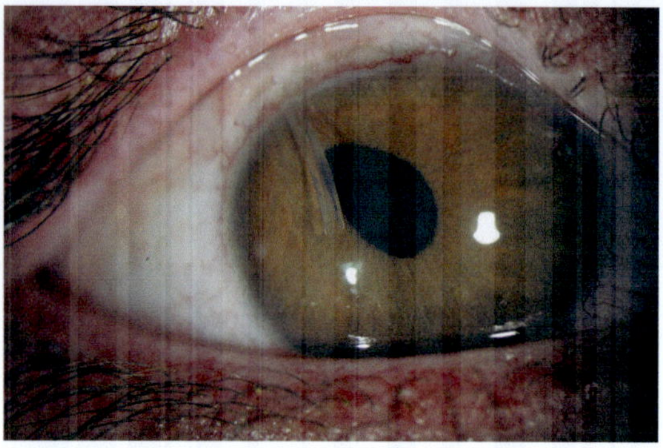

Fig. 7.12 Developmentally delayed teen with glaucoma associated with Sturge-Weber syndrome returned years later with a history of eye rubbing. IOP control was good and there was no erosion, but the plate had moved forward from its original position by about 3 mm so the tube was too long and risked causing corneal endothelial damage. The tube was everted through a small corneal incision 1 mm anterior to the limbus and shortened to about 2 mm in length. IOP control was maintained. Note that the pupil is drawn toward the tube entry point, a common late-term finding in eyes with Sturge-Weber syndrome. (Courtesy of James D. Brandt, MD)

Migration

Migration of the GDD may occur if the plate and tube are not securely sutured to the globe or the "wings" of a Baerveldt implant are placed above rather than behind the muscle insertions. As a consequence, the plate may end up advancing toward the limbus leading to "touch complications" or retracting toward the equator resulting in tube retraction out of the AC. With the device plate well secured, it is still possible for the tube to migrate out of the AC if it is not sutured securely to the sclera or with ocular growth (Fig. 7.12).

Changes in Intracameral Tube Length

Intracameral tube length may change with the IOP postoperatively. With a reduction in IOP, the dimensions of a child's eye may change with a reduction of the corneal diameter and the axial length. As a consequence, the intraocular portion of the tube may lengthen, and with that more "tube touch" complications are likely. Conversely, with elevated IOP following surgery, the corneal diameter and the axial length may increase, and the intraocular portion of the tube may retract from the anterior segment.

Ocular Motility Disturbances

Ocular motility disturbances may arise following GDD implantation, particularly when an eye has undergone prior strabismus surgery. Strabismus following GDD surgery should be managed by a surgeon familiar with both muscle surgery and pediatric GDD surgery, as these cases are very complex.

Outcomes

The World Glaucoma Association convened a Consensus Meeting on Childhood Glaucoma at its biennial global congress in 2013; the resulting monograph reported the results of a worldwide surgical consensus survey of glaucoma specialists and pediatric ophthalmologists with an interest in pediatric glaucoma surgery [46]. Almost half of experts (44%) preferred GDDs as the primary surgical procedure in glaucoma following cataract surgery (GFCS), with 30% preferentially using GDDs in uveitic glaucoma. Most stated they would use GDDs after failed trabeculectomy (82%) with the AGV being the most popular choice (63%) followed by the BGI (41%). Only 15% preferred to augment their surgery with adjunctive antimetabolites, and most preferred AC tube placement unless contraindicated.

Table 7.4 is a compilation of published studies on pediatric GDDs in the published literature from 1984 to 2017 which the reader may find useful [9, 12, 22, 35–44, 47–72].

The published success rates of GDDs in pediatric glaucoma vary widely between 54% and 90% [28, 40, 43, 73]. This is due largely to differences in the age of the child, underlying diagnosis, variation in surgical technique, and device employed as well as differences in the authors' definitions of success and failure. Despite these

Table 7.4 Published case series of glaucoma drainage devices in children, 1984–2017

	Study	Location(s)	Diagnosis	Implant	Eyes (*N*)	Mean follow-up (months)	1 year success (%)
1984	Molteno [47]	Otago (NZ)	Mixed	SP Molteno™	83	66	73
1988	Minckler [48]	Doheny Eye Institute (Los Angeles)	Mixed	SP Molteno™	13	22.8	54
1989	Billson [49]	Sydney	Mixed	DP Molteno	23	41.3	78
1991	Hill [35]	Doheny Eye Institute (Los Angeles)	Mixed	SP + DP Molteno	65	22.7	62
1991	Munoz [50]	KKESH (Riyadh)	Mixed	SP Molteno	53	18	68
1992	Lloyd [36]	Doheny Eye Institute (Los Angeles)	Mixed	SP Molteno	16	49.1	56
1992	Nesher [41]	Florida and Washington Univ.	Mixed	SP + DP Molteno	27	20	57
1993	Netland [51]	MEEI	Mixed	AGV + BGI	20	25	80
1995	Fellenbaum [37]	Doheny Eye Institute (Los Angeles)	Mixed	BGI	30	15	86
1995	Siegner [52]	MEEI and Univ California, Davis	Mixed	BGI	15	13.6	80
1997	Coleman [12]	UCLA	Mixed	AGV	21	16.3 ± 11.2	78
1997	Eid [38]	Wills Eye Institute (Philadelphia)	Mixed	Mixed	18	47.3	72
1997	Donahue [42]	Iowa	Mixed	BGI	23	19	61
1998	Cunliffe [53]	Otago (NZ)	Mixed	SP + DP Molteno	34	134.4	85
1999	Englert [39]	Duke University	Mixed	AGV	27	12.6 ± 8.2	85
1999	Hamush [54]	UCLA	Sturge-Weber	AGV	11	30.4 ± 19.1	79
1999	Huang [55]	Multiple	Mixed	AGV	11	13.4	91
2001	Djodeyre [43]	Madrid	Mixed	AGV	35	12.6	70
2002	Pereira [44]	Wills Eye Institute (Philadelphia)	Mixed	Mixed	10	50	80
2003	Morad [40]	Toronto	Mixed	AGV	60	24.3 ± 16	93
2004	Budenz [56]	Miami & Univ. of California, Davis	Mixed	BGI	62	23.4 ± 21.7	80
2004	Rodrigues [57]	Brazil	PCG	Susanna	24	24	88
2005	Chen [58]	MEEI	Mixed	AGV	52	26 ± 20	85
2005	Rolim De Moura [59]	Doheny Eye Institute (Los Angeles), Univ. of Southern California	Mixed	BGI	48	median 21 (4–95)	91
2005	Kafkala [60]	MEEI	Uveitic	AGV	7	36.8 (6–60)	69.9 IOP reduction rate
2006	Van Overdam [61]	Netherlands	Mixed	BGI	55	32 (2–78)	94

(continued)

Table 7.4 (continued)

	Study	Location(s)	Diagnosis	Implant	Eyes (*N*)	Mean follow-up (months)	1 year success (%)
2007	Autrata [62]	Czech Republic	Mixed	Molteno+ BGI	76	85 ± 78	91
2007	Souza [63]	UCLA	Mixed	AGV	78	61	80
2008	O'Malley Schotthoefer [22]	Duke Univ.	Mixed	AGV + BGI	70	66	92
2009	Sood [64]	Emory Univ.	Mixed	AGV + BGI	8	26.2 ± 9.5	75
2012	El Gendy [65]	USC	Mixed	BGI	20	46 ± 29	80
				AGV	11	33 ± 30	55
2014	Balekudaro [66]	India	Mixed	AGV	71	37.8 ± 32.1	97
2014	Razeghinejad [67]	Iran	PCG	AGV	33	32.6 ± 18.3	97
2014	Tai [68]	Univ. of Southern California	Mixed	BGI	45	??	87
2015	Chen [69]	UCLA	Mixed	AGV	119	73 ± 40	86
2015	Dave [70]	India	PCG	AGV	11	17.9 ± 9.3	91
2016	Mandalos [71]	United Kingdom	Mixed	Molteno+ BGI	69	45.7 ± 25.2	96
2017	Eksioglu [72]	Turkey	Uveitis	AGV	16	64.46 ± 33.56	56
2017	Vinod [9]	NYEEI	Mixed	PP BGI	37	78 ± 48.7	94.5

SP single plate, *DP* double plate, *AGV* Ahmed glaucoma valve, *BGI* Baerveldt® glaucoma implant, *PCG* primary congenital glaucoma, *KKESH* King Khaled Eye Specialist Hospital, *MEEI* Massachusetts Eye and Ear Infirmary, Boston, *NYEEI* New York Eye and Ear Infirmary limitations, a few general conclusions can be drawn. Firstly, although many studies report success rates around 80% after 1–2 years of follow-up [37, 74], longer-term studies consistently report a steady decline to ~50% success after 5 years of follow-up requiring reinstitution of medical therapy [22, 56, 59, 61, 73]. Secondly, while it is difficult to directly compare success rates between different GDDs, a number of studies have demonstrated equivalent results among devices [22, 51, 73, 75].

In most reported case series, GDDs have been reserved for use in refractory pediatric glaucoma of mixed etiology where other medical and surgical procedures have failed to optimally control IOP. Primary congenital glaucoma and secondary glaucoma particularly associated with aphakia form the bulk of cases analyzed. A small case series of GDDs in aniridia showed a success rate of up to 88% at 1 year [76]. The use of BGI [77] and AGV [54] in Sturge-Weber syndrome has also been shown to successfully improve IOP control in refractory cases, though meticulous hypotony prevention in the postoperative period is strongly advocated. A number of studies looking at surgical outcomes of GDDs in pediatric uveitic glaucoma have shown between 80% and 100% success rates up to 40 months of follow-up [60, 78, 79]. In these cases, however, GDDs of smaller surface areas were used to minimize the risk of hypotony. GDDs associated with corneal grafting procedures have demonstrated higher failure rates both in terms of IOP control and graft longevity [66], with higher complication rates particularly in simultaneous combined procedures [80]. Ideally, IOP should be controlled prior to considering corneal surgery. And while a pars plana approach may reduce corneal complications, it risks tube occlusion with vitreous.

While GDDs have demonstrated a high cumulative probability of long-term success, sight-threatening complications may occur at any stage postoperatively, requiring lifelong follow-up [71]. The most common complications relate either to hypotony or to the tube itself [28, 35, 37, 38, 43, 73, 81, 82].

Hypotony may occur at any stage during the early or late postoperative period, with the pediatric population at greater risk due to reduced scleral rigidity. The reported incidence of hypotony and flat AC varies, ranging from 0% to 25.7% in pediatric patients [12, 22, 34, 35, 37–41, 43, 50, 51, 73]. The results of different GDDs vary widely and are dependent on surgical technique and underlying diagnosis with underestimation also likely due to paucity of reliable IOP assessment in children. Early hypotony has been reported in AGVs to be as present in up to 7% of cases [66]. Rates of choroidal effusion range from 0% to 22% [12, 34, 35, 38–41, 43, 44, 53, 66, 73], while the most devastating complication of suprachoroidal hemorrhage has been documented to range from 0% to 13% [12, 34–38, 53, 73].

Tube-related complications are a heterogeneous group, encompassing erosion, occlusion, migration, iris or lens touch, and corneal decompensation related to corneal endothelial touch [73]. Interestingly, a recent retrospective comparative study of 69 pediatric eyes and 145 adult eyes found higher rates of corneal decompensating in the adult population occurring earlier in this group [83].

Tube migration and retraction may occur secondary to normalization or elevation of IOP, respectively, and tend to occur in younger patients with buphthalmic eyes. Rates of tube-cornea touch vary from 5.7% to 20% [37, 39, 40, 50, 73], with most identified cases requiring revision. Conversely, if tube retraction occurs, then a number of surgical options have been described including the use of a tube extender, a segment of 22-gauge intravenous catheter [84], or angiocatheter material [85].

Erosion of the tube or the scleral plate carries a significant risk of endophthalmitis and should be repaired immediately using a patch graft or where required explantation of the device in cases of plate erosion [74]. The reported incidence of erosion or extrusion of the tube or scleral plate ranges from 0% to 13% in pediatric patients [12, 34, 35, 37–44, 50, 51, 53, 56, 73]. Gedde and colleagues [86] noted that exposure of the tube was present in all cases of late-onset endophthalmitis associated with the BGI. Early and late postoperative endophthalmitis rates associated with GDDs in children have been reported between 0% and 5% [12, 34, 35, 37, 38, 40–43, 50, 51, 53, 56, 73].

Motility issues and strabismus should also be considered in children particularly where binocularity is present [22]. The incidence of this complication ranges from 0% to 11% in children with various devices [12, 34, 37, 38, 40, 43, 51, 56, 87]. Permanent motility disorders represent a late complication and may be due to mechanical restriction of the extraocular muscles secondary to adhesion or scarring or to a large bleb or episcleral plate.

Options After Failed Surgery

Elevated IOP after GDD insertion may be due to either tube obstruction at either the tube tip or in the valve mechanism or GDD failure due to bleb encapsulation. A number of treatment options are available once GDDs fail to control IOP effectively either through plate fibrosis, scarring, or bleb encapsulation. Recommencement of topical glaucoma medications is the usual first-line option. Failing this, of the pediatric glaucoma experts surveyed [46], 26% would proceed with cyclodestruction, 26% would revise the GDD (capsule excision with or without anti-scarring agent), and 23% would insert a second GDD. A nonrandomized chart review of 17 eyes suggests that secondary cyclodestruction versus secondary GDD has equivocal results at 2 years [64]. The amount of cyclodestructive treatment required to achieve the desired degree of IOP reduction may be difficult to titrate and may be associated with high rates of retinal detachment, phthisis bulbi, and other vision-threatening complications [74]. Shah et al. demonstrated that after failed GDD, an additional GDD offered better IOP control than revision by excision of an encapsulated bleb [88]. A further retrospective case series of 22 eyes did not demonstrate higher-than-expected rates of complications associated with GDDs [89]; however, both these studies were in an adult population.

Conclusion

Glaucoma drainage devices are increasingly useful in the management of childhood glaucoma. They can be used as a primary procedure in certain situations or as a secondary procedure where more conventional surgery (e.g., angle surgery) has been carried out and failed. We hope that this chapter has provided a comprehensive review of why, when, and how GDDs should be used in the treatment of childhood glaucoma.

The reader may be excused for coming away from this chapter with some pessimism, especially after the main conclusion above that these devices have a 50% failure rate at 5 years. We believe it is important to put this in perspective, however. The eyes in which GDDs are generally used are those same eyes that would have almost certainly gone blind prior to the introduction of these devices and are best implanted sooner than later to optimize long-term visual prognosis. The authors have patients who maintain useful and sometimes excellent vision many years (even decades) after implantation in early childhood. We encourage those caring for children with glaucoma to add the use of GDDs to their surgical portfolio. This recommendation is particularly important in resource-constrained settings now that low-cost GDDs are available worldwide. Successful GDD cases make all the hard work of managing these children among the most rewarding long-term aspect of childhood glaucoma care.

References

1. Barkan O. Operation for congenital glaucoma. Am J Ophthalmol. 1942;25(5):552–68.
2. Allen L, Burian HM. Trabeculotomy ab externo. A new glaucoma operation: technique and results of experimental surgery. Am J Ophthalmol. 1962;53:19–26.
3. Harms H, Dannheim R. Trabeculotomy 'ab externo'. Trans Ophthalmol Soc U K. 1970;89:589–90.
4. Minckler DS, Francis BA, Hodapp EA, Jampel HD, Lin SC, Samples JR, et al. Aqueous shunts in glaucoma: a report by the American Academy of ophthalmology. Ophthalmology. 2008;115(6):1089–98.
5. Britt MT, LaBree LD, Lloyd MA, Minckler DS, Heuer DK, Baerveldt G, et al. Randomized clinical trial of the 350-mm^2 versus the 500-mm^2 Baerveldt implant: longer term results: is bigger better? Ophthalmology. 1999;106(12):2312–8.

6. Gardiner BS, Smith DW, Coote M, Crowston JG. Computational Modeling of Fluid Flow and Intra-Ocular Pressure following Glaucoma Surgery PLoS ONE. 2010;5. (10) https://doi.org/:10.1371/journal.pone.0013178.
7. Molteno AC. New implant for drainage in glaucoma. Clinical trial. Br J Ophthalmol. 1969;53(9):606–15.
8. Molteno AC, Polkinghorne PJ, Bowbyes JA. The vicryl tie technique for inserting a draining implant in the treatment of secondary glaucoma. Aust N Z J Ophthalmol. 1986;14(4):343–54.
9. Vinod K, Panarelli JF, Gentile RC, Sidoti PA. Long-term outcomes and complications of pars Plana Baerveldt implantation in children. J Glaucoma. 2017;26(3):266–71.
10. Heuer DK, Lloyd MA, Abrams DA, Baerveldt G, Minckler DS, Lee MB, et al. Which is better? One or two? A randomized clinical trial of single-plate versus double-plate Molteno implantation for glaucomas in aphakia and pseudophakia. Ophthalmology. 1992;99(10):1512–9.
11. Coleman AL, Hill R, Wilson MR, Choplin N, Kotas-Neumann R, Tam M, et al. Initial clinical experience with the Ahmed Glaucoma valve implant. Am J Ophthalmol. 1995;120(1):23–31.
12. Coleman AL, Smyth RJ, Wilson MR, Tam M. Initial clinical experience with the Ahmed Glaucoma valve implant in pediatric patients. Arch Ophthalmol. 1997;115(2):186–91.
13. Kaushik S, Kataria P, Raj S, Pandav SS, Ram J. Safety and efficacy of a low-cost glaucoma drainage device for refractory childhood glaucoma. Br J Ophthalmol. 2017;101(12):1623–7.
14. Gedde SJ, Herndon LW, Brandt JD, Budenz DL, Feuer WJ, Schiffman JC, et al. Postoperative complications in the tube versus trabeculectomy (TVT) study during five years of follow-up. Am J Ophthalmol. 2012;153(5):804–14.
15. Gedde SJ, Schiffman JC, Feuer WJ, Herndon LW, Brandt JD, Budenz DL, et al. Treatment outcomes in the tube versus trabeculectomy (TVT) study after five years of follow-up. Am J Ophthalmol. 2012;153(5):789–803.
16. Swamynathan K, Capistrano AP, Cantor LB, WuDunn D. Effect of temporal corneal phacoemulsification on intraocular pressure in eyes with prior trabeculectomy with an antimetabolite. Ophthalmology. 2004;111(4):674–8.
17. Budenz DL, Barton K, Gedde SJ, Feuer WJ, Schiffman J, Costa VP, et al. Five-year treatment outcomes in the Ahmed Baerveldt comparison study. Ophthalmology. 2015;122(2):308–16.
18. Margeta MA, Kuo AN, Proia AD, Freedman SF. Staying away from the optic nerve: a formula for modifying glaucoma drainage device surgery in pediatric and other small eyes. J AAPOS. 2017;21(1):39–43.e1.
19. Suhr AW, Lim MC, Brandt JD, Izquierdo JC, Willits N. Outcomes of fornix-based versus limbus-based conjunctival incisions for glaucoma drainage device implant. J Glaucoma. 2012;21(8):523–9.
20. Cheng J, Abolhasani M, Beltran-Agullo L, Moss EB, Buys YM, Trope GE. Priming the Ahmed glaucoma valve: pressure required and effect of overpriming. J Glaucoma. 2015;24(4):e34–5.
21. Thakur S, Ichhpujani P, Kumar S. Grafts in glaucoma surgery: a review of the literature. Asia Pac J Ophthalmol (Phila). 2017;6:469–76.
22. O'Malley Schotthoefer E, Yanovitch TL, Freedman SF. Aqueous drainage device surgery in refractory pediatric glaucomas: I. Long-term outcomes. J AAPOS. 2008;12(1):33–9.
23. Vinod K, Panarelli JF, Gentile RC, Sidoti PA. Vitreous occlusion of a Glaucoma drainage implant-surgical management. J Glaucoma. 2017;26(7):669–72.
24. Tarantola RM, Agarwal A, Lu P, Joos KM. Long-term results of combined endoscope-assisted pars plana vitrectomy and glaucoma tube shunt surgery. Retina. 2011;31(2):275–83.
25. Costa VP, Azuara-Blanco A, Netland PA, Lesk MR, Arcieri ES. Efficacy and safety of adjunctive mitomycin C during Ahmed glaucoma valve implantation: a prospective randomized clinical trial. Ophthalmology. 2004;111(6):1071–6.
26. Cui QN, Hsia YC, Lin SC, Stamper RL, Rose-Nussbaumer J, Mehta N, et al. Effect of mitomycin c and 5-flurouracil adjuvant therapy on the outcomes of Ahmed glaucoma valve implantation. Clin Exp Ophthalmol. 2017;45(2):128–34.
27. Kirwan C, O'Keefe M, Lanigan B, Mahmood U. Ahmed valve drainage implant surgery in the management of paediatric aphakic glaucoma. Br J Ophthalmol. 2005;89:855–8.
28. Al-Mobarak F, Khan AO. Two-year survival of Ahmed valve implantation in the first 2 years of life with and without intraoperative mitomycin-C. Ophthalmology. 2009;116(10):1862–5.
29. Mahdy RA. Adjunctive use of bevacizumab versus mitomycin C with Ahmed valve implantation in treatment of pediatric glaucoma. J Glaucoma. 2011;20(7):458–63.
30. Nouri-Mahdavi K, Caprioli J. Evaluation of the hypertensive phase after insertion of the Ahmed Glaucoma valve. Am J Ophthalmol. 2003;136(6):1001–8.
31. Won HJ, Sung KR. Hypertensive phase following silicone plate Ahmed Glaucoma valve implantation. J Glaucoma. 2016;25(4):e313–7.
32. Law SK, Kornmann HL, Giaconi JA, Kwong A, Tran E, Caprioli J. Early aqueous suppressant therapy on hypertensive phase following Glaucoma drainage device procedure: a randomized prospective trial. J Glaucoma. 2016;25(3):248–57.
33. Pakravan M, Rad SS, Yazdani S, Ghahari E, Yaseri M. Effect of early treatment with aqueous suppressants on Ahmed glaucoma valve implantation outcomes. Ophthalmology. 2014;121(9):1693–8.
34. Hill R, Ohanesian R, Voskanyan L, Malayan A. The Armenian eye care project: surgical outcomes of

complicated paediatric glaucoma. Br J Ophthalmol. 2003;87(6):673–6.
35. Hill RA, Heuer DK, Baerveldt G, Minckler DS, Martone JF. Molteno implantation for glaucoma in young patients. Ophthalmology. 1991;98(7):1042–6.
36. Lloyd MA, Sedlak T, Heuer DK, Minckler DS, Baerveldt G, Lee MB, et al. Clinical experience with the single-plate Molteno implant in complicated glaucomas. Update of a pilot study. Ophthalmology. 1992;99(5):679–87.
37. Fellenbaum PS, Sidoti PA, Heuer DK, Minckler DS, Baerveldt G, Lee PP. Experience with the baerveldt implant in young patients with complicated glaucomas. J Glaucoma. 1995;4(2):91–7.
38. Eid TE, Katz LJ, Spaeth GL, Augsburger JJ. Long-term effects of tube-shunt procedures on management of refractory childhood glaucoma. Ophthalmology. 1997;104(6):1011–6.
39. Englert JA, Freedman SF, Cox TA. The Ahmed valve in refractory pediatric glaucoma. Am J Ophthalmol. 1999;127(1):34–42.
40. Morad Y, Donaldson CE, Kim YM, Abdolell M, Levin AV. The Ahmed drainage implant in the treatment of pediatric glaucoma. Am J Ophthalmol. 2003;135(6):821–9.
41. Nesher R, Sherwood MB, Kass MA, Hines JL, Kolker AE. Molteno implants in children. J Glaucoma. 1992;1(4):228–32.
42. Donahue SP, Keech RV, Munden P, Scott WE. Baerveldt implant surgery in the treatment of advanced childhood glaucoma. J AAPOS. 1997;1(1):41–5.
43. Djodeyre MR, Peralta Calvo J, Abelairas GJ. Clinical evaluation and risk factors of time to failure of Ahmed glaucoma valve implant in pediatric patients. Ophthalmology. 2001;108(3):614–20.
44. Pereira ML, Araujo SV, Wilson RP, Azuara-Blanco A, Moster MR, Schmidt CM. Aqueous shunts for intractable glaucoma in infants. Ophthalmic Surg Lasers. 2002;33(1):19–29.
45. Joos KM, Lavina AM, Tawansy KA, Agarwal A. Posterior repositioning of glaucoma implants for anterior segment complications. Ophthalmology. 2001;108(2):279–84.
46. Papadopoulos M, Edmunds B, Chiang M, Mandal A, Grajewski AL, Khaw PT. Glaucoma surgery in children. In: Weinreb RN, Grajewski A, Papadopoulos M, Grigg J, Freedman S, editors. Childhood glaucoma. WGA consensus series 9. Amsterdam: Kugler Publications; 2013. p. 95–134.
47. Molteno AC, Ancker E, Van Biljon G. Surgical technique for advanced juvenile glaucoma. Arch Ophthalmol. 1984;102(1):51–7.
48. Minckler DS, Heuer DK, Hasty B, Baerveldt G, Cutting RC, Barlow WE. Clinical experience with the single-plate Molteno implant in complicated glaucomas. Ophthalmology. 1988;95(9):1181–8.
49. Billson F, Thomas R, Aylward W. The use of two-stage Molteno implants in developmental glaucoma. J Pediatr Ophthalmol Strabismus. 1989;26(1):3–8.
50. Munoz M, Tomey KF, Traverso C, Day SH, Senft SH. Clinical experience with the Molteno implant in advanced infantile glaucoma. J Pediatr Ophthalmol Strabismus. 1991;28(2):68–72.
51. Netland PA, Walton DS. Glaucoma drainage implants in pediatric patients. Ophthalmic Surg. 1993;24(11):723–9.
52. Siegner SW, Netland PA, Urban RC Jr, Williams AS, Richards DW, Latina MA, et al. Clinical experience with the Baerveldt glaucoma drainage implant. Ophthalmology. 1995;102(9):1298–307.
53. Cunliffe IA, Molteno AC. Long-term follow-up of Molteno drains used in the treatment of glaucoma presenting in childhood. Eye (Lond). 1998;12(Pt 3a):379–85.
54. Hamush NG, Coleman AL, Wilson MR. Ahmed glaucoma valve implant for management of glaucoma in Sturge-weber syndrome. Am J Ophthalmol. 1999;128(6):758–60.
55. Huang MC, Netland PA, Coleman AL, Siegner SW, Moster MR, Hill RA. Intermediate-term clinical experience with the Ahmed glaucoma valve implant. Am J Ophthalmol. 1999;127(1):27–33.
56. Budenz DL, Gedde SJ, Brandt JD, Kira D, Feuer W, Larson E. Baerveldt glaucoma implant in the management of refractory childhood glaucomas. Ophthalmology. 2004;111(12):2204–10.
57. Rodrigues AM, Corpa MV, Mello PA, de Moura CR. Results of the Susanna implant in patients with refractory primary congenital glaucoma. J AAPOS. 2004;8(6):576–9.
58. Chen TC, Bhatia LS, Walton DS. Ahmed valve surgery for refractory pediatric glaucoma: a report of 52 eyes. J Pediatr Ophthalmol Strabismus. 2005;42(5):274–83. quiz 304-5
59. Rolim de Moura C, Fraser-Bell S, Stout A, Labree L, Nilfors M, Varma R. Experience with the baerveldt glaucoma implant in the management of pediatric glaucoma. Am J Ophthalmol. 2005;139(5):847–54.
60. Kafkala C, Hynes A, Choi J, Topalkara A, Foster CS. Ahmed valve implantation for uncontrolled pediatric uveitic glaucoma. J AAPOS. 2005;9(4):336–40.
61. van Overdam KA, de Faber JT, Lemij HG, de Waard PW. Baerveldt glaucoma implant in paediatric patients. Br J Ophthalmol. 2006;90(3):328–32.
62. Autrata R, Helmanova I, Oslejskova H, Vondracek P, Rehurek J. Glaucoma drainage implants in the treatment of refractory glaucoma in pediatric patients. Eur J Ophthalmol. 2007;17(6):928–37.
63. Souza C, Tran DH, Loman J, Law SK, Coleman AL, Caprioli J. Long-term outcomes of Ahmed glaucoma valve implantation in refractory glaucomas. Am J Ophthalmol. 2007;144(6):893–900.
64. Sood S, Beck AD. Cyclophotocoagulation versus sequential tube shunt as a secondary intervention following primary tube shunt failure in pediatric glaucoma. J AAPOS. 2009;13(4):379–83.
65. El Gendy NM, Song JC. Long term comparison between single stage Baerveldt and Ahmed glaucoma

implants in pediatric glaucoma. Saudi J Ophthalmol. 2012;26(3):323–6.
66. Balekudaru S, Vadalkar J, George R, Vijaya L. The use of Ahmed glaucoma valve in the management of pediatric glaucoma. J AAPOS. 2014;18(4):351–6.
67. Razeghinejad MR, Kaffashan S, Nowroozzadeh MH. Results of Ahmed glaucoma valve implantation in primary congenital glaucoma. J AAPOS. 2014;18(6):590–5.
68. Tai AX, Song JC. Surgical outcomes of Baerveldt implants in pediatric glaucoma patients. J AAPOS. 2014;18(6):550–3.
69. Chen A, Yu F, Law SK, Giaconi JA, Coleman AL, Caprioli J. Valved glaucoma drainage devices in pediatric glaucoma: retrospective long-term outcomes. JAMA Ophthalmol. 2015;133(9):1030–5.
70. Dave P, Senthil S, Choudhari N, Sekhar GC. Outcomes of Ahmed valve implant following a failed initial trabeculotomy and trabeculectomy in refractory primary congenital glaucoma. Middle East Afr J Ophthalmol. 2015;22(1):64–8.
71. Mandalos A, Tailor R, Parmar T, Sung V. The long-term outcomes of glaucoma drainage device in pediatric glaucoma. J Glaucoma. 2016;25(3):e189–95.
72. Eksioglu U, Yakin M, Sungur G, Satana B, Demirok G, Balta O, et al. Short- to long-term results of Ahmed glaucoma valve in the management of elevated intraocular pressure in patients with pediatric uveitis. Can J Ophthalmol. 2017;52(3):295–301.
73. Beck AD, Freedman S, Kammer J, Jin J. Aqueous shunt devices compared with trabeculectomy with mitomycin-C for children in the first two years of life. Am J Ophthalmol. 2003;136(6):994–1000.
74. Ishida K, Mandal AK, Netland PA. Glaucoma drainage implants in pediatric patients. Ophthalmol Clin N Am. 2005;18(3):431–42. vii
75. Tanimoto SA, Brandt JD. Options in pediatric glaucoma after angle surgery has failed. Curr Opin Ophthalmol. 2006;17(2):132–7.
76. Arroyave CP, Scott IU, Gedde SJ, Parrish RK, Feuer W. Use of glaucoma drainge devices in the managemnet of glaucoma associated with aniridia. Am J Ophthalmol. 2003;135(2):155–9.
77. Budenz DL, Sakamoto D, Eliezer R, Varma R, Heuer DK. Two-staged Baerveldt glaucoma implant for childhood glaucoma associated with Sturge-weber syndrome. Ophthalmology. 2000;107(11):2105–10.
78. Bohnsack BL, Freedman SF. Surgical outcomes in childhood uveitic glaucoma. Am J Ophthalmol. 2013;155(1):134–42.
79. Valimaki J, Airaksinen PJ, Tuulonen A. Molteno implantation for secondary glaucoma in juvenile rheumatoid arthritis. Arch Ophthalmol. 1997;115(10):1253–6.
80. Al-Torbak AA. Outcome of combined Ahmed glaucoma valve implant and penetrating keratoplasty in refractory congenital glaucoma with corneal opacity. Cornea. 2004;23(6):554–9.
81. Nassiri N, Nouri-Mahdavi K, Coleman AL. Ahmed glaucoma valve in children: a review. Saudi J Ophthalmol. 2011;25(4):317–27.
82. Al-Torbak AA, Al-Shahwan S, Al-Jadaan I, Al-Hommadi A, Edward DP. Endophthalmitis associated with the Ahmed glaucoma valve implant. Br J Ophthalmol. 2005;89(4):454–8.
83. Mandalos A, Sung V. Glaucoma drainage device surgery in children and adults: a comparative study of outcomes and complications. Graefes Arch Clin Exp Ophthalmol. 2017;255(5):1003–11.
84. Bansal A, Fenerty CH. Extension of retracted glaucoma drainage tube using a 22-gauge intravenous catheter in complex pediatric glaucoma. J Glaucoma. 2010;19(4):248–51.
85. Smith MF, Doyle JW. Results of another modality for extending glaucoma drainage tubes. J Glaucoma. 1999;8(5):310–4.
86. Gedde SJ, Scott IU, Tabandeh H, Luu KK, Budenz DL, Greenfield D, et al. Late endophthalmitis associated with glaucoma drainage implants. Ophthalmology. 2001;108(7):1323–7.
87. Christmann LM, Wilson ME. Motility disturbances after Molteno implants. J Pediatr Ophthalmol Strabismus. 1992;29(1):44–8.
88. Shah AA, WuDunn D, Cantor L. Shunt revision versus additional tube shunt implantation after failed tube shunt surgery in refractory glaucoma. Am J Ophthalmol. 2000;129(4):455–60.
89. Burgoyne JK, WuDunn D, Lakhani V, Cantor L. Outcomes of sequential tube shunts in complicated glaucoma. Ophthalmology. 2000;107(2):309–14.

Cyclodestruction

8

Ta Chen Peter Chang and Karen M. Joos

History

Cyclodestructive procedures are the only glaucoma procedures designed to reduce aqueous production and are generally reserved for cases in which the outflow-enhancing procedures have either failed or cannot be safely performed. The first cyclodestructive procedure, sclerocyclotomy with thermocautery, was described in 1929 by Fiore [1]. In the following six decades, the approach varied among diathermy, cryotherapy, photocoagulation, and cyclocoagulation using ultrasound (Table 8.1) [1–19]. Most were associated with high incidences of hypotony, phthisis, scleral necrosis, and uveitis [3, 20]. The risks of these complications decreased over time, as improved technologies and protocols were developed.

In general, the goal of cyclodestructive procedures is to achieve targeted destruction/inactivation of the inner, nonpigmented ciliary epithelium on the ciliary processes, which decreases the overall aqueous production and lowers the intraocular pressure (IOP). Treatment precision can be achieved with identification of anatomic landmarks and utilizing a modality that delivers energy with tissue specificity [21, 22]. The diode laser (wavelength of 810 nm) is absorbed to a greater degree by the melanin in the ciliary process compared to the surrounding tissues, whereas direct, endoscopic visualization of the ciliary body provides a more precise identification of anatomy compared to transscleral techniques, which rely on external landmarks to infer the location of the ciliary body [23]. Thus, endoscopic application of diode laser allows for the most targeted treatment of the ciliary processes, although it requires incisional surgery, and therefore is, in a sense, the most invasive approach. Laser delivery is commonly achieved in a continuous fashion, which results in both apoptosis and necrosis. Recent introduction of micropulse delivery, with bursts lasting 30 to 300 microseconds interrupted by longer (1700–2000 microseconds) intervals, may result in tissue apoptosis with less necrosis compared to continuous pulse delivery [21].

Of all modalities of cyclodestruction, those of cyclocryotherapy, transscleral cyclophotocoagulation, and endoscopic cyclophotocoagulation have been reported in the pediatric population [14, 17, 24–26, 28, 29, 31, 32, 34],

Electronic Supplementary Material The online version of this chapter (https://doi.org/10.1007/978-3-319-54003-0_8) contains supplementary material, which is available to authorized users.

T. C. P. Chang (✉)
Bascom Palemr Eye Institute, University of Miami Miller School of Medicine, Miami, FL, USA
e-mail: t.chang@med.miami.edu

K. M. Joos
Vanderbilt Eye Institute, Vanderbilt Univeristy Medical Center, Nashville, TN, USA

A. L. Grajewski et al. (eds.), *Surgical Management of Childhood Glaucoma*,
https://doi.org/10.1007/978-3-319-54003-0_8

Table 8.1 History of human cyclodestructive techniques

Date	Medium	Techniques	Application	Population	References
1929	Electrode	Sclerocyclotomy with thermocautery	Ab externo, contact	Adult	Fiore [1]
1933	Electrode	Diathermy	Ab externo, contact	Adult	Weve [2]
1950	Dry ice	Cryotherapy	Ab externo, contact	Adult	Bietti [3]
1961	Polychromatic xenon light	Photocoagulation	Ab externo, contact	Adult	Weekers et al. [4]
1972	Pulsed ruby laser	Photocoagulation	Ab externo, contact	Adult	Beckman et al. [5]
1973	Nitrous oxide gas	Cryotherapy	Ab externo, contact	Adult	Bellows and Grant [6]
1973	Neodymium-doped glass laser	Photocoagulation	Ab externo, contact	Adult	Beckman and Sugar [7]
1981	Xenon arc	Photocoagulation	Ab interno	Adult	Charles [8]
1985	Ultrasound	Other coagulation	Ab externo, contact	Adult	Coleman et al. [9]
1986	Argon laser	Photocoagulation	Ab interno	Adult	Patel et al. [10]
1989	Nd/YAG laser	Photocoagulation	Ab externo, contact	Adult	Shields et al. [11]
1990	Nd/YAG laser	Photocoagulation	Ab externo, noncontact	Adult	Hampton et al. [12]
1990	Nitrous oxide gas	Cryotherapy	Ab externo contact	Pediatric	al-Faran et al. [13]
1991	Nd/YAG laser	Photocoagulation	Ab externo, contact	Pediatric	Phelan and Higginbotham [14]
1992	Diode laser	Photocoagulation	Ab externo, contact	Adult	Hennis and Stewart [15]
1992	Diode laser	Photocoagulation	Ab interno, endoscopic	Adult	Uram [16]
1997	Diode laser	Photocoagulation	Ab externo, contact	Pediatric	Bock et al. [17]
1999	Diode laser	Photocoagulation	Ab interno, endoscopic	Pediatric	Plager and Neely [18]
2010	Micropulse diode laser	Photocoagulation	Ab externo, contact	Adult	Tan et al. [19]

Nd:YAG neodymium-doped yttrium aluminum garnet crystal

with cyclocryotherapy now rarely used with the widespread availability of cyclophotocoagulation [27]. A limited series of nine pediatric patients treated with the external micropulse diode laser reported initial IOP lowering, but reoperation was required in seven (78%) patients during the first year of follow-up [35].The remainder of this chapter will focus on ab externo and ab interno, continuous pulse delivery of cyclophotocoagulation.

Indications

In eyes with uncontrolled glaucoma where additional incisional surgery is thought to be unfeasible or unsafe, transscleral cyclophotocoagulation (TSCPC) is considered. Usually, the risk of complications should be justified with the potential benefit of preserving vision, although the level of visual function may not be easily tested in younger children. TSCPC can also be considered following inadequately functioning glaucoma drainage device (GDD) surgery on maximum medical treatment. In pseudophakic or aphakic eyes with uncontrolled or borderline-controlled glaucoma scheduled for another intraocular surgery, such as vitrectomy and membranectomy to clear an opacified visual axis, endoscopic cyclophotocoagulation (ECP) can be performed concurrently for additional pressure control.

Contraindications

Cyclodestructive procedures have low success rate in eyes with uveitis [28]. In eyes with scleral thinning, TSCPC is relatively contraindicated for concerns of anterior scleral staphyloma formation and perforation [29]. It should be avoided in children with pigmentation of the sclera (e.g., nevus of Ota), which can preferentially absorb the energy and cause conjunctival and scleral burns. ECP is usually preferred over TSCPC in eyes with abnormal anatomy, where the position of the ciliary processes cannot be determined accurately by external landmarks. Both TSCPC and ECP are usually performed under general anesthesia in a pediatric patient and would be contraindicated in children who are too ill for general anesthesia. The incidence of sympathetic ophthalmia (SO) in adults following TSCPC is estimated to be one in approximately 1500 [30], and pediatric cases have been reported [31, 32]. While it is not known if children are more susceptible to SO than adults, even a low risk of SO may be deemed unacceptable. Cyclodestruction is avoided in eyes with no light perception.

Risk Factors for Failure

Failure of cyclodestructive procedures is usually defined by inadequate IOP control, or sight-threatening complications, which may include chronic hypotony, cataract formation, post-laser inflammation, and choroidal and retinal detachment. Eyes with multiple prior incisional surgeries and/or prior cyclodestruction are at a higher risk of all complications [28–33].

Advantages and Disadvantages

The advantages and disadvantages of both TSCPC and ECP are outlined in Table 8.2.

Table 8.2 Advantages and disadvantages of cyclophotocoagulation techniques as compared to conventional glaucoma procedures

Advantages	Disadvantages
Short surgical time	Unpredictable response
Technically easy to perform	May require multiple treatment sessions
Prompt convalescence with fewer days of school missed	Ongoing medical treatment may be necessary
Fewer postoperative TSCPC precautions compared to incisional surgeries	Risk of sympathetic ophthalmia
ECP allows more targeted treatment	Increased risk of hypotony if subsequent incisional surgery were performed

TSCPC transscleral cyclophotocoagulation, *ECP* endoscopic cyclophotocoagulation

Preoperative Considerations and Preparation

When obtaining informed consent, it is useful to inform parents that in order to avoid hypotony and vision loss, treatment may be titrated over multiple sessions. This sets a reasonable expectation in case IOP is not sufficiently lowered after one session. Furthermore, parents must be advised that topical medical treatment may still be necessary after diode. The risks of postoperative vision loss from all causes and sympathetic ophthalmia are emphasized.

A list of instruments/devices is provided in Table 8.3.

Table 8.3 A list of instruments and devices needed to perform transscleral cyclophotocoagulation and endoscopic cyclophotocoagulation

Transscleral cyclophotocoagulation
Lid speculum
Semiconductor diode laser (Iris Medical Instruments, Mountain View, CA, USA)
G-probe (Iris Medical Instruments) or Ciliprobe (Katalyst Surgical, Chesterfield, MO, USA)
Fine-toothed forceps or squint hook
Transilluminator or ultrasound (for cases with difficult landmarks)
Optional IV ketorolac
Optional bupivacaine 0.25% (for subconjunctival injection)
Optional steroid (for subconjunctival injection, e.g., triamcinolone acetonide, betamethasone)
Prednisolone 1% (topical)
Atropine 1% (topical)
Endoscopic cyclophotocoagulation
Lid speculum
Microkeratome
Viscoelastic (for intraocular administration) or an AC maintainer
Mechanical vitrector (if pars plana approach and eye not fully vitrectomized)
Semiconductor diode laser (Endo Optiks, Little Silver, NJ, USA)
Endoscopic probe (Endo Optiks) – 20 or 23 gauge, straight or curved
Display monitor
Needle holder
Tying forceps
Fine-toothed forceps
Optional bupivacaine 0.25% (for subconjunctival injection)
Optional steroid (for subconjunctival injection, e.g., triamcinolone acetonide, betamethasone)
Prednisolone 1% (topical)
Atropine 1% (topical)

AC anterior chamber

Operation

Intraop Preparation General anesthesia is induced. A sterile preparation is not necessary for TSCPC, but mandatory and routine for ECP, whether or not it is combined with other intraocular procedures.

Surgical Technique For TSCPC, a speculum is introduced. A pair of fine-toothed forceps or squint hook can be used to stabilize and manipulate the eye. The footplate of the G-probe is applied to the limbus as specified by the manufacturer. However, transillumination to accurately identify the ciliary body is necessary in buphthalmic and anatomically abnormal eyes with the footplate adjusted as needed to treat the ciliary body. (Fig. 8.1) Initial settings are surgeon dependent. Consider 1100–1750 mW at 2-s duration (or 1250 mW at 4-s duration) for older children, while a power setting of 800–900 mW at 2-s duration may be appropriate for an infant. During the initial application, if a popping sound is heard (a marker of excessive tissue disruption), the power is adjusted downward at 50 mW or 100 msec increments until the sound is no longer heard or is barely audible. A reasonable initial treatment dose would be 18–30 laser spots dependent upon the energy levels over 270° (while avoiding areas of pre-existing glaucoma implants, scleral thinning, and long ciliary nerves at the 3- and 9-o'clock meridians). The treatment dose is titrated up or down based on the surgeon's experience, the preoperative IOP, and the patient's surgical history (Video 8.1).

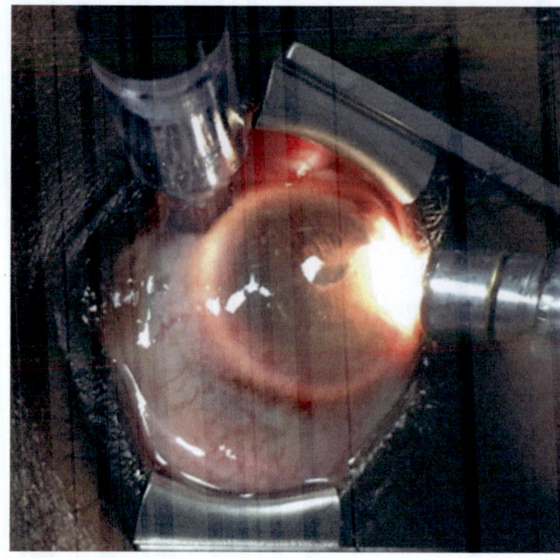

Fig. 8.1 Transillumination of a buphthalmic eye to identify the ciliary body. (Courtesy of Maria Papadopoulos, MBBS, FRCOphth)

ECP is essentially exclusively appropriate for aphakic or pseudophakic eyes, due to the difficulty reaching the target ciliary processes safely without injuring the native lens. After completion of the accompanying intraocular procedure, the pupils are pharmacologically dilated with intracameral administration of epinephrine. For pars plana approach, mechanical anterior vitrectomy is recommended to avoid traction on the vitreous base while performing the procedure. The endoscopic probe is made available, and the focus and orientation adjusted according to the manufacturer's instructions. The monitor is positioned within the surgeon's line of sight. The ciliary sulcus is inflated with viscoelastic or an anterior chamber (AC) maintainer is used. Under direct microscopic visualization, a 20- or 23-gauge endoscopic probe is introduced into the eye via a limbal (or pars plana) incision and advanced to the posterior chamber, with the tip of the probe positioned posterior to the contralateral iris border. The surgeon's attention is then turned to the monitor. The distance from the ciliary body is adjusted such that about four to five ciliary processes are visible on the screen at any given time. Too much distance will lead to insufficient photocoagulation, while too little distance will lead to excessive tissue disruption. With an initial power setting of 200 mW and continuous wave application, laser is applied to the ciliary processes until shrinkage and whitening occur without rupture of ciliary processes or bubble formation (Video 8.2). The power is adjusted up or down as needed for effective photocoagulation. A reasonable initial treatment dose would be one continuous coat of laser applied over 120–180°, titrated up or down based on the surgeon's experience, the target IOP, and the patient's surgical history. The viscoelastic is thoroughly irrigated from the eye, followed by meticulous closure of all incisions.

Intraoperatively, various strategies can be employed to minimize postoperative inflammation with steroids given intravenously or via the sub-Tenon or intraocular route. Sub-Tenon or peribulbar bupivacaine injections are useful for control of postoperative pain. Acetaminophen as directed on the bottle for a few days generally provides adequate pain relief.

Potential Modifications As previously mentioned, when performing TSCPC in buphthalmic eyes or in eyes where the limbus cannot be clearly identified, transillumination with a Finnoff illuminator or comparable light source should be performed through the pupil. The junction of light and dark areas denotes the scleral spur and the anterior attachment of uvea. In ECP, a second incision can be created in order to access and apply laser to a larger extent of ciliary processes; in some cases, the irrigation and laser ports can be exchanged if placed at least several clock hours apart from one another. In microphthalmic eyes, consider using lower total energy and number of burns.

Postoperative Management

The patient is evaluated on the first postoperative day to rule out any immediate intraocular complications and/or acute IOP spikes and again approximately 5–7 days later. Topical atropine (once to twice daily) and prednisolone or dexamethasone (four to six times daily) are used for 2 weeks, followed by cessation of atropine and tapering of prednisolone. Preoperative glaucoma medications are resumed as needed depending on the target and outcome IOP or continued and withdrawn if possible. The patient is examined again in 3–4 weeks, after discontinuation of steroid medications. In uncooperative pediatric patients, echography is used to rule out posterior pole complications due to hypotony or inflammation, and a repeat examination under anesthesia is scheduled at the surgeon's discretion to obtain new baseline optic nerve and biometric examinations. Repeat laser application is usually delayed at least 8 weeks to allow for resolution of inflammation, discontinuation of postoperative topical steroid, and a more accurate assessment of the results of the initial procedure on the eye's IOP.

Complications

The risks of chronic hypotony (including phthisis), cataract formation, visual loss, and choroidal and retinal detachment may be decreased with judicious laser dosing, while the risk of severe postoperative inflammation may be minimized with intraoperative administration of systemic dexamethasone, intraocular or sub-Tenon steroid (e.g., triamcinolone), and postoperative topical steroids. In one series, the risk of chronic hypotony following TSCPC was 10% over an average of 30 months, with number of treatment spots being the only statistically significant difference (54 vs 41 spots in hypotonous vs no hypotonous groups) [30].

To avoid marked thinning of the sclera in TSCPC, attempt to apply the laser only in areas with sclera of reasonably normal thickness as shown by transillumination and consider other glaucoma procedures rather than only multiple TSCPC procedures.

The incidence of sympathetic ophthalmia (SO) in children following cyclophotocoagulation is unknown. A recent review of published diode cases estimated the incidence of SO to be around 1 in 1500 or 0.07% [30].

Outcomes

In refractory childhood glaucoma (primary or secondary), success rate is approximately 62–66% with one treatment, and 72–70% with multiple treatments, where success is defined as IOP < 21 mmHg or a reduction of 30% from pretreatment baseline [23, 24]. Approximately 10% of patients had decreased vision and/or significant postoperative inflammation, and 4–6% had choroidal or retinal detachment [23, 24].

In a retrospective comparative series comprised of most secondary childhood glaucomas, TSCPC and ECP had similar efficacy, and approximately 46% of eyes were considered treatment successes, defined as IOP less than 21 mmHg at the most recent follow-up appointment, approximately 5 years following the procedure(s) [34]. Mean time to failure for TSCPC and ECP was approximately 1.7 and 1.0 years, respectively. In the subgroup who received TSCPC and ECP as initial glaucoma surgical therapy, 21% of TSCPC eyes and 45% of ECP eyes required subsequent incisional glaucoma surgery. Over 5 years, 23.4% (29/124) eyes lost vision, 5 eyes progressed to no light perception after complications from a corneal graft and retinal detachment, and 3 after GDD surgery [34].

Options After Failed Cyclophotocoagulation

The options after failed cyclophotocoagulation include:

- In eyes where additional incisional surgery is thought to be unfeasible or unsafe, repeat cyclophotocoagulation months to years later including any quadrant not previously treated.
- In eyes that have failed GDD surgery and diode, place a second GDD.
- In pseudophakic or aphakic eyes that have failed ECP combined with other surgery, consider GDD surgery.

Acknowledgment The authors thank Dr. Anna Junk (Bascom Palmer Eye Institute, Miami Veterans Affairs Healthcare System, Miami FL, USA) for sharing her intraoperative video of endocyclophotocogulation.

References

1. Fiore T. Cura radicale del glaucoma con la sclerociliarotomiaignea. Ann Ottal. 1929;57:820–57. [Article in Italian]
2. Weve H. Die Zyklodiatermie das Corpus Ciliare bei Glaukom. Zentralbl Ophthalmol. 1933;29:562–9. [Article in German]
3. Bietti G. Surgical intervention of the ciliary body. JAMA. 1950;142(12):889–97.
4. Weekers R, Lavergne G, Watillon M, Gilson M, Legros AM. Effects of photocoagulation of ciliary body upon ocular tension. Am J Ophthalmol. 1961;52:156–63.
5. Beckman H, Kinoshita A, Rota AN, Sugar HS. Transscleral ruby laser irradiation of the ciliary body in the treatment of intractable glaucoma. Trans Am Acad Ophthalmol Otolaryngol. 1972;76(2):423–36.
6. Bellows AR, Grant WM. Cyclocryotherapy in advanced inadequately controlled glaucoma. Am J Ophthalmol. 1973;75(4):679–84.
7. Beckman H, Sugar HS. Neodymium laser cyclophotocoagulation. Arch Ophthalmol. 1972;90:27–8.
8. Charles S. Endophotocoagulation. Retina. 1981;1(2):117–20.
9. Coleman DJ, Lizzi FL, Driller J, Rosado AL, Burgess SE, Torpey JH, et al. Therapeutic ultrasound in the treatment of glaucoma. II. Clinical applications. Ophthalmology. 1985;92(3):347–53.
10. Patel A, Thompson JT, Michels RG, Quigley HA. Endolaser treatment of the ciliary body for uncontrolled glaucoma. Ophthalmology. 1986;93(6):825–35.
11. Shields MB, Blasini M, Simmons R, Erickson PJ. A contact lens for transscleral Nd:YAG cyclophotocoagulation. Am J Ophthalmol. 1989;108(4):457–8.
12. Hampton C, Shields MB, Miller KN, Blasini M. Evaluation of a protocol for transscleral neodymium:YAG cyclophotocoagulation in one hundred patients. Ophthalmology. 1990;97(7):910–7.
13. al Faran MF, Tomey KF, al Mutlaq FA. Cyclocryotherapy in selected cases of congenital glaucoma. Ophthalmic Surg. 1990;21(11):794–8.
14. Phelan MJ, Higginbotham EJ. Contact transscleral Nd:YAG laser cyclophotocoagulation for the treatment of refractory pediatric glaucoma. Ophthalmic Surg Lasers. 1995;26(5):401–3.
15. Hennis HL, Stewart WC. Semiconductor diode laser transscleral cyclophotocoagulation in patients with glaucoma. Am J Ophthalmol. 1992;113(1):81–5.
16. Uram M. Ophthalmic laser microendoscope ciliary process ablation in the management of neovascular glaucoma. Ophthalmology. 1992;99(12):1823–8.
17. Bock CJ, Freedman SF, Buckley EG, Shields MB. Transscleral diode laser cyclophotocoagulation for refractory pediatric glaucomas. J Pediatr Ophthalmol Strabismus. 1997;34(4):235–9.
18. Plager DA, Neely DE. Intermediate-term results of endoscopic diode laser cyclophotocoagulation for pediatric glaucoma. J AAPOS. 1999;3(3):131–7.
19. Tan AM, Chockalingam M, Aquino MC, Lim ZI, See JL, Chew PT. Micropulse transscleral diode laser cyclophotocoagulation in the treatment of refractory glaucoma. Clin Exp Ophthalmol. 2010;38(3):266–72.
20. Krupin T, Mitchell KB, Becker B. Cyclocryotherapy in neovascular glaucoma. Am J Ophthalmol. 1978;86(1):24–6.
21. Amoozgar B, Phan EN, Lin SC, Han Y. Update on ciliary body laser procedures. Curr Opin Ophthalmol. 2017;28(2):181–6.

22. Chen TC, Chen PP, Francis BA, Junk AK, Smith SD, Singh K, Lin SC. Pediatric glaucoma surgery: a report by the American Academy of ophthalmology. Ophthalmology. 2014;121(11):2107–15.
23. Pastor SA, Singh K, Lee DA, Juzych MS, Lin SC, Netland PA, Nguyen NT. Cyclophotocoagulation: a report by the American Academy of ophthalmology. Ophthalmology. 2001;108(11):2130–8.
24. Autrata R, Rehurek J. Long-term results of trans-scleral cyclophotocoagulation in refractory pediatric glaucoma patients. Ophthalmologica. 2003;217(6):393–400.
25. Kirwan JF, Shah P, Khaw PT. Diode laser cyclophotocoagulation: role in the management of refractory pediatric glaucomas. Ophthalmology. 2002;109(2):316–23.
26. Carter BC, Plager DA, Neely DE, Sprunger DT, Sondhi N, Roberts GJ. Endoscopic diode laser cyclophotocoagulation in the management of aphakic and pseudophakic glaucoma in children. J AAPOS. 2007;11(1):34–40.
27. Vinod K, Gedde SJ, Feuer WJ, Panarelli JF, Chang TC, Chen PP, Parrish RK 2nd. Practice preferences for Glaucoma surgery: a survey of the American Glaucoma Society. J Glaucoma. 2017;26(8):687–93.
28. Heinz C, Koch JM, Heiligenhaus A. Transscleral diode laser cyclophotocoagulation as primary surgical treatment for secondary glaucoma in juvenile idiopathic arthritis: high failure rate after short term follow up. Br J Ophthalmol. 2006;90(6):737–40.
29. Sabri K, Vernon SA. Scleral perforation following trans-scleral cyclodiode. Br J Ophthalmol. 1999 Apr;83(4):502–3.
30. Aujla JS, Lee GA, Vincent SJ, Thomas R. Incidence of hypotony and sympathetic ophthalmia following trans-scleral cyclophotocoagulation for glaucoma and a report of risk factors. Clin Exp Ophthalmol. 2013;41(8):761–72.
31. Roberts MA, Rajkumar V, Morgan G, Laws D. Sympathetic ophthalmia secondary to cyclodiode laser in a 10-year-old boy. J AAPOS. 2009;13(3):299–300.
32. Jonas JB, Back W, Sauder G, Jünemann U, Harder B, Spandau UH. Sympathetic ophthalmia in vater association combined with persisting hyperplastic primary vitreous after cyclodestructive procedure. Eur J Ophthalmol. 2006;16(1):171–2.
33. Albahlal A, Al Dhibi H, Al Shahwan S, Khandekar R, Edward DP. Sympathetic ophthalmia following diode laser cyclophotocoagulation. Br J Ophthalmol. 2014;98(8):1101–6.
34. Kraus CL, Tychsen L, Lueder GT, Culican SM. Comparison of the effectiveness and safety of transscleral cyclophotocoagulation and endoscopic cyclophotocoagulation in pediatric glaucoma. J Pediatr Ophthalmol Strabismus. 2014;51(2):120–7.
35. Lee JH, Shi Y, Amoozgar B, Aderman C, De Alba Campomanes A, Lin S, Han Y. Outcome of micropulse laser transscleral cyclophotocoagulation on pediatric versus adult glaucoma patients. J Glaucoma. 2017;26(10):936–9.

9 Other Procedures for Pediatric Glaucoma Surgery: New Devices and Techniques

Elena Bitrian and Alana L. Grajewski

Introduction

In recent years, there have been multiple new devices developed in glaucoma surgery that target the angle and can be grouped in the category of minimally invasive glaucoma surgeries (MIGS). These procedures were mainly developed for adult glaucoma surgery, but by the very fact that they are variations on angle surgery, many may have application in pediatric glaucoma patients. With that being said, it should be noted that information regarding outcomes is limited for many of these devices in adults and even more so in children. Given the paucity of data regarding risk and/or benefit of these procedures in children, one should make the clinical decision for use of these newer techniques on an individual basis.

When considering new and novel techniques, it is always best to look back at the principal foundations that led to these innovations. The origin of pediatric glaucoma surgery dates back to 1938 with Barkan describing his goniotomy technique [1]. While classical angle surgery still continues to be a first-line treatment in primary congenital glaucoma (PCG) [2, 3], in recent years modifications in this technique and new devices have been developed. If the first angle surgery is not successful and the angle has not been treated 360°, many surgeons will further treat the angle before performing a filtering procedure (trabeculectomy) or glaucoma drainage device (GDD) [4]. Several instruments and techniques have been developed to extend the area of angle treated and/or to remove the trabecular meshwork (TM) from the eye or dilate Schlemm's canal.

This chapter presents these new surgical techniques and devices that target the angle via an ab interno approach. The following will be discussed: trabeculotomy with TRAB™360, viscodilation with VISCO™360, combined trabeculotomy and viscodilation with the OMNI™, gonioscopic-assisted transluminal trabeculotomy (GATT) with fiber optic or suture, and TM destruction and removal with Trabectome/Goniotome and the Kahook dual blade®. These devices share indications, complications, advantages, and limitations. We also introduce an ophthalmic surgery model eye (Bioniko, Miami, FL, USA) that can be used to teach angle surgery in a safe environment.

In PCG, the inhibited posterior sliding of the ciliary body (CB) from the Schwalbe line to scleral spur has been theorized to result in an

Electronic Supplementary Material The online version of this chapter (https://doi.org/10.1007/978-3-319-54003-0_9) contains supplementary material, which is available to authorized users.

E. Bitrian
Department of Ophthalmology, Mayo Clinic, Rochester, MN, USA

A. L. Grajewski (✉)
Samuel & Ethel Balkan International Pediatric Glaucoma Center, Bascom Palmer Eye Institute, University of Miami Miller School of Medicine, Miami, FL, USA
e-mail: agrajewski@med.miami.edu

A. L. Grajewski et al. (eds.), *Surgical Management of Childhood Glaucoma*, https://doi.org/10.1007/978-3-319-54003-0_9

anterior position of the CB and peripheral iris overlapping with the TM [5]. This arrest in maturation of the angle leads to a wide variation in appearance of the angle on gonioscopy and is felt to be the etiology of the obstruction to outflow. This anatomic anomaly in PCG and obstruction to outflow make the TM and the inner wall of Schlemm's canal the site of greatest resistance to aqueous outflow [6, 7]. Once opened, this allows aqueous humor flow from the anterior chamber (AC) to the collector channels in the external wall of Schlemm's canal [8–10].

Augmentation of the conventional (trabecular) outflow pathway can facilitate physiologic outflow and subsequently lower intraocular pressure (IOP). Recent techniques to enhance the conventional outflow pathway via an internal approach to the TM and Schlemm's canal fall into three novel surgical approaches:

1. Disruption of the TM and inner wall of Schlemm's canal via an internal approach (ab interno trabeculotomy) with the use of an illuminated microcatheter to perform gonioscopic-assisted transluminal trabeculotomy (GATT): iTrack™ catheter (Ellex iScience, Fremont, CA, USA) or with TRAB™360 (Sight Sciences, Menlo Park, CA, USA)
2. Dilation of Schlemm's canal with viscoelastic via an internal approach (ab interno canaloplasty): AbiC™ (iTrack™ catheter, Ellex iScience) VISCO™360 or with OMNI™ (Sight Sciences)
3. Removal of the TM and inner wall of Schlemm's canal by an internal approach (ab interno trabeculotomy) with the Trabectome®/Goniotome (NeoMedix, Tustin, CA, USA) and the Kahook dual blade® (New World Medical, Rancho Cucamonga, CA, USA)

In contrast to external filtration surgeries (trabeculectomy and GDD) and ab externo angle surgeries, the procedures above are performed from an internal approach via gonioscopic visualization of the angle and are aimed to remove obstruction to a natural outflow pathway. There are published reports of some of these techniques via an external approach, e.g., GATT for the treatment of selective types of glaucoma [10].

Indications and Contraindications (Table 9.1)

Given that these procedures are done from an ab interno approach on the same area of the outflow system, the indications and contraindications are similar to those of angle surgery. The common thread to all surgical procedures performed ab interno is the requirement to visualize the angle to safely complete the surgery. While areas of high insertion and iris adhesions can be overlooked, for the most part the angle must be identified [11].

Risks Factors for Failure

The risk factors for failure include the inability to clearly visualize the angle, a shallow AC, and the inability to fully cannulate Schlemm's canal.

Advantages and Disadvantages

Multiple studies describe the advantages of treatment of the TM in its entirety [12–15]. The unique advantage to the ab interno approach is similar to goniotomy, requiring only small corneal incisions leading to a significant reduction in surgical time and, in addition, the ability to treat the complete angle in one surgical event. While

Table 9.1 Indications and contraindications for ab interno procedures

Indications
Primary congenital glaucoma (PCG)
Juvenile open-angle glaucoma (JOAG)
Glaucoma following cataract surgery
Glaucoma associated with non-acquired ocular anomalies
Glaucoma associated with non-acquired systemic disease or syndrome
Some glaucoma associated with acquired conditions:
Uveitic glaucoma
Steroid-induced glaucoma
Contraindications
Corneal opacity of a degree that obscures the view of the angle
Complete secondary angle closure
Traumatic glaucoma
Neovascular glaucoma
Secondary glaucoma due to ciliary body or iris tumor

less clearly determined, there may also be an advantage to the simultaneous dilation and irrigation of the distal collecting system [16].

Similar to goniotomy, the disadvantage is manipulation in the AC with the attendant risk of damage to adjacent structures (lens, iris, and cornea).

Ab Interno Angle Surgery: Preoperative Surgeon Preparation

Ab interno angle surgery is becoming a more common procedure in the armamentarium of adult cataract and glaucoma surgeons. Glaucoma surgery for infants and children is not the same as glaucoma surgery for adults. The anterior segment of the child is a much different environment, and the task should not be taken lightly. Observation and training with skilled pediatric glaucoma surgeons is recommended. Wet labs and model eyes, while not perfect, do provide some level of competence for the surgeon who plans to do angle surgery in children. Bioniko (Miami, FL, USA) has developed an artificial eye with a canal that provides realistic access to the angle and practice for goniotomy, TRAB™ 360, VISCO™ 360, and GATT procedures (Fig. 9.1). The eye model is placed in a tilting holder that allows visualization with the goniolens at the same time as performing intraocular manipulation. Video 9.1 shows the SCHLEMM™ Model from Bioniko being used for TRAB™ 360 and GATT practice.

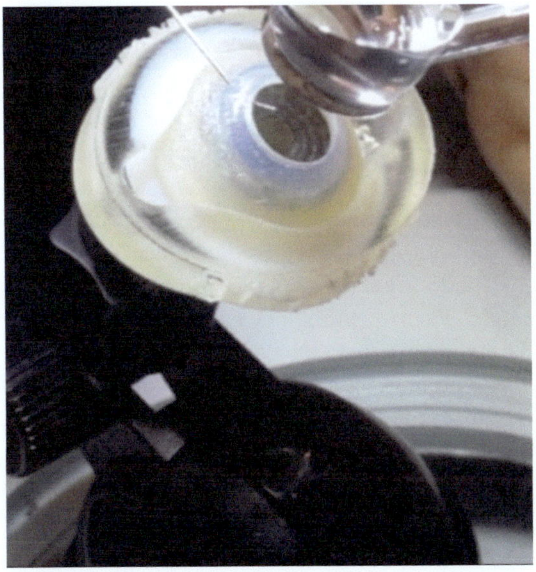

Fig. 9.1 Bioniko eye model for angle surgery simulation is a 3D printing model with Schlemm's canal that is held in a tilting holder and allows to visualize the angle and practice angle surgical procedures

Ab Interno Angle Surgery: Preoperative Patient Considerations and Preparation

In addition to surgeon preparation, careful patient selection and procedure selection are also key. Above all for ab interno surgery, one must be able to visualize the angle during the examination under anesthesia (EUA) preceding surgery. The examination in the office is often indicative of the ability to visualize the angle; a clear cornea or minimal corneal haze will often predict an adequate view of the angle. In some cases, the ability to see the angle at the time of surgery is improved if the cornea has cleared with interim topical treatment and/or the IOP is reduced with general anesthesia. At the time of the EUA, gonioscopy should be performed and the microscope and the child's head positioned appropriately to assist in the examination and incision of the angle. Once the decision to proceed with ab interno angle surgery is made, pilocarpine 1% or 2% may be instilled or a direct acting cholinergic (either acetylcholine chloride [Miochol™, Bausch & Lomb, Bridgewater, NJ, USA] or carbachol [Miostat®, Alcon Laboratories, Fort Worth, TX, USA]) at the time of surgery into the AC for miosis, before instillation of the viscoelastic. The surgeon sits temporally and the head of the patient is tilted 30° away from the surgeon. The microscope is tilted 40° towards the surgeon (Fig. 9.2). Table 9.2 shows the instruments and supplies needed for ab interno procedures.

Ab Interno Angle Surgery: Surgical Procedures

Intraoperative Preparation

- Position microscope: tilted approximately 40°
- Position child: head turn away from surgeon approximately 30°

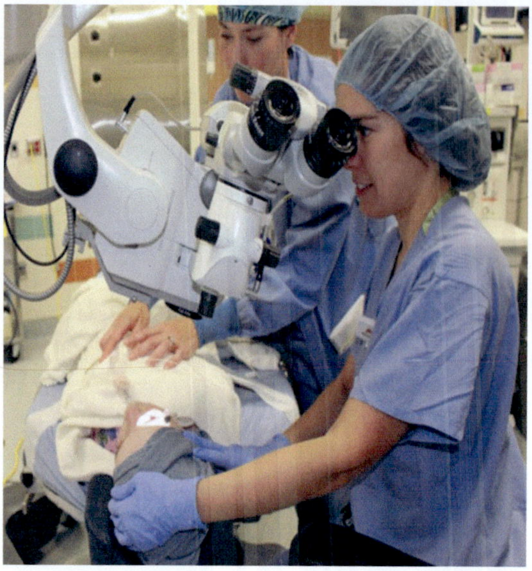

Fig. 9.2 Positioning for ab interno angle procedures. The surgeon sits temporally and the head of the patient is tilted 30° away from the surgeon. The microscope is tilted 40° towards the surgeon

Table 9.2 Surgical list of instruments and supplies for ab interno procedures

Instruments
Gonioscopic lens
Tying forceps
Microforceps (for GATT procedure)
Supplies
Balanced salt solution
75 blade or MVR blade or 2.2 mm keratome
Intraoperative miochol/miostat or preoperative pilocarpine 1%
Healon®
10-0 Vicryl® suture or 10-0 nylon

GATT gonioscopic-assisted transluminal trabeculotomy

- Position surgeon: temporal
- Review equipment (in particular intraoperative gonioprisms and device)

Ab Interno Angle Surgical Techniques

TRAB™360/VISCO™360/OMNI™ TRAB™360/VISCO™360/OMNI™ (Sight Sciences) are designed to treat the angle by disrupting 180°–360° of the internal wall of Schlemm's canal and TM by an ab interno approach. The VISCO™360 differs from the TRAB™360 in that there is the ability to use a microcatheter to inject and dilate the canal with viscoelastic (Healon®) simultaneous to the trabeculotomy. The OMNI™ also has the ability to perform both viscoelastic dilation and trabeculotomy.

Each of these devices is a handheld, single-use device that has a bent sharp needle tip to pierce the TM and inner Schlemm's canal wall and a nylon catheter that can be threaded 180° in Schlemm's canal (Fig. 9.3). After threading Schlemm's canal with the blue nylon catheter, the canal can then be unroofed. The same procedure can then be performed in the opposite direction, threading and unroofing Schlemm's canal 180° in the opposite direction. The VISCO™360 can be used just for irrigation and dilation of the canal with viscoelastic; however, there is no evidence in children that this procedure alone is efficacious (Fig. 9.4).

TRAB™360 Technique A 1 mm clear corneal incision is made with a paracentesis blade near the limbus and parallel to the iris. Acetylcholine chloride (Miochol™) is injected in the AC to achieve pupillary constriction and protect the lens. Ophthalmic viscoelastic (e.g., Healon®, Johnson & Johnson Vision, Santa Ana, CA, USA) is injected in the AC. The TRAB™360 instrument is unlocked by removing the safety pin at the base. After confirming the function and spinning the wheel minimally to advance and withdraw the blue filament, the instrument is introduced into the AC and advanced across the AC under direct visualization towards the nasal angle. Viscoelastic is placed on the corneal surface and a Swan-Jacob gonioprism lens is held by the nondominant hand of the surgeon and used to visualize the nasal angle. The TRAB™360 tip is used to pierce the TM and enter Schlemm's canal. The wheel in the handpiece is turned to allow the nylon inner filament to thread along Schlemm's canal until it comes to a stop. At this point, approximately 180° of the canal has been cannulated with the microfilament and the surgeon per-

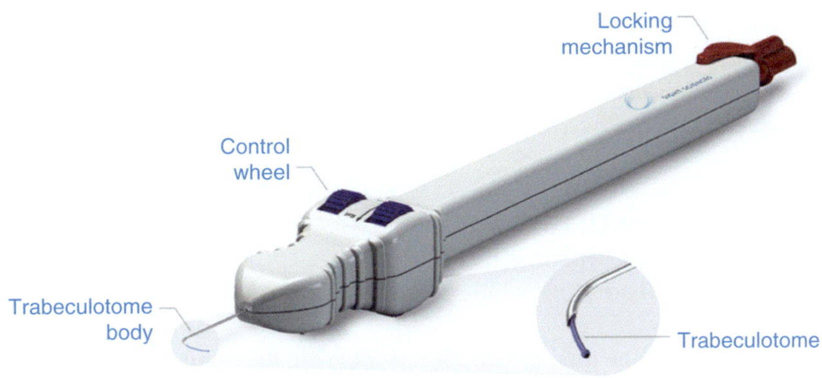

Fig. 9.3 The TRAB™360 is a single-use instrument with a bent sharp needle tip with a nylon filament to thread Schlemm's canal. It is advanced and withdrawn with a wheel mechanism. (Courtesy of Sight Sciences, Menlo Park, CA, USA)

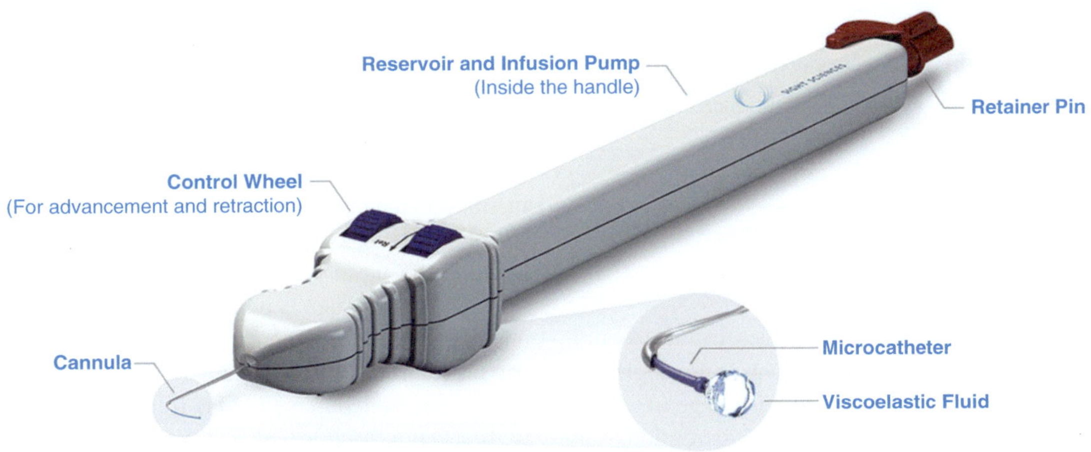

Fig. 9.4 The VISCO™360 is an instrument similar to TRAB™360 but also allows viscodilation of Schlemm's canal. (Courtesy of Sight Sciences, Menlo Park, CA, USA)

forms a maneuver to unroof Schlemm's canal by slowly withdrawing the handpiece through the corneal incision. If desired, the device is turned over and redirected to treat the opposite 180° of the angle after refilling the AC with viscoelastic (Video 9.2). At the time of writing, the filament can be advanced and withdrawn only two times before it locks and the instrument becomes nonfunctional.

VISCO™360 Technique Viscodilation with VISCO™360 is a surgical technique that intends to surgically restore the aqueous drainage system by catheterization and viscodilation of Schlemm's canal to decrease the resistance to aqueous outflow in the collector channels (see Fig. 9.4).

Surgical technique mirrors that for TRAB™360. Of note, the device is prepped with an ophthalmic viscoelastic and a small amount used to flush the instrument. As with the TRAB™360, the instrument is introduced into the eye and advanced across the AC until near the nasal angle. Using the gonioprism the angle is identified and the instrument is used to pierce the TM. Using the wheel on the handpiece, the microcatheter then advances in Schlemm's canal 180°. The wheel is turned in the opposite direction, and this allows the viscoelastic (usually Healon®) to be delivered in Schlemm's canal as the microcatheter is retracted and Schlemm's canal is incised. Then the instrument is removed from the AC, rotated, and inserted again in the eye to treat the remaining 180° of Schlemm's canal.

Both of these procedures result in some bleeding reflux into the AC.

Potential Modifications of TRAB™360, VISCO™360, and OMNI™: Combination Viscodilation-Trabeculotomy

The VISCO™360 device can be used to viscodilate 180° of Schlemm's canal and then reintroduced into the same region of the canal to disrupt the TM, creating a trabeculotomy. While this effectively treats only 180° of the angle, it combines the canal dilation and episcleral venous fluid wave irrigation with circumferential trabeculotomy [16]. Use of the OMNI™ actually allows 360° of both viscodilation and circumferential trabeculotomy.

GATT: Gonioscopic Ab Interno Assisted Trabeculotomy

Similar to the other techniques in this section, GATT is an ab interno approach to the angle. The technique offers the unique advantage of a small corneal incision to perform 360° disruption of the internal wall of Schlemm's canal with simultaneous infusion of viscoelastic [14, 17, 18]. Unlike TRAB™360, with GATT the treatment cannot be titrated into 180°. Similar to TRAB™360, GATT depends on successful ab interno access and cannulation of Schlemm's canal 360°.

GATT Surgical Technique

Following the standard surgeon and patient positioning discussed previously and confirmation of visualization of the angle, two clear cornea incisions are made at the temporal limbus: the first at the 3 or 9 o'clock position, depending on the surgical eye, and the second incision 2–3 clock hours to the right or left of this principal incision. The initial incision can be created with a 2.2 keratome angled incision, much like an entry for adult cataract extraction, and the second incision more like a paracentesis entry site. Miotic is instilled in the eye followed by a viscoelastic. An MVR blade or 30 g needle is used to cross the AC towards the nasal angle under direct visualization. The gonioprism is placed on the eye and the angle brought into focus. The blade/needle is used to unroof 1–2 clock hours of Schlemm's canal and then removed. The Iscience catheter with Healon® attached at the infusion site

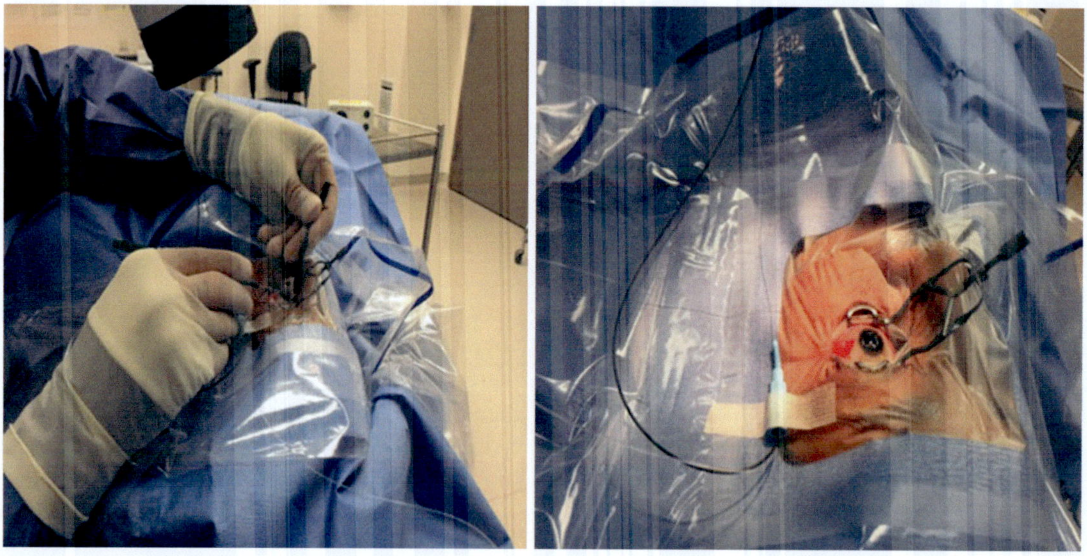

Fig. 9.5 Positioning and securing of the iTrack™ catheter and Healon® for gonioscopic-assisted transluminal trabeculotomy (GATT). (Courtesy of Davinder Grover MD, MPH, Glaucoma Associates of Dallas, Dallas, TX, USA)

(Fig. 9.5) is passed through the paracentesis incision into the AC. The gonioprism is placed on the cornea and the angle visualized. Using a microretinal forceps passed into the AC at the keratome incision site, the iScience catheter is grasped and directed to the opening in Schlemm's canal. The catheter is then fed into the canal with a grasp-regrasp technique to advance the iScience fiber optic around the canal. Once the end reappears, the micro forceps grasp the end and hold it in the AC while the external portion is grasped and pulled with a steady force until the catheter has incised the entire canal (Video 9.3).

Potential Modifications of GATT: Thermal Suture Modification with Dye-Stained Tip and Partial Angle Treatment

Grover and Fellman described a technique to perform the GATT procedure with a 4-0 or 5-0 nylon suture that is pretreated with a hand held cautery to blunt the tip before threading. In order to assist in the visualization of the suture as it advances, they also recommend staining the tip with a blue marker [19].

Another modification of the GATT procedure is partial angle treatment. There are occasions when the catheter or suture will not pass completely around the canal 360°. In these instances and depending on the location, one can attempt to go the other direction to see if the area that does not appear continuous can be passed or dilated with Healon®. If, however, the block persists, a small "cutdown" over the tip site, using the paracentesis blade, can be performed to grasp the catheter tip where it lies. Then, holding it, the catheter is pulled through to cannulate a portion of the canal. The catheter can then be threaded in the opposite direction to the cutdown area and the remaining angle incised.

Kahook Dual Blade

The Kahook dual blade® (KDB; New World Medical) was designed to perform a goniotomy and remove the TM and internal Schlemm's canal wall tissue of the treated area. The tip of the KDB has a special design that allows it to perforate the TM and the internal wall of Schlemm's canal. Once the KDB is correctly inserted in the canal, the instrument is advanced along the TM while the angulated metal at the tip of the instrument elevates the TM tissue and guides it towards the blades that are located at each side of the elevation. This allows cutting and removing the TM and inner Schlemm's canal tissue [20, 21]. The design of the KDB allows performing a precise incision without damaging the adjacent structures (Fig. 9.6).

Kahook Dual Blade Surgical Technique

As with all the ab interno angle surgery, positioning is an important step in this procedure: the microscope tilted, the head of the patient rotated away from the temporally positioned surgeon. A clear corneal incision is created (1.6 mm or bigger) close to the limbus and parallel to the iris. Cohesive viscoelastic is injected through the corneal incision to stabilize the AC. Bubbles need to be avoided in order to have a clear visualization of the angle structures. The KDB is introduced in the eye through the corneal incision and is advanced in the AC towards the nasal angle. Viscoelastic is placed on the corneal surface and then a gonioscopic lens is placed on the corneal surface to achieve direct visualization of the nasal angle. The tip of the KDB is inserted through the TM in Schlemm's canal. The surgeon makes a cut in the TM clockwise. Afterwards the surgeon returns to the original point of insertion and moves the blade counterclockwise in order to

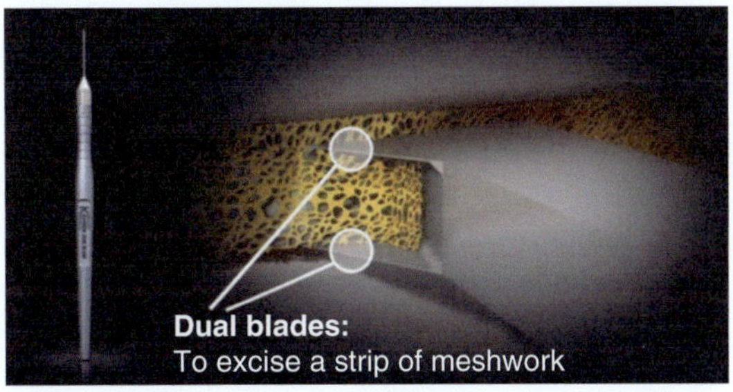

Fig. 9.6 The Kahook dual blade is designed to incise and remove the trabecular meshwork. (Courtesy of New World Medical, Rancho Cucamonga, CA, USA)

remove additional TM and inner Schlemm's canal wall tissue. The surgeon is able to remove this TM tissue out of the eye, since it remains in the instrument surface. Often, blood reflux is observed during the surgery, which confirms that Schlemm's canal has been unroofed.

Potential Modification of KDB: Viscoelastic Tamponade and Irrigation

As with most angle surgeries, there is reflux of blood into the AC at the time the canal is unroofed. The removal of tissue using the KDB makes the margins easily seen, and irrigation with the viscoelastic agent such as Healon® helps to tamponade the reflux of blood and can be seen clearing the episcleral venous veins around the limbus. The Healon® is left in the AC.

Trabectome/Goniotome

Trabeculotomy ab interno performed with Trabectome (NeoMedix) or the Goniotome (NeoMedix) is a technique that uses a bipolar electrode of 550 KHz to ablate the TM and the internal wall of Schlemm's canal. The ablation of tissue is mediated by plasma that ionizes and disintegrates the TM, dissipating the heat and minimizing surgical trauma [22–26].

The U.S. Food and Drug Administration cleared the Trabectome in 2004 for use in adults with open-angle glaucoma both phakic and pseudophakic. Outcomes of Trabectome have been published mainly for primary open-angle glaucoma and pseudoexfoliation glaucoma but also in pigmentary, uveitic, steroid-induced, and narrow-angle glaucoma [27–29]. Although studies include pediatric cases, there are no published outcomes of Trabectome in children. In general Trabectome has not found a place in the routine treatment of glaucoma in childhood, but there are some unique instances where the bipolar cutting electrode cautery applied to intraocular tissue in the AC (e.g., iridocorneal adhesions) has been helpful to create a better view of the angle without promoting bleeding from the iris, which would further obscure the view. The Goniotome is similar but is associated with irrigation and aspiration.

Trabectome/Goniotome Surgical Technique

Operative angle surgery positioning to allow adequate gonioscopic visualization of the nasal TM is again applied: the surgeon sitting temporally, the head of the patient rotated approximately 30° away from the surgeon, and the microscope inclined 40° towards the surgeon.

A 1.6–1.8 mm corneal incision is made close to the sclerocorneal limbus. Then the Trabectome is introduced through the corneal incision with active irrigation (AC maintainer) and a goniolens (a modified Swan-Jacob lens, Ocular Instruments, Bellingham, WA, USA) is placed on the corneal surface to allow visualization of the nasal angle. Then the triangular tip of the Trabectome is inserted in Schlemm's canal and the ablation of the TM tissue is performed in one direction; then the tip is turned and the other direction of the nasal angle is treated. Approximately 120°–180° of angle can be treated (Fig. 9.7).

The ablation is performed starting with 0.8 mW controlling the energy and aspiration rate through the pedal. The aspiration eliminates the remaining debrided tissue. The surgery is performed under continuous irrigation and after ablating the TM, the Trabectome is removed

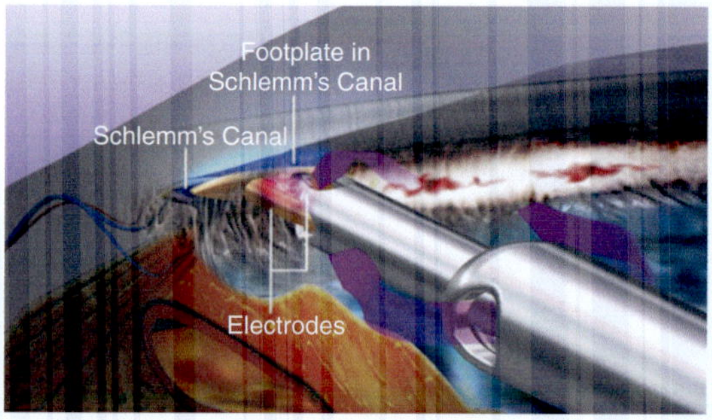

Fig. 9.7 Trabeculotomy ab interno with Trabectome uses a bipolar electrode to ablate the trabecular meshwork and the internal wall of Schlemm's canal. (Courtesy of NeoMedix, Tustin, CA, USA)

from the AC and viscoelastic is injected over the TM to minimize the postoperative hyphema. Then a 10-0 Vicryl® (Ethicon, Somerville, NJ, USA) or nylon corneal suture is placed and a bubble can be left in the AC as internal tamponade.

Potential Modification of Trabectome/ Goniotome: Goniosynechiolysis

The unique use of a bipolar electrode cautery tip to ablate tissue can be used to lyse iris adhesions to an anteriorly displaced Schwalbe line in Axenfeld-Riegers anomaly.

Ab Interno Angle Surgery: Postoperative Management

Postoperative management should be guided by treatment of the postoperative hyphema and inflammation. Each of these procedures results in a variable amount of bleeding and postoperative inflammation. Closure of the angle cleft by either peripheral anterior synechiae (PAS)—or, in some cases, iris strands—and membranes can result in less than satisfactory results. In general, postoperative medications are aimed at treating the postoperative bleeding. Steroids and often cycloplegia along with a topical antibiotic are used in the immediate postoperative period. Once the refluxed blood has cleared, pilocarpine 1% may help in pulling the iris away from the angle and assist in maintaining an open cleft.

Ab Interno Angle Surgery: Complications and Outcomes

The most common complication of ab interno angle surgery is intraoperative blood reflux and hyphema. Some patients following Trabectome can have recurrent spontaneous AC bleeding that can produce IOP spikes [29, 30]. Another complication is the formation of PAS in up to 24% of patients. Other uncommon but severe complications reported in adults are hypotony of <5 mmHg in 0.09% of cases, aqueous misdirection in 0.04%, cyclodyalisis 0.06%, and choroidal hemorrhage 0.01% [18, 24].

With respect to outcomes, Fellman et al. suggest that decompression and forceful irrigation of the AC to elicit an episcleral venous wave may indicate a functional collector channel system beyond Schlemm's canal and so be a predictor of angle surgery success [16].

Nevertheless, the fact remains that in children there is very little to no data regarding complications or outcomes from these newer procedures and devices. We are left to extrapolate from adult data along with the known pathophysiology of childhood glaucoma to access the risk and benefits of each of these surgical approaches.

Ab Interno Angle Surgery: Options After Failed Procedures

Depending on the time course, an unfavorable outcome following ab interno angle surgery may be approached in one of two ways after reexamining the amount of angle treated. The first option is to treat more angle if the first procedure did not treat 360°. If 360° were treated on the first procedure, we would then proceed with other surgical modalities. While this varies from region to region, for the most part either a GDD or a trabeculectomy with antimetabolite [31] are the procedures of choice following complete treatment of the angle.

References

1. Barkan O. Microsurgery in chronic simple glaucoma. Am J Opthalmol. 1938;21(4):403–5.
2. Morin JD, Merin S, Sheppard RM. Primary congenital glaucoma—a survey. Can J Ophthalmol. 1974;9:17–28.
3. Shaffer RN. Prognosis of goniotomy in primary infantile glaucoma (trabeculodysgenesis). Tans Am Ophthalmol Soc. 1982;80:321–5.
4. Papadopoulos M, Edmunds B, Chiang M, Mandal A, Grajewski AL, Khaw PT. Section 5: Glaucoma surgery in children. In: Weinreb RN, Grajewski AL, Papadopoulos M, et al., editors. World Glaucoma association consensus series – 9: childhood Glaucoma. Amsterdam: Kugler Publications; 2013.

5. Anderson DR. The development of the trabecular meshwork and its abnormality in primary infantile glaucoma. Trans Am Ophthalmol Soc. 1981;79:458–85.
6. Seiler T, Wollensak J. The resistance of the trabecular meshwork to aqueous humor outflow. Graefes Arch Clin Exp Ophthalmol. 1985;223(2):88–91.
7. Johnson MC, Kamm RD. The role of Schlemm's canal in aqueous outflow from the human eye. Invest Ophthalmol Vis Sci. 1983;24(3):320–5.
8. Godfrey DG, Fellman RL, Neelakantan A. Canal surgery in adult glaucomas. Curr Opin Ophthalmol. 2009;20(2):116–21.
9. Kaplowitz K, Bussel II, Honkanen R, Schuman JS, Loewen NA. Review and meta-analysis of ab-interno trabeculectomy outcomes. Br J Ophthalmol. 2016;100(5):594–600.
10. Sarkisian SR Jr. An illuminated microcatheter for 360-degree trabeculotomy [corrected] in congenital glaucoma: a retrospective case series. J AAPOS. 2010;14(5):412–41.
11. Jea SY, Francis BA, Vakili G, Filippopoulos T, Rhee DJ. Ab interno trabeculectomy for open-angle glaucoma. Ophthalmology. 2012;119(1):36–42.
12. Beck AD, Lynch MG. 360 degrees trabeculotomy for primary congenital glaucoma. Arch Ophthalmol. 1995;113(9):1200–2.
13. Sarkisian SR, Allan E. 360-degree ab interno trabeculotomy. In: Francis BA, Sarkisian SR, Tan JC, editors. Minimally invasive glaucoma surgery, a practical guide. New York: Thieme Medical Publishers Inc.; 2017.
14. Grover DS, Smith O, Fellman RL, Godfrey DG, Butler MR, Montes de Oca I, Feuer WJ. Gonioscopy assisted transluminal trabeculotomy: an ab interno circumferential trabeculotomy for the treatment of primary congenital glaucoma and juvenile open angle glaucoma. Br J Ophthalmol. 2015;99(8):1092–6.
15. Lim ME, Dao JB, Freedman SF. 360-degree trabeculotomy for medically refractory glaucoma following cataract surgery and juvenile open-angle glaucoma. Am J Ophthalmol. 2017;175:1–7.
16. Fellman RL, Feuer WJ, Grover DS. Episcleral venous fluid wave correlates with trabectome outcomes: intraoperative evaluation of the trabecular outflow pathway. Ophthalmology. 2015;122(12):2385–91.
17. Grover DS, Godfrey DG, Smith O, Feuer WJ, Montes de Oca I, Fellman RL. Gonioscopy-assisted transluminal trabeculotomy, ab interno trabeculotomy: technique report and preliminary results. Ophthalmology. 2014;121(4):855–61.
18. Grover DS, Fellman RL. Gonioscopy-assisted transluminal trabeculotomy. In: Francis BA, Sarkisian SR, Tan JC, editors. Minimally invasive glaucoma surgery, a practical guide. New York: Thieme Medical Publishers Inc.; 2017.
19. Grover DS, Fellman RL. Gonioscopy-assisted transluminal trabeculotomy (GATT): thermal suture modification with a dye-stained rounded tip. J Glaucoma. 2016;25(6):501–4.
20. Seibold LK, Soohoo JR, Ammar DA, Kahook MY. Preclinical investigation of ab interno trabeculectomy using a novel dual-blade device. Am J Ophthalmol. 2013;155(3):524–9.
21. Khouri AS, Wong SH. Ab interno trabeculotomy with a dual blade: surgical technique for childhood glaucoma. J Glaucoma. 2017;26(8):749–51.
22. Francis BA, See RF, Rao NA, Minckler DS, Baerveldt G. Ab intreno trabeculectomy: development of a novel device (Trabectome) and surgery for open angle glaucoma. J Glaucoma. 2006;15(1):68–73.
23. Francis BA, Akil H, Bert BB. Ab interno Schlemm's canal surgery. Dev Ophthalmol. 2017; 59(4):127–46.
24. Bussel II, Kaplowitz K, Schuman JS, Loewen NA, Trabectome Study Group. Outcomes of ab interno trabeculectomy with the trabectome by degree of angle opening. Br J Ophthalmol. 2015;99(7):914–9.
25. Mosaed S, Rhee DJ, Filippopoulos T, Tseng H, Deokule S, Weinreb RN. Trabectome outcomes in adult open angle glaucoma patients- one year follow up. Clin Surg Ophthal. 2010;28(8):5–9.
26. Bailey AK, Vold SD, Sarkisian SR Jr. Ab interno approach to Schlemm canal: ab interno trabecular ablative procedures. J Cataract Refract Surg. 2014;40(8):1281–4.
27. Mosaed S. The first decade of global Trabectome outcomes. Clin Surg Ophthalmol. 2014;32:21–9.
28. van Oterendorp C, Ness T, Illerhaus G, Neuburger M, Jordan JF. The trabectome as treatment option in secondary glaucoma due to intraocular lymphoma. J Glaucoma. 2014;23(7):482–4.
29. Ahuja Y, Ma Khin Pyi S, Malihi M, Hodge DO, Sit AJ. Clinical results of ab interno trabeculotomy using the trabectome for open-angle glaucoma: the Mayo Clinic series in Rochester, Minnesota. Am J Ophthalmol. 2013;156(5):927–35.
30. Minckler D, Baerveldt G, Ramirez MA, Mosaed S, Wilson R, Shaarawy T, Zack B, Dustin L, Francis B. Clinical results with the Trabectome, a novel surgical device for treatment of open-angle glaucoma. Trans Am Ophthalmol Soc. 2006;104:40–50.
31. Wang Q, Harasymowycz P. Goniopuncture in the treatment of short-term post-trabectome intraocular pressure elevation: a retrospective case series study. J Glaucoma. 2013;22(8):e17–20.

Surgical Considerations in Children with Corneal Opacities and Cataracts

10

Alexander Foster, Anne Ko, and Michael R. Banitt

Introduction

Corneal opacities in children have been classified as congenital versus acquired or as traumatic versus nontraumatic in nature. While these categories may offer some insight into prognosis, the evolution of corneal surgery beyond penetrating keratoplasty suggests that more attention should also be directed toward the anatomic location of the corneal pathology. In Peters anomaly, many congenital corneal opacities are typically treated with penetrating keratoplasty, while congenital hereditary endothelial dystrophy (CHED) can now be treated with endothelial keratoplasty. This chapter discusses surgical treatment options for pediatric corneal opacities, including penetrating, endothelial, and lamellar keratoplasties. Attention will also be given to Boston keratoprostheses (KPro), as well as to a less frequently reported procedure, optical iridectomy. The management of coincident glaucoma will also be discussed.

Electronic Supplementary Material The online version of this chapter (https://doi.org/10.1007/978-3-319-54003-0_10) contains supplementary material, which is available to authorized users.

A. Foster · A. Ko · M. R. Banitt (✉)
Department of Ophthalmology, University of Washington, Seattle, WA, USA
e-mail: mrbanitt@uw.edu

Indications and Timing of Corneal Transplantation

One of the rewards of caring for pediatric patients is the ability to limit or avoid lifelong visual disability. Since there is great variability in how pediatric corneal disorders are expressed, no two pediatric cornea cases are ever the same, which, in turn, makes it difficult to make blanket statements about whether, when, or which specific surgery is advisable.

Indications for pediatric keratoplasty vary by region. In North America, congenital corneal opacities and dystrophies are the most common [1]. Opacities that result from infectious keratitis, ulceration, and traumatic scar predominate in Asia and Africa [2, 3].

Although the timing of surgical interventions has been studied, when best to operate remains unclear. Early interventions intended to minimize amblyopia may be associated with increased risks from general anesthesia and graft rejection. However, studies have not always demonstrated worse outcomes for surgery at a younger age [1]. Early surgery should be considered in cases of bilateral involvement, particularly when there are concerns about bilateral deprivational amblyopia.

Due to the heterogeneity of corneal opacities and varying study sizes and follow-up periods, it is difficult to make firm conclusions from the literature regarding the outcomes of penetrating keratoplasty in children related to age. A study

A. L. Grajewski et al. (eds.), *Surgical Management of Childhood Glaucoma*,
https://doi.org/10.1007/978-3-319-54003-0_10

from Lowe and co-workers of 765 grafts in individuals younger than 20 years of age revealed that the grafts of children 5 years of age and younger did worse than did those in the older age groups [4]. Grafts did best in the oldest subjects. However, adolescents aged 13 to 19 tended to undergo penetrating keratoplasty for keratoconus, which carries a more favorable prognosis (due to its limited clinical associations) than does, for instance, Peters anomaly. Dana and coauthors reported on over 160 grafts for which visual outcome was not affected by the timing of surgery [1]. And, finally, Low and colleagues studied 105 children for whom graft survival tended to improve in patients over 12 months of age [2], although the difference was not statistically significant. The effect of the patient's age and ideal timing of surgery on prognosis is not clear cut.

The ability of a patient's family to comply with treatment and follow-up should also inform decisions regarding the timing and type of surgery performed. Furthermore, as some corneal opacities present as part of a syndrome, the general health of a patient (and his/her ability to undergo serial examinations under anesthesia [EUA]) must be taken into consideration. Comorbidities, including developmental delay, can affect daily care and drop administration. The potential for self-inflicted trauma should also be considered, particularly if penetrating keratoplasty is to be performed.

The decision to perform a corneal transplant should be carefully considered, weighing various factors including the bilateral or unilateral nature of the disease, the density of the opacity(ies), intraocular pressure (IOP) control, anesthetic and surgical risks, and risks for early or delayed complications, including amblyopia. In general, we tend to be surgically less aggressive in children with unilateral opacities. Children with bilateral central opacities typically warrant early surgery. For example, a child with congenital hereditary endothelial dystrophy who undergoes bilateral endothelial keratoplasty can expect to do well. On the other hand, a child with a unilateral type 2 Peters anomaly presenting with no clear peripheral cornea and glaucoma would require a penetrating keratoplasty and glaucoma surgery with a more complicated postoperative course and a guarded visual prognosis. Preoperative discussions should include a reasonable estimation of visual potential, particularly in unilateral cases, as a well as a thorough discussion of medication and appointment regimens to be expected postoperatively.

Pediatric Penetrating Keratoplasty

At all stages, penetrating keratoplasty in a child is more challenging than when undertaken in an adult. Concomitant ocular abnormalities, such as anterior segment dysgenesis and glaucoma, are common. Reduced scleral rigidity and positive posterior pressure can make surgery more difficult. Depending on the ability of the child to cooperate, routine postoperative evaluations and suture removal may not be able to be performed in a clinic setting and therefore require multiple serial EUAs. For patients who are unable to articulate complaints, parents may only become aware of problems after symptoms and findings become severe. Since the pediatric immune response is robust, children experience higher rates of allograft rejection compared to adults [1, 5]. Even when graft clarity is maintained, visual outcomes can be disappointing due to amblyopia. Despite these difficulties, the art of pediatric keratoplasty has evolved considerably.

Surgical Technique

The surgical technique for penetrating keratoplasty in pediatric populations is similar to adult surgery with a few notable exceptions. To reduce the risk of damage to the lens, pilocarpine can be administered preoperatively in cases where the iris is not adherent to the cornea. Placement of a Flieringa or McNeill-Goldman ring (Katena Products, Denville NJ, USA) can assist with reduced scleral rigidity, a characteristic of young eyes. Preoperative use of a Honan balloon or intravenous mannitol can mitigate positive posterior pressure that might otherwise cause the lens to come forward. Rather than oversizing grafts by 0.25–0.5 mm as we typically do in adults, larger grafts (oversized by 0.75–1.0 mm) can aid in securing the wound over the lens and iris. Larger grafts also offer the advantage of deepening the anterior chamber (AC) and limiting or preventing the formation of iridocorneal adhesions and glaucoma [6, 7].

For young children, host buttons are often punched to a diameter of 5–6 mm. Although these wounds can be closed with fewer sutures than in larger grafts, sutures loosen frequently and early in children, so we feel it is best to place roughly 16 interrupted sutures. The use of a running suture is discouraged due to the possibility of uneven wound healing and suture loosening.

Postoperative Management

Younger patients often require frequent EUAs to monitor graft health, IOP, and axial length. As the likelihood of graft rejection is higher in the first year after transplant, close follow-up will be necessary during this period [8]. Suture removal tends to occur earlier than it does in adults due to faster healing. Unlike in adults, all sutures should ultimately be removed to minimize the risk of suture-related infections. These children are often best managed by a team of specialists able to attend to amblyopia and patching as well as congenital and secondary glaucoma.

Outcomes

Pediatric corneal opacities are a heterogenous group of disorders, which makes it difficult to make firm statements about outcomes after penetrating keratoplasty. The prognosis after pediatric penetrating keratoplasty (PKP) depends on several factors, most important of which might be the presence of other ocular anomalies.

Table 10.1 summarizes selected series of pediatric PKP and highlights the heterogeneity of the patients and outcomes [1, 2, 4, 9–15]. Yang and coauthors found that corneal staphylomas and adhesions between the lens and cornea conferred a 7.93-fold increase in the rate of graft failure [5]. In reviewing the literature, Bhandari and coauthors noted a similar finding in Peters anomaly patients with the more severe, lens-involving form of Peters having significantly worse graft survival than type 1 patients, 14.2% compared to 87.5% [16]. Not surprisingly, several studies have indicated that concurrent surgical procedures, including lensectomy and vitrectomy, are also associated with poorer graft survival [11, 13, 16, 17]. A series reported by Low et al. also identified deep corneal neovascularization, active inflammation, preexisting glaucoma drainage device, and ocular surface disease as factors associated with poor graft survival [2].

Subsequent intraocular surgery, including cataract extraction with intraocular lens placement, has also been found to negatively affect graft survival [1]. In a study that involved 164 grafts, Dana and colleagues found that only 19% of 27 eyes that underwent repeat grafting remained clear. Of the six eyes that underwent a third graft, none maintained clarity, suggesting that prior grafting may be strongly associated with graft failure [1].

Age at the time of first surgery has been variably implicated as a prognostic factor [8, 10, 11, 15, 18]. With a mean age at first transplant of 42.4 months and 83% of children undergoing their first surgery after 12 months of age, Chang et al. noted graft failure rates at 1, 3, 5, and 10 years of 30%, 39%, 70%, and 77%, respectively [10]. They concluded that delaying PKP was not inferior to earlier surgery in children with Peters anomaly. Rao and coauthors determined that children with Peters anomaly younger than 6 months of age had a 2.2-fold higher risk of graft failure than did older children [8]. However, the poor outcomes in these studies may be less related to age at the time of surgery than to the underlying pathology.

While it is likely that delaying PKP increases the incidence and depth of deprivational amblyopia, a large study from Dana and associates found that amblyopia treatment (and not timing of surgery) was the only independently significant prognostic factor for postoperative visual improvement [1]. In a small study from Al-Rajhi

Table 10.1 Summary of selected studies of pediatric penetrating keratoplasty, demonstrating the varying indications and outcomes in such a heterogenic group of patients

Series	Number of grafts	Indications for surgery	Age at time of surgery	Follow-up	Results and conclusions
Al-Ghamdi et al. [9]	165	78.8% congenital opacity (27% CHED), traumatic opacity 10.9%, acquired nontraumatic opacity 10.3%	Not documented	50 months for clear grafts, 6 months for failed grafts	44.2% of grafts remained clear, 55.8% failed. Graft survival, likelihood of ambulatory vision significantly higher in CHED than other indications. Worst prognosis was non-CHED congenital opacities
Chang et al. [10]	23	Peters anomaly	42.4 months	1–10 years	30% failure rate at 1 year, 39% at 3 years, 70% at 5 years, 77% 10 years. Mean final acuity in clear graft group was 1.883 LogMAR, failed graft group 2.767 LogMAR
Cowden [11]	66	33% congenital opacification, 30% corneal decompensation, 18.5% keratoconus, 18.5% failed grafts		1–10 years	32 clear grafts, 30 failed grafts, 4 enucleations. Acquired scars, corneal decompensation, older children had best prognosis. Perforations, active inflammation, or multiple abnormalities did worse
Dana et al. [1]	164	64% congenital opacities, 17% traumatic, 19% acquired nontraumatic	45.3 months	45 months	80% graft survival at 12 months, 67% at 24 months. When quantifiable, 33% had better than 20/200 vision. Vitrectomy/lensectomy, regrafting associated with poor survival. Amblyopia treatment associated with better outcomes
Karadag et al. [12]	46	89.1% congenital opacity, 4.3% traumatic opacity, 6.5% acquired nontraumatic opacity	24.6 ± 39.9 months	36.4 ± 28.8 months	Mean graft survival time 45.2 ± 5.8 months (survival rate 75.7% at 1 year). 1-year graft survival was 51.9% and 90.7% with and without glaucoma, respectively. Concomitant vitrectomy was a poor prognostic factor. Age at surgery not associated with poorer survival
Low et al. [2]	105	22.9% corneal scar, 21.9% limbal dermoid, 15.2% anterior segment dysgenesis, 14.3% keratoconus	8.38 ± 5.63 years	34.6 ± 39.1 months	Penetrating keratoplasty survival was 92.8% at 1 year, 88.9% at 2–4 years, 80.9% 5–16 years. Deep corneal vascularization, preexisting glaucoma drainage implant, preexisting ocular surface disease associated with worse prognosis

Lowe et al. [4]	765	Infant group: 44% Peters anomaly, 21% corneal deformity; 5–12-year age group: keratoconus 35%, scar or opacity 27%; adolescent group: keratoconus 86%			Graft survival 16 years postoperatively was 40% in infants compared to 70% in 5–12-year-old age group. 14 of 32 grafts done for Peters' anomaly failed. Graft survival reduced by history of failed graft, graft neovascularization, post-graft operative procedure, 1 or more rejection episodes. Best survival was seen in host-bed size 7.5–8.5 mm
Majander et al. [13]	42	Injury (27%), acquired nontraumatic opacity (23%), keratoconus (17%), corneal dystrophy (14%), congenital opacity (13%), aniridia (6%)	4.5 months to 16 years (median 12 years)		46% of grafts clear at 5 years. Simultaneous intraocular surgery at time of graft, corneal neovascularization, and regrafting were independent risk factors for failure. When none of these factors were present, survival was 84% at 5 years
Patel et al. [14]	65	Congenital (14%), acquired nontraumatic (66%), acquired traumatic (9%)	10.6 ± 4.3 years	1 year	82% survival at 1 year. Congenital indications had lower rates of survival and worse visual outcome
Stulting et al. [15]	152	Congenital (30%), acquired nontraumatic (20%), acquired traumatic (20%)	30 months in congenital group, 97 months for acquired nontraumatic, 98 months for acquired traumatic	30.1 months	Clarity rates at 1 year were 60% for congenital opacities, 70% for acquired traumatic opacities, and 73% for nontraumatic acquired opacities. Rates of 20/400 vision or better were 29%, 45%, and 67%, respectively. Preoperative corneal vascularization, persistent epithelial defects, and concomitant lensectomy/vitrectomy associated with poor survival

CHED congenital hereditary endothelial dystrophy

and coauthors, children who presented with the delayed-onset form of CHED had better postoperative acuity and graft survival (92 vs 56.4%) than did those with the congenital form of CHED [19]. In one of the largest studies of PKP in children, Lowe et al. attributed the better outcomes attained by their adolescent patients to their primary indication for surgery, keratoconus [4]. None of their Peters anomaly patients saw 20/40 or better. The majority of these patients saw 20/240 or worse. For all other indications, a nearly equal number of children saw 20/120 or better (mostly with 20/40 or better vision) or 20/240 or worse. In the end, amblyopia was seen to have a major impact on visual outcome, affecting 8% of the total cohort with infants accounting for over 40% of the group.

Pediatric PKP and Glaucoma

It is common for glaucoma to develop or worsen after PKP due to synechial angle closure. The postoperative use of topical steroids can also play a role.

Glaucoma negatively affects graft survival in adults, and it appears that the same holds true in children. Huang et al. reported a 1-year graft survival rate of 32% in eyes with glaucoma compared to 70% in eyes without glaucoma [17]. Karadag and colleagues corroborated this finding in their series of 46 grafts in which 51.9% of patients with glaucoma had a clear graft at 1 year compared to 90% of patients with clear grafts in those without glaucoma [12]. The mechanism for this discrepancy is unclear. It is not solely attributable to endothelial failure secondary to raised IOP, as children with controlled glaucoma also had a higher likelihood of graft failure. In a series of 66 PKPs performed in 50 children, Cowden noted higher rates of failure in the setting of preoperative glaucoma. His recommendation that IOP be controlled prior to PKP [11] aligns with other studies that indicate that children who undergo combined procedures tend to have poorer long-term success rates.

Autorotational Penetrating Keratoplasty

For patients with smaller corneal opacities and 4–5 mm of clear peripheral cornea, a rotational graft fashioned from the patient's own cornea can be effective in producing a clear central visual axis. This technique is best employed in patients with static corneal scars whose opacities do not extend more than 10–20% (3–4 mm area of clear peripheral cornea present) of the corneal diameter beyond the corneal center [19]. Although fundamentally a PKP, autorotational grafts offer a large advantage over PKP in that there is little need for chronic, topical steroid use to suppress rejection. Therefore, autorotational grafts are most appropriate for patients at high risk for rejection. The aim of rotational autokeratoplasty is to achieve a clear central visual axis of approximately 3 mm, if possible, with rotation of the scar [20]. Those in resource-poor countries where there is scarce access to optical-grade corneal tissue may also benefit.

Children who undergo rotational grafts are at risk for suture-related problems and infections. These grafts seem to result in a significant increase in postoperative astigmatism when compared to traditional, centered, penetrating keratoplasty. Jonas and coauthors have suggested that planning for a clear central axis of 3–4 mm permits better postoperative acuity [20]. Patients with induced, irregular astigmatism will likely benefit postoperatively from rigid gas permeable contact lens wear, if tolerated. Consultations with pediatric ophthalmologists and optometrists are warranted with regard to irregular astigmatism, contact lens use, and amblyopia assessment and treatment in children.

Endothelial Keratoplasty

Endothelial keratoplasty is the procedure of choice for adults with endothelial dysfunction, but it has also been adapted to pediatric cases. Pediatric Descemet stripping endothelial keratoplasty (DSEK) was first reported in 2008 by

Fernandez and Jeng and their colleagues [21, 22]. Since then, the indications for pediatric DSEK have expanded to include other causes of relatively isolated endothelial dysfunction, such as CHED, primary corneal graft failure, Descemet breaks caused by forceps delivery, and posterior polymorphous dystrophy (PPMD).

The advantages of DSEK over PKP are well documented and include early stabilization of refractive error (6 weeks versus 1 year for PKP) and a lower risk of traumatic wound dehiscence. For children in particular, DSEK requires fewer EUAs for suture removal (and fewer suture-related complications) as well as less induced astigmatism and, therefore, a reduced dependence on contact lenses.

Surgical Technique

In children, positive posterior pressure from the vitreous pushes the lens-iris diaphragm forward, further shallowing the AC of eyes that are usually small and often phakic. To mitigate the effect of posterior pressure, we employ many of the techniques discussed earlier with regard to pediatric PKP: use of a Honan balloon, administration of intravenous mannitol, and administration of pilocarpine (to protect the lens from inadvertent damage). In these cases, the cardinal sutures are often extremely difficult to place and care should be taken to observe for incarceration of iris within the wound.

In eyes with CHED, the view into the AC may be limited by severe edema. Removal of the epithelium often improves visualization. The application of topical glycerin may also be helpful.

The corneas of CHED patients are characterized by thickened Descemet membranes and few endothelial cells [23]. In these patients, Descemet membrane is firmly adherent to stroma and can be difficult to identify and remove. To avoid iatrogenic damage to the lens and iris, non-Descemet stripping endothelial keratoplasty (nDSEK) has been performed. Eliminating this step has not been shown to affect visual outcomes [24–26]. However, there is some indication that children who undergo nDSEK are subject to higher rates of postoperative graft dislocation [27]. Poor compliance with postoperative positioning may also have contributed to this finding.

Donor tissue can be inserted into the eye in a variety of ways. The method of tissue insertion must be compatible with a comparatively shallow AC in an eye that is often phakic. In pull-through techniques, where instruments reach across the eye, shifting incision sites to either side of the pupil can help to avoid reaching over the lens with instruments [23].

Poor cooperation with postoperative positioning is likely in young patients and may suggest a role for a larger air bubble with an inferior iridotomy. Postoperative assessments of graft adherence and IOP will also be difficult. Use of imaging to assess graft adherence may not be possible due to patient positioning and cooperation.

Outcomes

In the largest series of DSEK performed for CHED, Busin and coauthors showed visual outcomes that were superior to published results for PKP, with eight out of nine patients (88%) achieving visual acuities of 20/40 or better [23]. In a paired-eye analysis of five children with CHED [28], Ashar and colleagues directly compared DSEK to PKP. Despite the presence of residual anterior stromal haze in the corneas that underwent DSEK, the final visual acuities were comparable. The authors postulated that the haze was a result of differences in the ultrastructure of the stroma.

Advances in endothelial keratoplasty are promising. Gonnerman and colleagues have reported on the case of a 12-year-old boy who underwent Descemet membrane endothelial keratoplasty (DMEK) for corneal endothelial dysfunction secondary to Kearns-Sayre syndrome [29]. They observed an excellent anatomic result. The final visual acuity of 20/100 was achieved within 1 week after surgery and was thought to be limited by retinal dysfunction.

Endothelial Keratoplasty and Glaucoma

Glaucoma after endothelial keratoplasty can occur immediately after surgery as a result of pupillary block caused by a large air bubble. Alternatively, air that has travelled behind the iris can occlude the angle by pushing the iris forward. Both forms of air bubble-induced angle-closure glaucoma should be recognized early and treated promptly to minimize long-term effects.

Standard glaucoma surgeries can be performed in eyes that have undergone endothelial keratoplasty, namely, angle-based, trabeculectomy, and glaucoma drainage devices. If an angle-based surgery is planned, areas of iridocorneal adhesions and synechial angle closure should be mapped out, with careful consideration to the possible necessity of goniosynechialysis. Some types of iridocorneal adhesions after endothelial keratoplasty can be broken and the angle can be reopened, but frequently the anterior synechiae can reform again postoperatively, thereby undoing or negating any IOP reduction from the angle surgery. Glaucoma drainage devices can be performed before, concurrently, or after endothelial keratoplasty. In children who are pseudophakic, we prefer posterior chamber tube insertion to avoid ongoing damage to the corneal graft.

Lamellar Keratoplasty

Keratoconus is the most common indication for lamellar keratoplasty in the pediatric population. With a later age of onset, adolescents who undergo surgery are typically well outside of the amblyopic period. The limited nature of the disease also confers an excellent visual prognosis. If the stroma is successfully dissected from the Descemet membrane, surgery in this population should proceed as it does in an adult.

Keratoprosthesis

Keratoprosthesis surgery involves the implantation of an artificial cornea with a clear central visual zone. The Boston keratoprosthesis (KPro) is most commonly used. The 7.0 mm backplate version is approved for pediatric use.

Published indications for the KPro have included multiple graft failures, congenital glaucoma with corneal decompensation, keratitis-ichthyosiform-deafness syndrome, and congenital opacities [30]. In contrast to grafts, the KPro's rigid, clear optic allows for rapid visual improvement without concern for astigmatism, rejection, or tissue edema. However, the postoperative course can be challenging and fraught with unique complications. The most common of these are the formation of retroprosthetic membranes, which required surgical removal in 26% of children in the largest published series to date with a mean follow-up of 9.7 months [30]. Crowding of the angle results in high incidence (up to 100% in some series) of glaucoma, which we prefer to proactively manage with Baerveldt glaucoma implants (Abbott Laboratories, Abbott Park IL, USA) [31]. Endophthalmitis with predictably devastating consequences has also been reported after pediatric keratoprosthesis [32]. The postoperative management of these patients has traditionally involved the use of a protective contact lens and prophylactic antibiotics. Although keratoprosthesis may have a role in the pediatric population, it should likely be considered as a last resort due to its significant complication profile. This view is supported by a more recent publication with a mean follow-up of 42 months where the authors recommended against the use of the KPro (type 1) in the pediatric population due to its significantly higher rate of complications, device failure, and worse visual outcomes than adults [33].

Optical Iridectomy

Optical iridectomy was first described in 1932 by Foster [34]. It is an alternative to penetrating keratoplasty in children who have a central corneal opacity with an adjacent clear area [34]. The goal of optical iridectomy, as with keratoplasty, is to provide a clear visual axis. It offers significant advantages over PKP, including no need for suture management and no risk from suture-related complications or rejection.

Optical iridectomy should be considered in cases of Peters anomaly, where central opacities are bordered by clear cornea and the lens is clear. From the experience of the authors, in Peters anomaly the peripheral clear areas of cornea can become slightly larger over weeks to years, especially if the IOP is normal range and the iris adhesions are swept from the posterior cornea (Figs. 10.1 and 10.2).

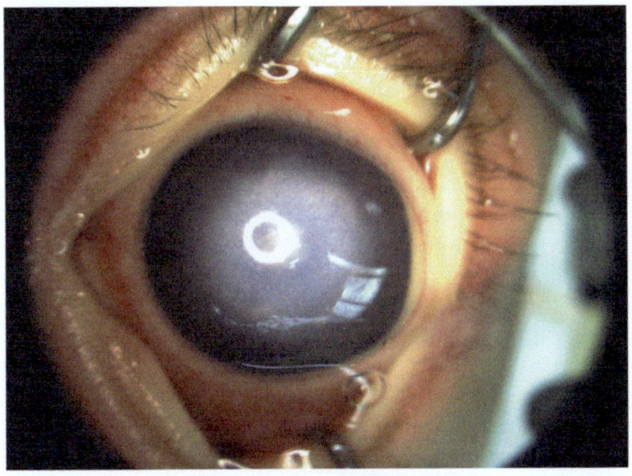

Fig. 10.1 Photo before surgery on 20-day-old infant with Peters anomaly and cloudy cornea. (Courtesy of Alana L. Grajewski, MD)

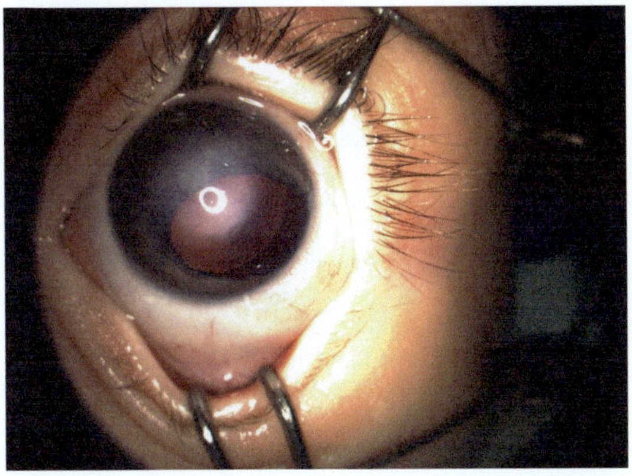

Fig. 10.2 Photo of the same patient after iridocorneal adhesions lysed, 360° trabeculotomy, and optical sector iridectomy. Notice the significant corneal clearing. (Courtesy of Alana L. Grajewski, MD)

Surgical Technique

The site at which an optical iridectomy is made is important. Ideally the size of the peripheral clear zone will equal or surpass the diameter of a normal pupil (3 mm). Medial or temporal sites are preferred, as the upper eyelid tends to encroach on the superior quadrants.

A conjunctival peritomy is typically created in the area of the planned iridectomy so that a near limbal incision can be created. A relatively vertical, anteriorly placed (anterior surgical limbus) incision is constructed with the width of the incision being proportional to the size of the iridectomy desired. The verticality of the wound facilitates pulling of the iris up through the wound. Typically non-toothed forceps are used in a hand-over-hand technique to externalize the iris until the pupillary border is just outside of the wound. The iris is then excised with scissors as close as possible to the incision, as is done during trabeculectomy surgery. The AC is reformed using balanced salt solution. Making sure there are no iris fibers within the wound, the incision should be closed with a 10–0 nylon or polyglactin suture. Ophthalmic viscoelastic devices can be used but must be removed from the eye before concluding. It can be used during the procedure to stabilize the AC, especially if sweeping of the iridocorneal adhesions will be performed in an attempt to increase the clear peripheral cornea. Video 10.1 demonstrates optical iridectomy as described above. Video 10.2 shows a similar approach but combined with an ab externo 360° trabeculotomy, iridocorneal adhesion lysis, and temporal optical sector iridectomy, demonstrating a combined procedure.

Alternatively the procedure can be performed through smaller incisions accommodating an AC maintainer and a vitrector. The vitrectomy cutter is applied to the iris to create the iridectomy. Agarwal et al. described placing the vitrectomy cutter between the iris and lens with the cutter facing anteriorly to avoid cutting the lens [35].

Outcomes

In a series from Sundaresh and colleagues, 22 children with corneal opacities underwent optical iridectomy [36]. Preoperative acuity ranged from 6/60 to light perception. Postoperative best-corrected acuity was variable, ranging from 6/60 to 6/12, but improved in all but two patients. Agarwal et al. published a series of 15 patients who underwent vitrectomy-facilitated iridectomy [35]. There were no intraoperative complications and no cases of cataract formation. The median best-corrected visual acuity improved from 1/60 to 6/24.

While less studied, optical iridectomy is an excellent option for children with corneal opacities. In good candidates, it offers visual results comparable to PKP with far fewer potential complications and easier postoperative care. It is unlikely to cause glaucoma, nor will it worsen preexisting glaucoma, as opposed to PKP, optical iridectomy has no suture related complications or concerns about rejection. Recovery is rapid and a clear visual axis is established much faster than after PKP, allowing retinoscopy and the initiation of amblyopia treatment soon after surgery.

If unsuccessful, an optical iridectomy does not preclude later PKP, if necessary. Since patients with type 2 Peters anomaly have a guarded prognosis with PKP, we prefer to attempt optical iridectomy if there is peripheral clear cornea. For these children, optical iridectomy also offers the advantage of potentially not having to disturb the central lens-cornea attachments.

Conclusion

Pediatric keratoplasty demands skill and postoperative vigilance. It can be humbling, yet immensely rewarding. The care of these patients is often complicated by glaucoma. Traditional penetrating keratoplasty in the pediatric population has given some ground to the same anatomically selective keratoplasty options being performed in adults. We believe that optical iridectomy should not be overlooked as an effective option with few potential complications for the treatment of children with corneal opacities.

References

1. Dana MR, Moyes AL, Gomes JAP, Rosheim KM, Schaumberg DA, Laibson PR, et al. The indications for and outcome in pediatric keratoplasty. Ophthalmology. 1995;102(8):1129–38.
2. Low JR, Anshu A, Tan AC, Htoon HM, Tan DT. The outcomes of primary pediatric keratoplasty in Singapore. Am J Ophthalmol. 2014;158(3):496–502.
3. Trief D, Marquezan MC, Rapuano CJ, Prescott CR. Pediatric corneal transplants. Curr Opin Ophthalmol. 2017 Sep;28(5):477–84.
4. Lowe MT, Keane MC, Coster DJ, Williams KA. The outcome of corneal transplantation in infants, children, and adolescents. Ophthalmology. 2011;118(3):492–7.
5. Yang LL, Lambert SR, Lynn MJ, Stulting RD. Long-term results of corneal graft survival in infants and children with peters anomaly. Ophthalmology. 1999;106(4):833–48.
6. Michaeli A, Markovich A, Rootman DS. Corneal transplants for the treatment of congenital corneal opacities. J Pediatr Ophthalmol Strabismus. 2005;42(1):34–44.
7. Vajpayee RB, Vanathi M, Tandon R, Sharma N, Titiyal JS. Keratoplasty for keratomalacia in preschool children. Br J Ophthalmol. 2003;87(5):538–42.
8. Rao KV, Fernandes M, Gangopadhyay N, Vemuganti GK, Krishnaiah S, Sangwan VS. Outcome of penetrating keratoplasty for Peters anomaly. Cornea. 2008;27(7):749–53.
9. Al-Ghamdi A, Al-Rajhi A, Wagoner MD. Primary pediatric keratoplasty: indications, graft survival, and visual outcome. J AAPOS. 2007;11(1):41–7.
10. Chang JW, Kim MK, Kim JH, Kim SJ, Wee WR, Yu YS. Long-term visual outcomes of penetrating keratoplasty for Peters anomaly. Graefes Arch Clin Exp Ophthalmol. 2013;251(3):953–8.
11. Cowden JW. Penetrating keratoplasty in infants and children. Ophthalmology. 1990;97(3):324–8. discussion 8-9
12. Karadag R, Chan TC, Azari AA, Nagra PK, Hammersmith KM, Rapuano CJ. Survival of primary penetrating keratoplasty in children. Am J Ophthalmol. 2016;171:95–100.
13. Majander A, Kivela TT, Krootila K. Indications and outcomes of keratoplasties in children during a 40-year period. Acta Ophthalmol. 2016;94(6):618–24.
14. Patel HY, Ormonde S, Brookes NH, Moffatt LS, McGhee CN. The indications and outcome of paediatric corneal transplantation in New Zealand: 1991-2003. Br J Ophthalmol. 2005;89(4):404–8.
15. Stulting RD, Sumers KD, Cavanagh HD, Waring GO 3rd, Gammon JA. Penetrating keratoplasty in children. Ophthalmology. 1984;91(10):1222–30.
16. Bhandari R, Ferri S, Whittaker B, Liu M, Lazzaro DR. Peters anomaly: review of the literature. Cornea. 2011;30(8):939–44.
17. Huang C, O'Hara M, Mannis MJ. Primary pediatric keratoplasty: indications and outcomes. Cornea. 2009;28(9):1003–8.

18. Beauchamp GR. Pediatric keratoplasty: problems in management. J Pediatr Ophthalmol Strabismus. 1979;16(6):388–94.
19. Al-Rajhi AA, Wagoner MD. Penetrating keratoplasty in congenital hereditary endothelial dystrophy. Ophthalmology. 1997;104(6):956–61.
20. Jonas JB, Rank RM, Budde WM. Autologous ipsilateral rotating penetrating keratoplasty. Am J Ophthalmol. 2001;131(4):427–30.
21. Fernandez MM, Buckley EG, Afshari NA. Descemet stripping automated endothelial keratoplasty in a child. J AAPOS. 2008;12(3):314–6.
22. Jeng BH, Marcotty A, Traboulsi EI. Descemet stripping automated endothelial keratoplasty in a 2-year-old child. J AAPOS. 2008;12(3):317–8.
23. Busin M, Beltz J, Scorcia V. Descemet-stripping automated endothelial keratoplasty for congenital hereditary endothelial dystrophy. Arch Ophthalmol. 2011;129(9):1140–6.
24. Caldwell MC, Afshari NA, Decroos FC, Proia AD. The histology of graft adhesion in descemet stripping with endothelial keratoplasty. Am J Ophthalmol. 2009;148(2):277–81.
25. Kobayashi A, Yokogawa H, Sugiyama K. Non-Descemet stripping automated endothelial keratoplasty for endothelial dysfunction secondary to argon laser iridotomy. Am J Ophthalmol. 2008; 146(4):543–9.
26. Price FW Jr, Price MO. Endothelial keratoplasty to restore clarity to a failed penetrating graft. Cornea. 2006;25(8):895–9.
27. Anwar HM, El-Danasoury A. Endothelial keratoplasty in children. Curr Opin Ophthalmol. 2014;25(4):340–6.
28. Ashar JN, Ramappa M, Vaddavalli PK. Paired-eye comparison of Descemet's stripping endothelial keratoplasty and penetrating keratoplasty in children with congenital hereditary endothelial dystrophy. Br J Ophthalmol. 2013;97(10):1247–9.
29. Gonnermann J, Klamann MK, Maier AK, Bertelmann E, Schroeter J, von Au K, et al. Descemet membrane endothelial keratoplasty in a child with corneal endothelial dysfunction in Kearns-Sayre syndrome. Cornea. 2014;33(11):1232–4.
30. Aquavella JV, Gearinger MD, Akpek EK, McCormick GJ. Pediatric keratoprosthesis. Ophthalmology. 2007;114(5):989–94.
31. Nguyen P, Chopra V. Glaucoma management in Boston keratoprosthesis type I recipients. Curr Opin Ophthalmol. 2014;25(2):134–40.
32. Rachitskaya AV, Moysidis SN, Miller D, Perez VL, Banitt MR, Alfonso EC, et al. Streptococcal endophthalmitis in pediatric keratoprosthesis. Ophthalmology. 2013;120(7):1506–7 e1.
33. Fung SSM, Jabbour S, Harissi-Dagher M, Tan RRG, Hamel P, Baig K, et al. Visual outcomes and complications of type i Boston keratoprosthesis in children: a retrospective multicenter study and literature review. Ophthalmology. 2018 Feb;125(2):153–60.
34. Foster J. Optical iridectomy, indications, method and value. Br J Ophthalmol. 1932;16(8):476–84.
35. Agarwal T, Jhanji V, Dutta P, Tandon R, Sharma N, Titiyal JS, et al. Automated vitrector-assisted optical iridectomy: customized iridectomy. J Cataract Refract Surg. 2007;33(6):959–61.
36. Sundaresh K, Jethani J, Vijayalakshmi P. Optical iridectomy in children with corneal opacities. J AAPOS. 2008;12(2):163–5.

11 Childhood Glaucoma Surgery in Developing Countries

Anil K. Mandal and Sirisha Senthil

Introduction

The surgical management of childhood glaucoma is one of the biggest challenges in the field of glaucoma and an even greater challenge in the developing world. Despite its rarity, childhood glaucoma is one of the leading causes of admission to schools for the blind in both developed and developing countries. Glaucoma accounts for 3–5% of blindness in children worldwide [1, 2], but in certain regions such as Latin America and the Caribbean, it is the cause of blindness in 7% of cases. Overall, the number of blind children in the world is estimated to be 1.4 million, with a disproportionate number, approximately three-quarters, living in the poorest regions of Africa and Asia [3].

Surgery is the main modality of treatment for childhood glaucoma, and a proportion of patients need multiple surgical interventions for long-term control of intraocular pressure (IOP). While early diagnosis and appropriate surgical technique are important in the management of this condition, the treatment does not end there. It is almost a lifelong commitment for both the parents and doctors caring for these children. Childhood glaucoma blindness in the developing world can be minimized by earlier detection and treatment and by strategies to reduce cases that are lost to follow-up.

Although therapies have improved the prognosis of many childhood glaucomas, the number of complex glaucoma cases being seen has increased, needing expert care and multiple interventions. Although there is paucity of data on the surgical management of childhood glaucoma from the developing world, the aim of this chapter is to highlight the challenges of managing childhood glaucoma in developing countries, the different surgical options available, and their outcomes.

Challenges of Managing Childhood Glaucoma in Developing Countries

Several problems and issues are associated with the effective management of childhood glaucoma in developing countries [4] and include:

1. The burden of disease is greater in the developing world. Primary congenital glaucoma (PCG) is the most common form of childhood glaucoma. A recent published report from an urban center in Miami, Florida, USA, reported that PCG constituted the largest group (32%) among

Electronic Supplementary Material The online version of this chapter (https://doi.org/10.1007/978-3-319-54003-0_11) contains supplementary material, which is available to authorized users.

A. K. Mandal · S. Senthil (✉)
Department of Glaucoma and Pediatric Ophthalmology, L. V. Prasad Eye Institute, Hyderabad, Telangana, India
e-mail: sirishasenthil@lvpei.org

A. L. Grajewski et al. (eds.), *Surgical Management of Childhood Glaucoma*,
https://doi.org/10.1007/978-3-319-54003-0_11

all types of childhood glaucoma [5]. However, its incidence varies widely, occurring in approximately 1 in 20,000 in Western populations [6, 7] but more frequently in the developing world. PCG is often transmitted in an autosomal recessive pattern and may occur up to ten times more frequently in certain ethnic and religious populations where consanguineous marriage is socially and culturally acceptable. The highest reported prevalence is found in Slovakian gypsies at 1 in 1250 [8], and among Saudi Arabians, it is 1 in 2500 [9]. In southern India, prevalence of PCG is estimated at 1 in 3300 live births, accounting for 4.2% of overall childhood blindness [10].

2. More severe disease phenotype and late presentation of the disease in an advanced stage when it is less amenable to successful surgical treatment.
3. Limited number of trained personnel with the appropriate skill sets (surgeon, anesthesiologist, nursing staff, and other professionals) for microsurgical treatment and postoperative care.
4. Cultural fear of surgical treatment, which must be overcome.
5. Incurable disease that needs ongoing follow-up, which is often inadequate in treated cases leading to poor prognosis. So the initial benefits of glaucoma surgery may be lost if there is no continuity of care for these children.
6. Limited access to health care and long travel distances to health-care centers.
7. Poor socioeconomic status of the family and lack of affordability of health care.
8. Barriers to affordability and availability in rural areas of topical medications along with variable nature and efficacy (quality) of available generic medication.

Surgical Therapy of Childhood Glaucoma in Developing Countries

Goniotomy

The classic surgery for PCG is goniotomy as described by Barkan [11]. PCG, which occurs in India, the Middle East, South Africa, and several other parts of the developing world, is mostly familial compared to the West and responds less favorably to goniotomy [4]. Furthermore, in developing countries, the disease is of a more severe phenotype and presents late with severe corneal edema precluding goniotomy [12, 13]. Compared to Western and European populations, a large number of Indian children (>80%) present with a severely cloudy cornea at birth, thus in whom goniotomy is technically impossible [14]. In such cases trabeculotomy ab externo is advocated as the initial surgical procedure of choice by several authors [15–19]. However, if corneal clarity and diameter of the cornea permit, goniotomy may be attempted by surgeons who are trained and competent in performing the surgery (see Chap. 4).

Trabeculotomy Ab Externo

Trabeculotomy ab externo was simultaneously and independently described by Burian [20, 21] and by Smith [22] in 1960 and is our preferred angle surgical technique due to a number of advantages [19, 23] over goniotomy in the management of childhood glaucomas in our part of the world. The popularity of trabeculotomy ab externo as an initial procedure in the surgical management of PCG has been championed by a number of authorities [23, 24] (see Chap. 4).

Trabeculectomy with or Without Antiscarring Therapy

Trabeculectomy is a procedure that most ophthalmologists are familiar with and is technically easier than goniotomy or trabeculotomy. Hence some surgeons in developing countries perform only trabeculectomy. However, many others do not consider it as a first-line procedure for PCG in view of the higher incidence of complications and lower success rates reported in the early literature [25–27]. Nevertheless, several subsequent reports documented successful results following primary trabeculectomy for PCG that are comparable to goniotomy or external trabeculotomy [28–32]. In refractory PCG following failed angle surgery or combined trabeculotomy-trabeculectomy (CTT), trabeculectomy with mitomycin C (MMC) [33, 34] may be an option (see Chap. 5).

Combined Trabeculotomy-Trabeculectomy (Ab Externo)

The prevalence of children presenting with glaucoma and opaque corneas precluding goniotomy, coupled with encouraging reports of primary trabeculectomy in PCG, prompted Indian surgeons to combine trabeculotomy ab externo with trabeculectomy as the initial surgery for PCG in the Indian patient population [35]. In mild forms of PCG, i.e., mild angle anomaly and corneal haze, we perform trabeculotomy ab externo in isolation. However, in most cases of PCG with megalocornea and associated significant corneal edema, we prefer CTT. In secondary childhood glaucomas, if Schlemm canal is technically possible to explore, we perform CTT. However, if Schlemm canal is difficult to dissect or is anatomically absent, we perform trabeculectomy alone.

Surgical Technique:

1. A limbus-based conjunctival flap is raised 7 mm from the superior limbus with blunt-tipped Westcott scissors and plain forceps. The dissection is normally done in the episcleral plane. Hemostasis is meticulously maintained throughout the dissection of the conjunctival flap with bipolar wet-field cautery.
2. Retracting the conjunctival flap gently toward the pupil, *light cautery is applied on the sclera to outline the sides of a 4 mm equilateral triangle* with its base at the limbus. *The authors prefer triangular flap* as it allows adequate exposure of Schlemm canal and involves less scleral dissection than a rectangular flap.
3. *A one-half thickness scleral incision* is then made with a no. 11 blade. Here we must bear in mind that the sclera in a buphthalmic eye is usually much thinner than in the adult eye.
4. *The partial thickness scleral flap is then dissected* toward the limbus using a no. 15 blade. The flap is held with Pierse-Hoskin forceps during the dissection. Care should be taken to maintain the same plane while dissecting the scleral flap, especially near the limbus.
5. *Surgical landmarks and anatomy of the limbal region should be carefully identified* before one can proceed to the next step. Closest to the limbus is a transparent band of deep corneal lamellae, behind which is a narrow grayish-blue band, which is an external landmark of the trabecular meshwork. The grayish-blue band is followed by white, opaque sclera. The junction of the posterior border of the grayish-blue band and the opaque sclera is the external landmark for finding Schlemm canal. In most eyes, this is situated between 2 and 2.5 mm behind the surgical limbus. The second landmark is one or more perforator vessels entering the sclera, indicating the area of Schlemm canal. Another landmark is a depression or dip at the area of Schlemm canal—the continuity of the two zones is not smooth; there is a dip between blue and white zone, which marks the junction.
6. *A 2 × 2-mm-deep block is outlined* without penetrating the anterior chamber (AC), which marks the area of the sclerostomy.
7. *A central radial incision is then made across the scleral spur.* The objective of this radial incision is to cut the external wall of Schlemm canal and to avoid entering the AC. It is important to bear in mind that Schlemm canal is separated from the AC only by the trabecular meshwork.

   This is the most delicate step in the surgery and demands utmost microsurgical skill. Under high magnification the radial incision is gradually deepened with a no. 11 blade until it is carried through the external wall of Schlemm canal, at which point there is a gush of aqueous, occasionally mixed with blood. *In our experience, a drop of aqueous is more common than a drop of blood.* The dissection is carefully continued through the external wall until the inner wall is characteristically slightly pigmented and is composed of criss-crossing fibers. Vannas scissors are used to enlarge the lumen of the canal. Some surgeons confirm passage into the canal by passing a 6-0 nylon/prolene suture into the canal, as described by Smith [22].

8. *The internal arm of the trabeculotome is introduced into the canal* with external parallel arm as a guide. Once 90% of the trabeculotome is within the canal, *it is rotated into the* AC until 75% of the probe arm length has entered, and the instrument is withdrawn. About 2–2½ clock hours of the internal wall of Schlemm canal and trabecular meshwork are disrupted by rotation of the trabeculotome into the AC. The same procedure is repeated on the other side. In total, about 100–120° of trabecular meshwork is opened by this technique.
9. *Excess force should not be used while introducing the probe into the canal*, to avoid creating a false passage. If the probe does not slip easily down the canal, it should be withdrawn and dissection of the outer wall continued until the surgeon is satisfied that all fibers of the outer wall are severed. The probe is then reintroduced into the canal to complete trabeculotomy.

   As the probe passes into the AC, minimal resistance is felt while disrupting the inner wall of the canal. *There may be minimal intracameral bleeding from the inner wall,* leaving a small hyphema that often resolves in a few days.
10. *The probe is swept in a plane parallel to the iris.* If done incorrectly, this may cause iridodialysis. Anterior rotation can cause trauma to the Descemet membrane.
11. *The trabeculotomy has been completed and now trabeculectomy has to be performed.* The deep block is excised using Vannas scissors.
12. *An iridectomy is then completed.* It is imperative that the base of the iridectomy opening is wider than the trabeculectomy opening to prevent ostium block and iris pillar attachment to the ostium causing pupillary peaking.
13. *The scleral flap is then closed* with one to three 10-0 nylon sutures, one at the apex and one on each lateral side of the triangular flap. The knots should be buried to avoid later exposure through the conjunctival tissue.
14. *Conjunctiva and Tenon capsule are then closed* with a running suture of an absorbable material (e.g., 8-0 vicryl).
15. In highly buphthalmic eyes, Schlemm canal may not be located with certainty. In such cases it is possible to convert the procedure to a trabeculectomy despite the lack of successful trabeculotomy.
16. *Some surgeons prefer to perform a paracentesis opening* with a beveled corneal incision at the beginning of the surgery. In such a situation, the anterior chamber is reformed with balanced salt solution, and patency of the trabeculectomy can be tested at the conclusion of the surgery. The authors, however, do not prefer making a paracentesis opening.
17. If bilateral surgery is needed, both procedures are performed at the same operating sessions, although an entirely different set of draping, gloves, drops, instruments, and irrigating solutions for each eye is necessary.
18. Subconjunctival dexamethasone injection (0.2 ml) is given, and a drop of cycloplegic and antibiotic is instilled into the conjunctival sac before a patch and shield are applied to the eye.

Refer to Video 11.1 for the surgical technique of primary CTT on a 3-month-old child with primary congenital glaucoma.

When primary surgery fails, medical treatment may be initiated with topical carbonic anhydrase inhibitors, beta-blockers, and prostaglandin analogues (in that order) after ruling out contraindications. If the medical treatment is ineffective, either trabeculectomy with antiscarring agents or a GDD is our next choice based on the health of the conjunctiva and severity of the disease. We consider trabeculectomy with MMC (0.4 mg/ml for 2 min) in the superotemporal or superonasal quadrant with unscarred conjunctiva. When trabeculectomy fails, bleb needling with adjunctive antimetabolite use is an option, especially if the sclerostomy is patent and the flap edge is visible [36].

Glaucoma Drainage Device (GDD) Surgery

GDDs are indicated when primary surgery fails or in certain secondary glaucomas even as a primary procedure. However, in certain parts of the developing world, the cost of these devices prohibits their regular use. Although the Ahmed glaucoma valve (AGV) (New World Medical, Rancho Cucamonga, CA, USA) has been available in India for the past 1–2 decades, the Baerveldt implant has never been made available. Since 2014, we have been using a prototype similar to the Baerveldt, the Aurolab aqueous drainage implant (AADI), developed by the Aravind Group (Madurai, Tamil Nadu, India). We use both flow-restricted, e.g., AGV, and non-flow-restricted, e.g., AADI, implants. The choice of device is dependent on the surgeon's comfort and the availability of the GDD. Both types of GDD are equally effective in controlling IOP. However, studies in adults suggest that the need for medications is higher with flow-restricted GDDs, and hypotony-related problems are higher with non-flow-restricted GDDs [37]. One has to weigh the benefits and risks on an individual patient basis and choose the procedure that is safe and effective. Our indications for GDD surgery are failed CTT surgery in PCG as a primary procedure or after failed trabeculectomy surgery in eyes with aniridia, Sturge–Weber syndrome, and other secondary childhood glaucomas and as primary surgery for secondary glaucomas following congenital cataract surgery, uveitis, trauma, steroid use, post-keratoplasty, and post-vitreoretinal surgery or in eyes with severely scarred conjunctiva.

Proper planning, patient selection, and meticulous surgery are important for safe and successful surgery. With regard to technique, we prefer a superotemporal location and most often or always a limbal-based conjunctival flap (6 mm limbal-based conjunctival opening, 6 mm posterior to the limbus to reduce the size of the conjunctival opening). We prefer double ligature of the tube using 6/0 Vicryl. We use a 24G needle to perform 3–4 mm needle track, and the AC is entered parallel to the limbus. For eyes having a pars plana GDD, a 25G needle entry is preferred. We prefer to place the tube in the ciliary sulcus in pseudophakic eyes, leaving a long tube to allow visualization of the tube tip through the pupil and to avoid the tube blocking. In eyes with aniridia, a short tube with oblique entry into the AC oriented away from the crystalline lens can help prevent lenticular touch. We leave longer tubes in uveitic eyes to decrease the risk of occlusion from peripheral anterior synechiae. Pars plana tube insertion is preferred in vitrectomized eyes or eyes with shallow anterior chamber or those with penetrating keratoplasty. The conjunctiva is closed with 8/0 Vicryl in a continuous fashion with a mattress suture, ensuring traction-free closure. Continuous mattress conjunctival closure provides a posterior suture line, watertight closure, and with minimal discomfort. Refer to Videos 11.2 and 11.3 for the surgical technique of an AADI and AGV implant.

We find the use of ICare tonometer (Icare Finland Oy, Vantaa, Finland) for IOP estimation and ultrasound biomicroscopy to evaluate the bleb dimensions and the fluid pocket very useful in decreasing the number of examinations under anesthesia in these children. Ultrasound also helps to identify posterior segment complications that may occur in the immediate or late postoperative period.

A hypertensive phase occurs at 3–4 weeks after AGV implantation and the 9–10th week following an AADI implant. Hypertensive phase is defined as elevated IOP >21 mmHg after initial low or normal IOP in the presence of cystic and tense bleb. Starting prophylactic glaucoma medications post AGV implantation can decrease the rate of hypertensive phase. The high IOP during the hypertensive phase is managed with topical and oral glaucoma medications. In our experience the number of eyes needing medications for the hypertensive phase was close to 46% with flow-restricted and 26% with non-flow-restricted implants (unpublished data). With IOP control, the majority of the corneas are clear (Fig. 11.1); however, aftercare includes frequent follow-up,

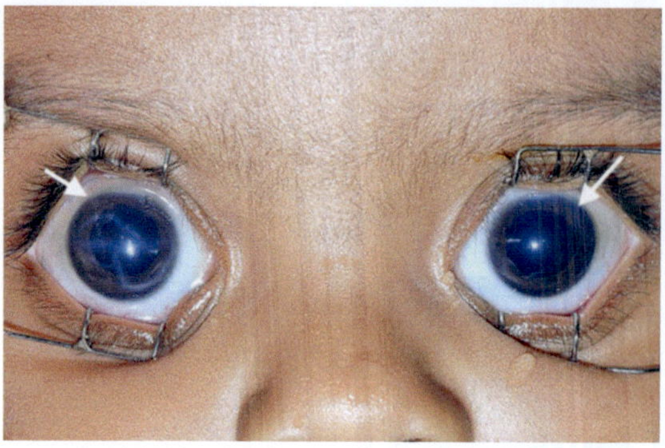

Fig. 11.1 Postoperative appearance after Ahmed glaucoma valve implantation in a child with primary congenital glaucoma. Both eyes show clear corneas and Haab striae in the right eye and well-placed tubes (*arrows*) in a child with failed combined trabeculotomy and trabeculectomy

not just for IOP evaluation but for tube- and plate-related complications, which are much higher in children compared to adults [38, 39].

Laser Surgery

Cyclodestructive procedures are preferred in patients with limited visual potential, with high risk of intraocular complications with incisional surgery, and with severely scarred conjunctiva precluding GDD surgery or as an adjunct when the GDD surgery is failing. The commonly used cycloablative procedure is contact transscleral cyclophotocoagulation (TSCPC) using Nd:YAG and 810 nm diode laser with a G-probe [40]. The power used is 1500–2000 mW with a soft pop. In children we limit the treatment to 180° or to 20–25 shots to prevent hypotony and phthisis. The laser can be repeated if needed, and repeat laser is not done earlier than 3–4 months after first laser. The placement of the G-probe and laser delivery is based on the limbal anatomy and the globe enlargement. Transillumination to identify the area of the ciliary body helps to deliver the laser appropriately. We avoid the areas of thinning and staphyloma, as well as pigmented areas, to help prevent inadvertent perforations. We also avoid delivering laser at the 3 and 9 o'clock position to avoid ciliary nerve damage increasing risk of subsequent corneal anesthesia and corneal complications. We restrict using TSCPC to eyes with refractory glaucomas and poor visual potential. We also use it as adjunct in treating eyes with failed implants before a second implant is planned. The IOP control is not uniform, with a proportion of children requiring repeat interventions. In conditions where vitreoretinal surgery is needed with refractory glaucoma or those with ciliary staphylomas or in eyes with sclerocorneas, we prefer intraocular cycloablation with endocyclophotocoagulation. We use a straight or a curved laser probe with endoscopic visualization using much lower energy (250–300 mW) and treat 270° of the ciliary processes.

Surgical Outcomes of Primary Congenital Glaucoma in Developing Countries

There are very few reports on the outcomes of goniotomy in PCG eyes with corneal clouding. Bowman et al. presented the results of goniotomy to treat advanced PCG with late presentation in Tanzania, demonstrating a 60% success rate after one goniotomy and an 89% success rate after two goniotomies in 36 eyes followed up for only 12 months [41]. Al-Hazmi et al. reviewed 532 children with PCG and stratified them into mild, moderate, and severe disease based on IOP, corneal diameter, and corneal clarity [42]. Patients with milder form of the disease had good surgical outcomes with goniotomy; however, outcomes were poor in the advanced stage of the disease irrespective of the surgical procedure. They concluded that surgical success decreased with disease severity and that CTT with MMC would provide best results in advanced cases. Similar results have been published by several authors from different parts of United Arab Emirates, Africa, and India. Ben-Zion et al. reported that advanced stage of the disease and late presentation at surgery are related to poor surgical outcomes [43]. They used trabeculotomy and the AGV to treat 20 patients (38 eyes) with PCG in Ethiopia. They also detailed problems of surgery in the advanced stages of the disease with extremely buphthalmic eyes. Furthermore, authors reporting on a series of West African children with PCG described poor results from CTT, with probability of success falling from 83% at 6 months to 44% at 1 year, possibly due to severe disease at presentation, racial influences, and no use of antiscarring agent [44].

Elder reported poor long-term success (IOP ≤ 21 mmHg and no medication) in Palestinian Arab children with PCG undergoing goniotomy and trabeculotomy as compared to primary trabeculectomy without antiscarring agents [45]. In a subsequent study by the same author comparing retrospective trabeculectomy data to prospectively collected CTT data, both without antiscarring agents, the cumulative chance of success for CTT was 93.5% compared to trabeculectomy, which was 72% after a 24-month follow-up [46]. For a similar follow-up in the same population, trabeculotomy had only a 51% cumulative chance of success. Mullaney et al. reported that CTT was superior to trabeculotomy or trabeculectomy alone; however, they did use MMC [47].

Whether primary CTT is superior to trabeculotomy or trabeculectomy alone is a subject of considerable debate. In a small series of seven Arab Bedouin infants, Biender and Rothkoff found no difference between trabeculotomy and CTT in patients with PCG [48]. Dietlein et al. investigated retrospectively the outcome of trabeculotomy, trabeculectomy, and combined procedure as initial surgical treatment in PCG [49]. Although the combined procedure seemed to have favorable outcome, the advantage of this procedure over trabeculotomy or trabeculectomy was not significant after 2 years when assessed by life table analysis. The authors concluded that the prognosis of primary ab externo glaucoma surgery in PCG seemed to be governed more by the individual course and severity of the disease than by modification of surgical techniques. In a retrospective, comparative study, Lawrence and Netland concluded that trabeculectomy and CTT with MMC were equally effective at lowering average IOP in children [50]. However, CTT was associated with greater long-term success. In a prospective comparative study conducted in Egypt, Khalil and Abdelhakim concluded that both primary trabeculotomy and CTT with MMC had similar outcomes, which could mean that trabeculotomy could be resorted to first [51].

The argument in favor of primary CTT in some ethnic populations is the higher incidence of successful IOP control with a single operative procedure, as has been reported from India and the Middle East (Fig 11.2) [42, 49, 52]. In the largest Indian series of 624 eyes of 360 consecu-

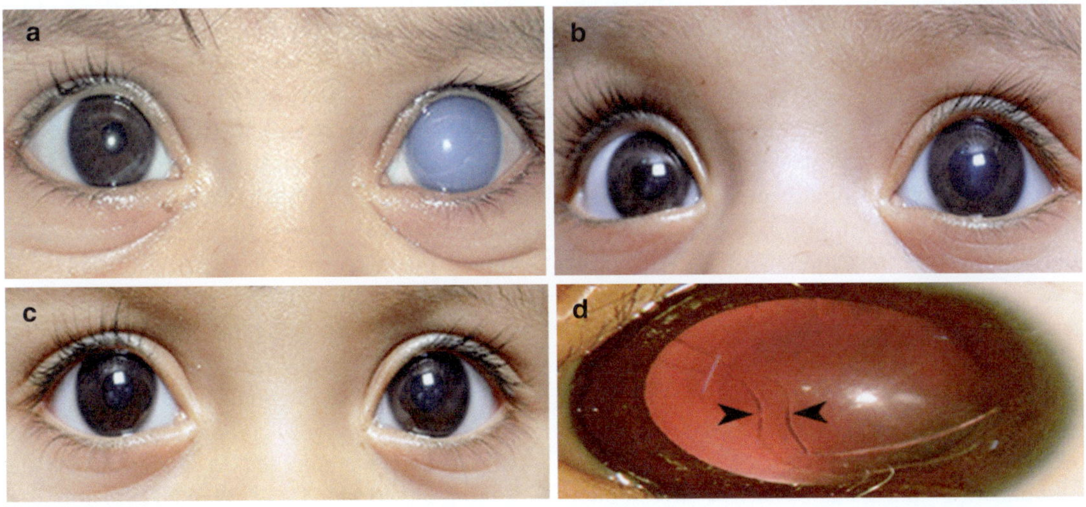

Fig. 11.2 (**a**) Preoperative appearance of the left eye in a 3-month-old child with primary congenital glaucoma who presented with acute corneal hydrops. (**b**) Two-week postoperative appearance of the left eye showing dramatic improvement of corneal edema. (**c**) Six-month postoperative appearance showing normal corneal clarity of the left eye. (**d**) Photomicrograph of the left cornea showing Haab striae (*arrows*)

tive Indian children with PCG undergoing CTT without MMC, IOP control was achieved in 85% of children after 1 year, reducing to 58% after 6 years. Forty-two percent of patients achieved vision of ≥20/60 [52]. Furthermore, primary CTT is a promising surgical technique for the management of different forms of childhood glaucoma in the developing world.

Although CCT offers the advantage of the dual mechanism of IOP control (trabeculotomy-trabeculectomy) and good long-term results have been reported by authors from India and various other parts of the developing world, there is always a search for the best surgical technique that should be employed in the given patient. Recently 360° trabeculotomy has emerged as an attractive choice that can be performed with a blunted 6/0 Prolene suture or with the help of an illuminated microcatheter. Shi et al. retrospectively studied 43 consecutive cases of Chinese eyes with childhood glaucoma undergoing trabeculotomy performed using either an illuminated microcatheter or a rigid probe trabeculotome [53]. They found microcatheter-assisted circumferential trabeculotomy to be significantly more effective at 1 year and as safe as traditional trabeculotomy with a rigid probe. Similarly, Shakrawal et al. from India performed a randomized clinical trial and concluded that in PCG, illuminated microcatheter-assisted circumferential trabeculotomy performed better than conventional partial trabeculotomy at 1-year follow-up and resulted in significantly lower IOP measurements [54]. However, a steep learning curve and the cost of therapy using disposable illuminated microcatheter is a limiting factor, especially in the context of the developing world. In a prospective study from India, illuminated microcatheter-assisted circumferential trabeculotomy achieved comparable results to primary CTT with MMC [55]. Hence, it appears that primary CTT may be the procedure of choice for advanced cases of PCG in developing countries.

Following failed angle surgery investigators have compared CTT to GDD. Helmy et al. reported their results of CTT versus AGV (FP8) in children with PCG (80% parental consanguinity) who had failed previous goniotomy or trabeculotomy [56]. They included 66 eyes with 33 eyes in each group. Success rates were 97% at 1 year in both groups, which decreased to 61% in the CTT group and 66% in the AGV group at 4 years. They concluded that AGV had slightly better long-term survival; however, doing a CTT first would allow a future implant in these patients. In their series 24.2% of the eyes in AGV group had hypertensive phase. Our results show a 90% success rate in PCG with the Ahmed device following failed CTT at 1 year [57].

With regard to the surgical outcomes of GDD surgery in the developing world, Al-Mobarak et al. have reported their results with AGV in PCG and secondary glaucoma and found success rates of 54.8% at 2 years with polypropylene implant versus 90.9% with silicone implant [58]. They also found poor success rates with AGV when MMC was used (31.3% at 2 years), although there may have been selection bias between the two groups. Better outcomes have been reported by Balekudaru et al. from India with AGV (both silicone and polypropylene) in refractory pediatric glaucoma, with cumulative success rates of 97% at 1 year and 80% at 2 years [59]. Reoperations for tube-related complications were needed in 12.6% of eyes and 13% of eyes needed repeat surgery for IOP control. In their study, post-keratoplasty glaucoma was a significant risk factor for failure. In our unpublished data, the success rates with silicone AGV implantation are 91% in refractory PCG and 83% in secondary glaucomas with 4-year follow-up; our success rates with AADI are 91% at 1 year and 81% at 2 years (unpublished data). A recent study by Kaushik et al. from India has prospectively studied the outcomes of the AADI implant in refractory pediatric glaucomas and reported success rates of 81.7% at 2 years [60].

Although PCG accounts for the majority of pediatric glaucomas, glaucoma following congenital cataract surgery is the next most common childhood glaucoma and is important in the developing world [61–64]. Mandal et al. reported complete success probability with trabeculectomy with or without MMC (IOP between 6 and 21 mmHg without medication/additional surgery/sight-threatening complication) in only

37% eyes, and an additional 21% eyes had qualified success after a mean follow-up of 2 years [65]. So this group of patients has a higher risk of failure of trabeculectomy and may need GDD or other surgery.

Refractory Childhood Glaucomas in Developing Countries

Some children with glaucoma have a poor surgical prognosis with uncontrolled IOP despite surgery and/or with maximum tolerated medical treatment. The majority of studies show surgical failure is higher in eyes with greater severity of disease at presentation and increases with time. However, in the developing world, this is further compounded by the fact that most children with PCG are born to consanguineous parents [66] with more severe disease at presentation and usually with delayed diagnosis [42, 67]. Causes of late presentation in the developing world are thought to include delayed diagnosis (lack of awareness of disease) and the limited access to and unaffordability of health care. Furthermore, the majority of cases require repeat surgical intervention to control IOP. Hence, it is not surprising that children in the developing world who are blind from glaucoma have a high degree of consanguinity [56, 68]. Furthermore, the initial benefits of glaucoma surgery may be lost if there is no continuity of care for these children when they fail to attend follow-up appointments. There may also be issues with continuing medical therapy due to the inability to prescribe or afford medications [41, 43]. Therefore, the burden of blindness due to pediatric glaucoma in the developing world is significant with three-fourths of the world's blind children living in developing countries [69].

The above points are illustrated by a number of studies. Ben-Zion et al. reported the average age at diagnosis of congenital glaucoma in Ethiopia to be 3.3 years [43] compared to Western counterparts, where the average age was less than 1 year of age [6, 70]. Close to 50% of the eyes continued to have elevated IOP beyond 22 mmHg even after surgery, and the majority needed second intervention for IOP control. Also Mandal et al. showed that the success rate of CTT in advanced glaucoma (with corneal diameter ≥ 14 mm) was 75.5% at 1 year but decreased to 60.5% at 6 years [67]. Furthermore, Al-Hazmi reported a retrospective review of 820 eyes of 532 PCG patients with variable degrees of severity and less than 1 year of age who underwent goniotomy, trabeculotomy, or CTT with MMC [42]. The mild form of PCG had high success rates with all techniques (81–100%). Eyes with moderate glaucoma following CTT with MMC had an 80% success rate, and those with advanced PCG (corneal diameter of >14.5 mm) 70% at 1–3 years. In moderate to advanced PCG, the other techniques had poor outcomes. A study from Northern Tanzania reporting the outcomes in secondary childhood glaucoma of TSCPC (18%) compared to trabeculectomy (48%, with higher rate of complications) noted that a third of children did not return for follow-up after 1 year [71]. Distance to the hospital of greater than 100 km was a significant risk factor for trabeculectomy failure and was also speculated to contribute to late presentation and erratic follow-up. The same group published results in children with PCG comparing various surgical techniques. Their conclusion recommended that for early disease, goniotomy and trabeculotomy were options and for severe disease trabeculectomy showed moderate success. TSCPC had poor success rate of 17% at 1 year [72].

A number of strategies have been initiated in the developing world to expedite diagnosis and improve prognosis. For example, in India the training of pediatricians and neonatologists for timely referral is in progress, along with public education and childhood glaucoma awareness programs through the media. To alleviate the fear surrounding the diagnosis of glaucoma, potential blindness, and surgery, various education strategies and special support groups for children with glaucoma and families have also been implemented.

Quality of Life of Children Afflicted with Glaucoma and that of their Caregivers

Good quality of life (QoL) is a key outcome for children afflicted with glaucoma, an outcome parents want most for their children. Patient-based assessment of the impact of disease is now widely advocated [73, 74]. However, little is known about the QoL of children with congenital glaucoma in the developing world. It is necessary to assess the health-related QoL (HR-QoL) of the children with congenital glaucoma who undergo surgery and to compare it with an age-matched control group.

Children with PCG undergo surgery at a very early age and undertake multiple, frequent hospital visits over a long period of time, during which there can be uncertainty about visual prognosis. In advanced cases, children with glaucoma require several surgical interventions to achieve satisfactory IOP control, and treatment of such cases is often challenging. In a cross-sectional study at LV Prasad Eye Institute, Hyderabad, India, we assessed the HR-QoL of 121 children with PCG (mean age, 11.8 years) who underwent glaucoma surgery (mean time since surgery, 10 months–2 years) by a single surgeon and 204 age-matched healthy controls. Despite undergoing successful glaucoma surgery, children with PCG reported significantly compromised HR-QoL as compared with their typically developing peers (unpublished data). Younger children with PCG and those belonging to families from lower socioeconomic status were more likely to experience decreased HR-QoL. Ophthalmologists need to be alert to the impact of glaucoma on the QoL of children and efforts must be made to improve it.

Caregivers of children with PCG have significant emotional and psychological burdens; moderate to severe depression may be present in a third of such caregivers [75].

Recently Gothwal et al. designed, developed, and validated the first novel Caregivers Congenital Glaucoma Quality of Life (carCGQoL) questionnaire for use in helping caregivers of children with PCG. It is psychometrically robust, short (20 items), and relatively easy to complete [76]. It has excellent psychometric properties: unidimensionality, good reliability, good targeting, and well functional rating scale. In a cohort, which included 111 consecutive caregivers, Gothwal et al. demonstrated a large improvement in the caregivers QoL scores from preoperative (baseline) to the 6–8-week postoperative period [77]. In a subsequent study, the same authors demonstrated that this significant improvement in the caregivers QoL was maintained up to 2 years following surgery (unpublished data). Hence, successful PCG surgery can improve not only the child's clinical condition but also the caregiver's quality of life (see Chap. 11).

Conclusion

The prevalence and severity of childhood glaucoma are higher in developing countries and a significant number of these children are blind. Delayed diagnosis from lack of awareness (among other factors leading to late presentation), more severe disease, and poor follow-up are probably the reasons for this increased blindness rate. Surgery is the primary treatment option in managing childhood glaucomas. However, due to the severity of disease at presentation, repeat interventions with a combination of different surgical techniques may be needed to manage these complex glaucomas.

The responsibility of the surgeon does not stop with surgery and good surgical control of IOP. Visual rehabilitation is as important in the management of the disease as is IOP control. Visual rehabilitation involves correction of refractive errors, correction of opacities in the media (e.g., corneal scarring and cataract), and amblyopia therapy (when necessary). Amblyopia must also be aggressively managed to give these children the best chance for good vision in both eyes. These measures should be undertaken as early as possible.

One of the major concerns in the developing countries, despite improvement with early recognition and appropriate treatment, is the problem of poor follow-up. The emphasis on childhood glaucoma as a serious chronic disease with need for lifelong follow-up is needed. Creating awareness is the first step to tackling this problem and patient support groups play an important role in helping this cause. Furthermore, to provide appropriate care as well as to follow these children, pediatric glaucoma specialists must be appropriately trained and their skill and knowledge updated periodically.

It must be recognized that in some eyes the prognosis for long-term vision is poor regardless of the technical skill and heroic efforts of patients, caregivers, and physicians. Preservation of even limited amounts of vision in these children can improve their ability to function as adults. However, children with glaucoma resulting in moderate to severe visual loss require the combined resources of a team that extends well beyond the patient-caregiver-physician triad, including those who can provide counseling and help with training, education, integration into the schools, and later into society. These needs are great in all societies but perhaps greatest in developing countries.

References

1. Rahi JS, Gilbert CE. Epidemiology and the worldwide impact of visual impairment in children. In: Lambert SR, Lyons CJ, editors. Taylor and Hoyt's pediatric ophthalmology and strabismus. 5th ed. Philadelphia: Elsevier; 2016. p. 7–16.
2. World Health Organization/International Agency for the Prevention of Blindness. Global initiative for the elimination of avoidable blindness. Geneva: WHO; 1998.
3. World Health Organization. Preventing blindness in children: report of a WHO/IAPB scientific meeting, Hyderabad, India, 13–17 April 1999, WHO/PBL/00.77.
4. Beck AD. Primary congenital glaucoma in the developing world. Ophthalmology. 2011;118(2):229–30.
5. Hoguet A, Grajewski A, Hodapp E, Chang TC. A retrospective survey of childhood glaucoma prevalence according to Childhood Glaucoma Research Network classification. Indian J Ophthalmol. 2016;64(2):118–23.
6. Papadopoulos M, Cable N, Rahji J, Khaw PT. The British infantile and childhood glaucoma (BIG) eye study. Invest Ophthalmol Vis Sci. 2007;48:4100–6.
7. Gencik A, Gencikova A, Ferak V. Population genetical aspects of primary congenital glaucoma. I. Incidence, prevalence, gene frequency, and age of onset. Hum Genet. 1982;61(3):193–7.
8. Gencik A. Epidemiology and genetics of primary congenital glaucoma in Slovakia. Description of a form of primary congenital glaucoma in gypsies with autosomal-recessive inheritance and complete penetrance. Dev Ophthalmol. 1989;16:76–115.
9. Bejjani BA, Lewis RA, Tomey KF, Anderson KL, Dueker DK, Jabak M, et al. Mutations in CYP1B1, the gene for cytochrome P4501B1, are the predominant cause of primary congenital glaucoma in Saudi Arabia. Am J Hum Genet. 1998;62(2):325–33.
10. Dandona L, Williams JD, Williams BC, Rao GN. Population-based assessment of childhood blindness in southern India. Arch Ophthalmol. 1998;116(4):545–6.
11. Barkan O. Operation for congenital glaucoma. Am J Ophthalmol. 1942;25(5):552–68.
12. deLuise VP, Anderson DR. Primary infantile glaucoma (congenital glaucoma). Surv Ophthalmol. 1983;28(1):1–19.
13. Mandal AK. Current concepts in the diagnosis and management of developmental glaucomas. Indian J Ophthalmol. 1993;41(2):51–70.
14. Agarwal HC, Sood NN, Kalra BR. Clinical presentation of congenital glaucoma. Indian J Ophthalmol. 1983;31(5):619–22.
15. Harms H, Dannheim R. Epicritical consideration of 300 cases of trabeculotomy 'ab externo'. Trans Ophthalmol Soc UK. 1970;89:491–9.
16. Dannheim R. Symposium: microsurgery of the outflow channels. Trabeculotomy. Trans Am Acad Ophthalmol Otolaryngol. 1972;76(2):375–83.
17. McPherson SD Jr. Results of external trabeculotomy. Am J Ophthalmol. 1973;76(6):918–20.
18. Luntz MH, Livingston DG. Trabeculotomy ab externo and trabeculectomy in congenital and adult-onset glaucoma. Am J Ophthalmol. 1977;83(2):174–9.
19. Luntz MH. The advantages of trabeculotomy over goniotomy. J Pediatr Ophthalmol Strabismus. 1984;21(4):150–3.
20. Burian HM. A case of Marfan's syndrome with bilateral glaucoma. With description of a new type of operation for developmental glaucoma (trabeculotomy ab externo). Am J Ophthalmol. 1960;50:1187–92.
21. Allen L, Burian HM. Trabeculotomy ab externo. A new glaucoma operation: technique and results of experimental surgery. Am J Ophthalmol. 1962;53:19–26.
22. Smith R. A new technique for opening the canal of Schlemm. Preliminary report. Br J Ophthalmol. 1960;44:370–3.
23. Luntz MH. Congenital, infantile, and juvenile glaucoma. Ophthalmology. 1979;86(5):793–802.
24. Kiffney GT Jr, Meyer GW, SD MP Jr. The surgical management of congenital glaucoma. South Med J. 1960;53:989–93.

25. Beauchamp GR, Parks MM. Filtering surgery in children: barriers to success. Ophthalmology. 1979;86(1):170–80.
26. Cadera W, Pachtman MA, Cantor LB, Ellis FD, Helveston EM. Filtering surgery in childhood glaucoma. Ophthalmic Surg. 1984;15(4):319–22.
27. Levene RZ. Glaucoma filtering surgery: factors that determine pressure control. Ophthalmic Surg. 1984;15(6):475–83.
28. Debnath SC, Teichmann KD, Salamah K. Trabeculectomy versus trabeculotomy in congenital glaucoma. Br J Ophthalmol. 1989;73(8):608–11.
29. Rao KV, Sai CM, Babu BV. Trabeculectomy in congenital glaucoma. Indian J Ophthalmol. 1984;32(5):439–40.
30. Burke JP, Bowell R. Primary trabeculectomy in congenital glaucoma. Br J Ophthalmol. 1989;73(3):186–90.
31. Miller MH, Rice NS. Trabeculectomy combined with beta irradiation for congenital glaucoma. Br J Ophthalmol. 1991;75(10):584–90.
32. Fulcher T, Chan J, Lanigan B, Bowell R, O'Keefe M. Long-term follow up of primary trabeculectomy for infantile glaucoma. Br J Ophthalmol. 1996;80(6):499–502.
33. Mandal AK, Walton DS, John T, Jayagandan A. Mitomycin C-augmented trabeculectomy in refractory congenital glaucoma. Ophthalmology. 1997;104(6):996–1001. discussion 2–3
34. Mandal AK, Prasad K, Naduvilath TJ. Surgical results and complications of mitomycin C-augmented trabeculectomy in refractory developmental glaucoma. Ophthalmic Surg Lasers. 1999;30(6):473–80.
35. Sood NN, Aggarwal HC, Kalra BR. Evaluation of surgery for congenital glaucoma. Indian J Ophthalmol. 1983;31(5):609–11.
36. Elsayed TH, El-Raggal TM. Mitomycin-C needle bleb revision in congenital glaucoma. Middle East Afr J Ophthalmol. 2010;17(4):369–73.
37. Christalkis PG, Zhang D, Budenz DL, Barton K, Tsai JC, Ahmed IIK, ABC-AVB Study Groups. Five-year pooled data analysis of the Ahmed Baerveldt comparison study and the Ahmed versus Baerveldt study. Am J Ophthalmol. 2017;176:118–26.
38. Khan AO, Almobarak FA. Comparison of polypropylene and silicone Ahmed valve survival 2 years following implantation in the first 2 years of life. Br J Ophthalmol. 2009;93(6):791–4.
39. Netland PA, Walton DS. Glaucoma drainage implants in pediatric patients. Ophthalmic Surg. 1993;24(11):723–9.
40. Kirwan JF, Shah P, Khaw PT. Diode laser cyclophotocoagulation: role in the management of refractory pediatric glaucomas. Ophthalmology. 2002;109(2):316–23.
41. Bowman RJ, Dickerson M, Mwende J, Khaw PT. Outcomes of goniotomy for primary congenital glaucoma in East Africa. Ophthalmology. 2011;118(2):236–40.
42. Al-Hazmi A, Awad A, Zwaan J, Al-Mesfer SA, Al-Jadaan I, Al-Mohammed A. Correlation between surgical success rate and severity of congenital glaucoma. Br J Ophthalmol. 2005;89(4):449–53.
43. Ben-Zion I, Tomkins O, Moore DB, Helveston EM. Surgical results in the management of advanced primary congenital glaucoma in a rural pediatric population. Ophthalmology. 2011;118(2):231–235.e1.
44. Essuman VA, Braimah IZ, Ndanu TA, Ntim-Amponsah CT. Combined trabeculotomy and trabeculectomy: outcome for primary congenital glaucoma in a West African population. Eye. 2011;25(1):77–83.
45. Elder MJ. Congenital glaucoma in the West Bank and Gaza Strip. Br J Ophthalmol. 1993;77(7):413–6.
46. Elder MJ. Combined trabeculotomy-trabeculectomy compared with primary trabeculectomy for congenital glaucoma. Br J Ophthalmol. 1994;78(10):745–8.
47. Mullaney PB, Selleck C, Al-Awad A, Al-Mesfer S, Zwaan J. Combined trabeculotomy and trabeculectomy as an initial procedure in uncomplicated congenital glaucoma. Arch Ophthalmol. 1999;117(4):457–60.
48. Biedner BZ, Rothkoff L. Combined trabeculotomy-trabeculectomy compared with primary trabeculotomy for congenital glaucoma. J Pediatr Ophthalmol Strabismus. 1998;35(1):49–50.
49. Dietlein TS, Jacobi PC, Krieglstein GK. Prognosis of primary ab externo surgery for primary congenital glaucoma. Br J Ophthalmol. 1999;83(3):317–22.
50. Lawrence SD, Netland PA. Trabeculectomy versus combined trabeculotomy-trabeculectomy in pediatric glaucoma. J Pediatr Ophthalmol Strabismus. 2012;49(6):359–65.
51. Khalil DH, Abdelhakim MA. Primary trabeculotomy compared to combined trabeculectomy-trabeculotomy in congenital glaucoma: 3-year study. Acta Ophthalmol. 2016;94(7):e550–4.
52. Mandal AK, Gothwal VK, Nutheti R. Surgical outcome of primary developmental glaucoma: a single surgeon's long-term experience from a tertiary eye care centre in India. Eye. 2007;21(6):764–74.
53. Shi Y, Wang H, Yin J, Li M, Zhang X, Xin C, et al. Microcatheter-assisted trabeculotomy versus rigid probe trabeculotomy in childhood glaucoma. Br J Ophthalmol. 2016;100(9):1257–62.
54. Shakrawal J, Bali S, Sidhu T, Verma S, Sihota R, Dada T. Randomized trial on illuminated-microcatheter circumferential trabeculotomy versus conventional trabeculotomy in congenital glaucoma. Am J Ophthalmol. 2017;180:158–64.
55. Temkar S, Gupta S, Sihota R, Sharma R, Angmo D, Pujari A, et al. Illuminated microcatheter circumferential trabeculotomy versus combined trabeculotomy-trabeculectomy for primary congenital glaucoma: a randomized controlled trial. Am J Ophthalmol. 2015;159(3):490–497.e2.
56. Helmy H. Combined trabeculotomy-trabeculectomy versus Ahmed valve implantation for refractory primary congenital glaucoma in Egyptian patients: a long-term follow-up. Electron Physician. 2016; 8(2):1884–91.

57. Dave P, Senthil S, Choudhari N, Sekhar GC. Outcomes of Ahmed valve implant following a failed initial trabeculotomy and trabeculectomy in refractory primary congenital glaucoma. Middle East Afr J Ophthalmol. 2015;22(1):64–8.
58. Al-Mobarak F, Khan AO. Two-year survival of Ahmed valve implantation in the first 2 years of life with and without intraoperative mitomycin-C. Ophthalmology. 2009;116(10):1862–5.
59. Balekudaru S, Vadalkar J, George R, Vijaya L. The use of Ahmed glaucoma valve in the management of pediatric glaucoma. J AAPOS. 2014;18(4):351–6.
60. Kaushik S, Kataria P, Raj S, Pandav SS, Ram J. Safety and efficacy of a low-cost glaucoma drainage device for refractory childhood glaucoma. Br J Ophthalmol. 2017;101(12):1623–7.
61. Magnusson G, Abrahamsson M, Sjostrand J. Glaucoma following congenital cataract surgery: an 18-year longitudinal follow-up. Acta Ophthalmol Scand. 2000;78(1):65–70.
62. Baden C, Shija F, Lewallen S, Courtright P, Hall A. Glaucoma after pediatric cataract surgery in a population with limited access to care. J AAPOS. 2013;17(2):158–62.
63. Ashaye A, Ashaolu O, Komolafe O, Ajayi BG, Olawoye O, Olusanya B, et al. Prevalence and types of glaucoma among an indigenous African population in southwestern Nigeria. Invest Ophthalmol Vis Sci. 2013;54(12):7410–6.
64. Swamy BN, Billson F, Martin F, Donaldson C, Hing S, Jamieson R, et al. Secondary glaucoma after paediatric cataract surgery. Br J Ophthalmol. 2007;91(12):1627–30.
65. Mandal AK, Bagga H, Nutheti R, Gothwal VK, Nanda AK. Trabeculectomy with or without mitomycin-C for paediatric glaucoma in aphakia and pseudophakia following congenital cataract surgery. Eye. 2003;17(1):53–62.
66. Panicker SG, Reddy AB, Mandal AK, Ahmed N, Nagarajaram HA, Hasnain SE, et al. Identification of novel mutations causing familial primary congenital glaucoma in Indian pedigrees. Invest Ophthalmol Vis Sci. 2002;43(5):1358–66.
67. Mandal AK, Matalia JH, Nutheti R, Krishnaiah S. Combined trabeculotomy and trabeculectomy in advanced primary developmental glaucoma with corneal diameter of 14 mm or more. Eye. 2006;20(2):135–43.
68. Dorairaj SK, Bandrakalli P, Shetty C, R V, Misquith D, Ritch R. Childhood blindness in a rural population of southern India: prevalence and etiology. Ophthalmic Epidemiol. 2008;15(3):176–82.
69. Gilbert C, Foster A. Childhood blindness in the context of VISION 2020--the right to sight. Bull World Health Organ. 2001;79(3):227–32.
70. Zagora SL, Funnell CL, Martin FJ, Smith JE, Hing S, Billson FA, et al. Primary congenital glaucoma outcomes: lessons from 23 years of follow-up. Am J Ophthalmol. 2015;159(4):788–96.
71. Fieβ A, Shah P, Sii F, Godfrey F, Abbott J, Bowman R, et al. Trabeculectomy or transscleral cyclophotocoagulation as initial treatment of secondary childhood glaucoma in Northern Tanzania. J Glaucoma. 2017;26(7):657–60.
72. Fieβ A, Furahini G, Bowman R, Bauer J, Dithmar S, Philippin H. Outcomes of surgical interventions for primary childhood glaucoma in Northern Tanzania. Br J Ophthalmol. 2017;101(2):126–30.
73. Freedman BL, Jones SK, Lin A, Stinnett SS, Muir KW. Vision-related quality of life in children with glaucoma. J AAPOS. 2014;18(1):95–8.
74. Dahlmann-Noor A, Tailor V, Bunce C, Abou-Rayyah Y, Adams G, Brookes J, Khaw PT, Papadopoulos M. Quality of life and functional vision in children with glaucoma. Ophthalmology. 2017;124(7):1048–55.
75. Dada T, Aggarwal A, Bali SJ, Wadhwani M, Tinwala S, Sagar R. Caregiver burden assessment in primary congenital glaucoma. Eur J Ophthalmol. 2013;23(3):324–8.
76. Gothwal VK, Bharani S, Mandal AK. Quality of life of caregivers of children with congenital glaucoma: development and validation of a novel questionnaire (CarCGQoL). Bull World Health Organ. 2015;56(2):770–7.
77. Gothwal VK, Bharani S, Mandal AK. Impact of surgery on the quality of life of caregivers of children with congenital glaucoma. Ophthalmology. 2016;123(5):1161–2.

Impact of Childhood Glaucoma and Glaucoma Surgery on Quality of Life

12

Shveta Bali and Tanuj Dada

Defining Quality of Life

Quality of life (QoL) is defined as "an overall general well-being that comprises objective indicators and subjective evaluations of physical, material, social and emotional well-being together with the extent of personal development and purposeful activity, all weighted by a personal set of values" [1]. Chronic and irreversible health conditions have been shown to have a significant negative impact on one's QoL. The World Health Organization recognizes that the measurement of health and the effects of health care must include not only an indication of changes in the frequency and severity of diseases but also an estimation of well-being which can be assessed by measuring the improvement in the QoL related to health care [2].

The concept of QoL finds equal if not greater application in the pediatric population. The United Nations Convention on the Rights of the Child (UNCRC) declares that children at a minimum have the rights and freedoms of all human beings [3]. Every child has a right to a standard of living adequate for that child's physical, mental, spiritual, moral, and social development. Also, children have a right to have their views taken into account in matters that affect them [4]. Within the field of QoL, a great deal of effort has gone into attempting to distinguish "health-related" QoL (HR-QoL), as described above, from holistic QoL. It is hard to disagree with some researchers who favor evaluation of holistic QoL, with the premise that it is unjust to segregate one's life into what is influenced by a disease from what is influenced by current and past experiences [5]. However, the value of disease-specific, self-reported outcome measures lies in providing understanding about the specific limitations faced by young people with a particular illness. For example, in young people with visual impairment, "vision-related" QoL (VR-QoL) assessment could give an insight into an individual's subjective impression of various aspects of their life such as physical, emotional, social, and schooling as it relates to their vision [6]. In contrast, "functional vision" relates to the impact of an individual's vision on their activities of daily living.

Children are a vulnerable group. They are dependent on adults to identify and address their needs and act on behalf of their rights, including the right to quality of life. The implications of this aspect are manifold. Firstly, it is common for adults, typically parents, to report or "proxy-report" on the child's functioning and perception,

S. Bali
Department of Ophthalmology, The Ottawa Hospital, University of Ottawa, Ottawa, ON, Canada

T. Dada (✉)
Glaucoma Services, Department of Ophthalmology, Dr. Rajendra Prasad Centre for Ophthalmic Sciences, All India Institute of Medical Sciences, New Delhi, India

A. L. Grajewski et al. (eds.), *Surgical Management of Childhood Glaucoma*, https://doi.org/10.1007/978-3-319-54003-0_12

either in addition to or in place of the child's self-report [5, 7]. Eiser and Jenney reported generally greater parent-child agreement for ill as compared to healthy children and greater for objective observable behaviors (i.e., physical health) than cognitive and emotional attributes [8]. Subsequently, researchers have found parents of children in a nonclinical sample tended to report higher HR-QoL scores for their children than the children themselves, while parents of children with health conditions tended to underestimate their child's HR-QoL [9–11]. Secondly, caring for children with chronic illnesses has been proven to have a significant impact on QoL of their parents as primary caregivers [12–14]. Caregiver burden has been defined as the type of stress or strain that caregivers experience related to the problems and challenges they face as a result of the status of the care recipient [15]. Andolsek et al. described caregivers as hidden patients, who may carry enormous emotional burden in their task [16]. Caregivers of patients with chronic systemic and mental illnesses carry significant burden as a result of this role [17–21]. Caregiver burden has also been shown to have a negative impact on behavioral aspects and QoL of affected patients [12, 13, 19, 22]. In the pediatric population, parents being the primary caregivers also have an added component of significant worry related to their child's illness. Therefore, evaluation of the caregivers' QoL should form an important aspect of holistic management of patients—especially children—with chronic medical illnesses.

Impact of Adult-Onset Glaucoma on Quality of Life

The effect of adult-onset glaucoma on QoL is multifaceted and has been more extensively investigated than childhood-onset glaucoma. Visual dysfunction from glaucoma has been proven to have a negative influence on several aspects of QoL. Mere diagnosis of glaucoma could cause significant worry and fear of blindness [23, 24]. A greater prevalence of anxiety and depression has been found in patients with glaucoma as compared to control population [25–27]. Limitation in driving [28], fear of falling, and imbalance resulting from glaucoma make a significant contribution to the aforementioned psychological effects [26–29].

Even early glaucoma without significant visual changes has been shown to affect physical, financial, psychological, social, and emotional health [30, 31]. However, some studies have failed to support this hypothesis finding better QoL scores in patients with suspected or early glaucoma compared to controls [32]. This could however be influenced by the educational and socioeconomic level as suggested by the authors, as well as the sensitivity of the instrument used to measure QoL. Some studies also found that glaucomatous changes exert greater influence on physical functioning than psychosocial domains in the long term, as patients may adapt to their feelings over time [33]. As the responsible physician, it is paramount to know from the patient's perspective which of his/her activities are affected in a worse manner resulting from glaucoma. Not only do the "patient-reported outcomes" provide better understanding of the limitations faced by the patients themselves, but these measures can also help devise management strategies tailored to the patient's disability. This better understanding, in turn, could go a long way toward true "holistic management" of our patients.

In adult glaucoma, the QoL scores correlate to visual acuity especially in the better eye and visual field damage [34]. A drop in visual acuity in better eye has been found to cause a corresponding drop in QoL scores [34]. Both the severity and location of visual field defects have also been shown to correlate to QoL scores [35, 36]. Patients with inferior visual field changes are more likely to have a slower walking speed and higher risk of falls [37]. Although mean deviation scores have been correlated to VR-QoL, studies have shown that visual field index (or glaucoma progression index) that better represents central visual field has better correlation to VR-QoL [38]. Specific limitations self-reported by patients include difficulty in bright lights, light and dark adaptation, and visual distortion [39].

Impact of Childhood Glaucoma on Quality of Life

Visual impairment can also cause a significant negative short-term and long-term effect on an affected child's functioning. Strabismus, congenital cataract, amblyopia, and primary brain tumors affecting vision are some of the conditions that have been shown to impact physical, social, and emotional aspects of a child's development. Unlike in the adult population, fewer studies have been reported in the pediatric population that assess these effects in an elaborate manner. This may be due to the fact that the primary focus for childhood visual conditions has heretofore been the visual outcome. Also, there has been a deficiency of child-specific, vision-specific, and age-appropriate tools to measure QoL related to vision. However, recently there has been an interest in identifying the relevant content in assessing VR-QoL in pediatric population.

The management of childhood glaucoma is a challenging process for affected children, family, and treating physicians. Firstly, the initial diagnosis of a sight-threatening and life-changing diagnosis is stressful to most families, including parents and especially older children. These children often require multiple examinations under anesthesia, surgeries, and long-term IOP-lowering medications. Management also entails multiple appointments, requiring time off from work for caregivers and absence from school for older children. The other important aspect of managing childhood glaucoma is treating ametropia, amblyopia, and other primary or secondary associated ocular conditions. All these facets may have a significant effect on the development, education, social integration, and independence of the child. Thus, it is crucial to assess and address both HR- and VR-QoL as outcome variables in the management of children with glaucoma.

At the time this chapter was written, only four studies evaluating the QoL in childhood glaucoma had been published (Table 12.1) [11, 40–42]. Freedman et al. conducted a cross-sectional study to evaluate the VR-QoL in 43 children with glaucoma and the factors that influence it [41]. Neither age, number of glaucoma surgeries, nor number of prescribed eye drops seemed to impact VR-QoL. Another research group, Dahlmann-Noor et al., conducted a study to measure functional vision, HR-QoL, and VR-QoL in childhood

Table 12.1 Quality of life studies in childhood glaucoma

Authors, journal	Type of study	Participants (*n*)	Age	Questionnaire used	Self/proxy	Results
Zhang et al. [40] *Chinese J Ophthal* (2009)	Cross-sectional	51 children with primary congenital glaucoma 50 controls	5–20	PCG-QOL scale	Unclear	PCG-QOL: 60.22 vs. 71.41 in controls ($P < 0.01$)
Freedman et al. [41] *J AAPOS* (2014)	Descriptive	43 children with glaucoma	5–17	IVI-C	Self	Mean score: 24
Tailor et al. [42] *J AAPOS* (2015)	Descriptive	180 children with glaucoma, cataract, aphakia, pseudophakia	2–16	CVAQC PedsQL	Self and proxy	CVAQC: −1.65 PedsQL: Parental report: 69 Self-report: 78
Dahlmann-Noor et al. [11] *Ophthalmology* (2017)	Descriptive	119 children with glaucoma	2–16	CVAQC IVI-C PedsQL	Self + proxy	Marked impact on VR-, HR-QoL, and functional visual ability CVAQC: −1.24 IVI-C: 67.3 PedsQL self-report:78.8

CVAQC, Cardiff Visual Ability Questionnaire for Children (functional vision); IVI-C, Impact of Vision Impairment on Children (VR-QoL); PCG-QOL scale, primary congenital glaucoma quality of life scale; PedsQL (HR-QoL)

glaucoma [11]. They analyzed responses from 119 children aged 2–16 years and their parents. It was found that glaucoma and its management have a marked influence on a child's functional vision and both HR- and VR-QoL. They also found that older children had better HR-QoL scores than the younger population, possibly reflecting coping strategies and adjustment over time by the older children to manage their visual disability. As in the adult glaucoma literature, one consistent factor in most of these studies that was found to reliably correlate to higher QoL in children was better visual acuity.

Parent Perception, Caregiver Burden, and Quality of Life

The target effect of a childhood illness extends beyond the child himself. Especially in the very young pediatric population, the immediate burden of the disease is borne by the primary caregiver, usually the mother/parents and the family. The type and extent of the impact may vary with the type of illness [43]. Studies have shown that caregivers have to cope not only with psychological strain, i.e., anxiety and depression related to the child's condition [44, 45], but also with changes in their normal routine, extended time necessary for the child's care [44, 46], absenteeism from work in relation to the child's illness and medical appointments, financial burden, social isolation, and increased responsibility [44, 46–48]. There are documented negative effects in people caring for children with chronic systemic conditions like diabetes [49], human immunodeficiency virus [47], asthma [50], dermatitis, and congenital conditions [44, 51].

These concepts find parallel application in chronic pediatric ophthalmic conditions. Ocular conditions also bring an added concern of threat to the child's visual development. Even adult individuals with impaired vision require more help with their activities of daily living and additional hours of close supervision per day, leading to significant burden to their primary caregivers [52]. There is evidence of significant time-dependent, emotional, existential, and physical burden and depression among individuals caring for legally blind patients. Hours of close supervision and intensity of caregiving have been identified as factors related to the overall burden. In the same study, depression was found to be prevalent in 16–48% of the population caring for legally blind individuals [52]. Mothers of children with visual impairment experience more stress than mothers of children with no disability, particularly in areas involving the children's behavior and especially when the children have multiple disabilities [53]. Since childhood glaucoma commonly affects younger children, the caregivers (commonly parents and family) have to take the onus of providing constant care to the child over many years. Also, the diagnosis of this vision-threatening condition could induce significant emotional strain to the parents, leading to significant emotional stress.

However, there is a paucity of literature investigating this issue of caregiver stress. We conducted a study where we interviewed caregivers providing care to children with childhood glaucoma for assessment of emotional, socioeconomic, perceived, and aggregate stress from caregiving [14]. It was noted that while all subjects experienced some degree of burden, 71% individuals faced moderate burden related to caring for their child with glaucoma. We also found that one third of these caregivers reported symptoms of moderate or severe depression. Similarly, another study by Gothwal et al. showed that 60% of individuals caring for children with primary congenital glaucoma reported moderate to severe amounts of impact on their QoL [54]. All the examined subjects showed feelings of anger, powerlessness, anxiety, depression, decreased appetite and self-confidence, and lack of interest in pursuing their leisure activities [54].

Tools to Measure Quality of Life in Adult-Onset Glaucoma

The standard tools to measure QoL include WHOQOL-100 and the WHOQOL-BREF questionnaires [55, 56]. These tools have been applied to a wide variety of cultures and diseases and have been found to be comparable among populations in different socioeconomic settings. SF-36 is a short general health questionnaire evaluating different health concepts and has been shown to be sensitive enough to separate symptomatic and asymptomatic patients, distinguish stages and severity of a disease, and classify treatment effects [32, 57]. Another widely used generic instrument is EuroQOL-5D (EQ5D) multidimensional questionnaire that inspects five dimensions: mobility, self-care, usual activities, pain/discomfort, and anxiety/depression [58].

Lately, there has been an increasing international emphasis on patient-led assessment of the impact of illness and health care. This has led to a proliferation of questionnaires also known as patient-reported outcome measures (PROMs), intended to measure the impact of illness or disability and treatment from the patient's perspective. Generic instruments capture a broad range of health-related aspects and give a comparison between different disease states; however, they do not capture patient's perceptions and specific limitations that patients with a particular condition encounter. Disease-specific PROMs are immensely helpful to understand the impact of illness and treatment from patient's perspective and are more sensitive to detect small changes in condition-specific health status. Furthermore, they may be more acceptable for patients than generic instruments because of clear relevance to their condition.

The effect of adult glaucoma on QoL has been well studied. This is evidenced by the development of various PROMs designed to measure the patient's perspectives in adult glaucoma. While some of them are considered vision-specific, there are also several instruments that are specific for the evaluation of glaucoma-related impact. These have been classified into three different categories: PROMs addressing functional vision, PROMs addressing quality of life, and PROMs assessing other factors related to disease and treatment [59]. Table 12.2 gives an overview of these different instruments available for evaluation of adult individuals with glaucoma [60–74].

Table 12.2 Commonly used patient-reported outcome questionnaires for evaluation of adult patients with glaucoma

Questionnaire	Concept assessed	Content
Glaucoma Quality of Life-15 (GLQ-15) [60]	Effect of binocular visual field loss on visual function	15 items related to central and near vision, peripheral vision, glare and dark adaptation, outdoor mobility
Independent mobility [61]	Patient-based assessment of difficulty in mobility	35 items related to mobility situations
Glaucoma Symptom Identifier (GSI) [62]	Functional status relating to vision, impact of glaucoma symptoms on vision	34 items related to visual activities
Glaucoma Utility Index [63]	Patient-reported effects related to glaucoma and preference-based status in glaucoma	32 items related to central and near vision, lighting and glare, mobility, activities of daily living, eye discomfort
Glaucoma Quality of Life (Glau-QoL) [64]	Glaucoma health-related quality of life	36 items related to psychological well-being, self-image, daily life, burden of treatment, driving, anxiety, and confidence in health care
Glaucoma Health Perceptions Index (GHPI) [65]	Glaucoma health-related quality of life, perceived impact of glaucoma	Six items; perception about physical, emotional, social, and cognitive health; and stress attributable to glaucoma and treatment
National Eye Institute Visual Function Questionnaire-51 items (NEI-VFQ-51) [66]	Vision-targeted functioning and socio-emotional issues	51 items related to general health, general vision, ocular pain, near vision, distance vision, social functioning, mental health, expectations, role functioning, dependency, driving, peripheral vision, color vision
National Eye Institute Visual Function Questionnaire-25 items (NEI-VFQ-25) [67, 68]	Vision-related functioning and socio-emotional issues	25 items related to visual functioning and socio-emotional traits

Table 12.2 (continued)

Questionnaire	Concept assessed	Content
Nursing Home Vision-Targeted Health-Related Quality of Life (NHVQoL) [69]	Vision-targeted health- related quality of life in nursing home residents	57 items related to reading, ocular symptoms, general vision, ADL, mobility, social activities/hobbies, psychological distress, adaptation/coping, social interaction
Low Vision Quality of Life (LVQOL) [70]	Effect of visual impairment on quality of life	25 items/activities: basic aspects of vision, mobility, adjustment, reading, and fine works
Impact of Vision Impairment Questionnaire [71]	Impact of vision impairment on a person's ability	28 items related to common daily activities mobility and independence, emotional well-being, reading, and accessing information
Treatment Satisfaction Survey for Intraocular Pressure (TSS-IOP) [72]	Patient satisfaction with topical treatment	15 items related to effectiveness, hyperemia, eye irritation, convenience of use, ease of use
Comparison of Ophthalmic Medications for Tolerability (COMTO) [73]	Frequency and common side effects and its effect on quality of life, adherence, and satisfaction with the medication	15 items related to frequency of side effects; 15 items related to bothersomeness of side effects; 7 items related to limitation of activities; 5 items related to global impact as a result
Glaucoma Symptom Scale (GSS) [74]	Symptoms and side effects of glaucoma or eye drop treatment	10 items related to symptoms of side effects

Tools to Measure Vision-Related Quality of Life in the Pediatric Population

In contrast to adult literature, there is a dearth of conceptually grounded, psychometrically robust, self-reporting questionnaires suitable for use with children and young individuals. As previously mentioned, the use of generic instruments could help understand how the impact of certain ophthalmic conditions affects QoL as compared to unaffected fully sighted children. However these instruments are not sensitive enough to detect changes in QoL experienced by the children over the course of their management, hence causing the clinicians and researchers to miss essential disease and treatment information [75]. QoL measurement tools have only been developed for a few ophthalmic conditions, e.g., amblyopia (amblyopia treatment index, ATI [76]; Children's Amblyopia Treatment Quality of Life Questionnaire, CAT-QoL [77]; Emotional Impact of Amblyopia Questionnaire, EIAQ [78]), juvenile idiopathic arthritis-associated uveitis (Effects of Youngsters' Eyesight on Quality of Life, EYE-Q [79]), refractive error (Pediatric Refractive Error Profile, PREP [80]), intermittent exotropia (Intermittent Exotropia Questionnaire, IXTQ [81]), and vernal keratoconjunctivitis (Quality of Life in Children with Vernal Keratoconjunctivitis, QUICK [82]). Due to a relative paucity of disease-specific instruments in the world of childhood ophthalmology, most pediatric studies have used vision-specific instruments to measure QoL in children with pediatric glaucoma and other various eye-related conditions. The deficiency of disease-specific instruments could reflect a limited understanding of the conceptual framework necessary to develop such instruments, coupled with challenges of child-centered methodology necessary to drive development of such measures.

Table 12.3 [83–88] summarizes the various instruments available and commonly used to measure "generic" PROMs in children. Some of the instruments intend to measure QoL related to visual impairment as perceived by the children (VR-QoL), and others actually measure functional vision. The concept of QoL rests on the "individual's perception" of their position in life in the context of the culture and value systems in which they live and in relation to their goals, expectations, standards, and concerns. While it seems intuitive to assume that visual acuity would correlate to one's QoL, the existence of "disability paradox," whereby people with disabilities have

Table 12.3 Commonly used questionnaires for assessing vision-related quality of life in pediatric population

Questionnaire and year of development	Age range (y)	Items (no.)	Concept being assessed	Respondents
	2 versions			
Children's Visual Function Questionnaire (CVFQ) 2004 [83, 84]	Younger 0–3 Older 3–7	 34 39	Vision-related quality of life. Measures four QoL-related subscales: competence, personality, family impact, and treatment difficulty	Proxy
Cardiff Visual Ability Questionnaire for Children (CVAQC) 2010 [85]	5–18	25	Functional vision. Measures difficulty with education, near vision, distance vision, getting around, social interaction, entertainment, and sports	Child
The Impact of Vision Impairment on Children (IVI_C) 2011 [86]	8–18	24	Vision-related quality of life	Child
Vision-Related Quality of Life of Children and Young People (VR-QoL_CYP) 2011 [87]	10–15	35	Vision-related quality of life. Evaluates the impact of living with a visual impairment from the affected child's perspective	Child
LV Prasad-Functional Vision Questionnaire Second Version (LVP-FVQ II) 2012 [88]	8–16	23	Functional vision. Measures level of difficulty in performing activities of daily living, academic, and leisure activities	Child

been reported to have a better QoL, does not fully support this concept [89]. Therefore, although visual function may be one of the dominant factors correlating to VR-QoL, other factors, e.g., physical health, personality, personal circumstances (wealth, living conditions, etc.), social relationships, and functional activities and pursuits, also make a significant impact on the measured constructs. Thus, efforts toward improving a child's VR-QoL should not only include visual rehabilitation but also an assessment and improvement of other domains of life.

Tools to Evaluate Quality of Life of Caregivers

Awareness about stress related to caregiving has led to development of several instruments for assessment of the burden experienced by caregivers and their QoL. One of the definitions of caregiver burden is the impact of providing care on the caregiver's physical, psychological, emotional, social, and financial situation that either results from the perception that caregiving demands exceed the informal caregiver's physical and mental capacity or jeopardizes this capacity [90–93]. Tools for identification and measurement of caregiver stress may be categorized into those measuring caregiver: burden [91, 92, 94–96], QoL [56–58], management and coping [97–99], emotional and mental health [100–104], psychosocial impact [105, 106], and physical health [107].

The tools most widely employed for evaluating burden are the Zarit Burden Interview (ZBI), also called the Zarit Burden Inventory, Zarit (Carer) Burden scale, and Zarit scale [91–95]. Dada et al. used the caregiver burden questionnaire (CBQ) to evaluate the impact of caregiving for children with glaucoma [14]. This questionnaire allows for separate identification of the caregiver burden into socioeconomic, emotional, and psychological and perceived burden. Tools available to measure the emotional and psychological aspects of caregiver health are mainly generic instruments. The application of these instruments is limited by their lower specificity and sensitivity than disease-specific instruments. These instruments treat individuals as patients rather than caregivers and may not be completely applicable in context of caregiving.

As every childhood disease may bring different challenges to caregiving, efforts have been made to develop disease-specific questionnaires to evaluate the impact of caregiving for children [107, 108]. Gothwal et al. developed Caregivers Congenital Glaucoma Quality of Life (CarCGQoL) questionnaire to provide insight into challenges faced as the primary caregiver for children with primary congenital glaucoma [109]. The instrument was generated after literature review and focus group discussions with caregivers and pediatric glaucoma experts. After subsequent phases of item refinement, cognitive debriefing, and validation, CarCGQoL was developed as a 20-item instrument that can be used as an assessment of QoL of caregivers of children with PCG [109].

Impact of Glaucoma Treatment on Quality of Life of Child and Caregiver

Medical or surgical management of childhood glaucoma improves prognosis for visual preservation for affected children. However, it is important to evaluate and understand the impact of our interventions on the QoL of children, their caregivers, and family. Identification of such measures may guide us as to what factors influence one's perception of their limitations and hence could function as key elements in treatment planning and research.

In the Collaborative Initial Glaucoma Treatment Study (CIGTS) trial for adult patients with glaucoma, patients undergoing surgical treatment were bothered by local symptoms to a greater extent than those started on medical management [110]. However, these symptoms were found to decline with time. In another study conducted by Arora et al., initiating medical treatment was found to be associated with worsening of quality of life, possibly from psychological impact of a sight-threatening condition and adverse effects of medications [111].

Very few studies have sought to evaluate the impact of medical or surgical treatment on QoL in childhood glaucoma. Dahlmann-Noor et al. found that HR-QoL scores in children with glaucoma did not correlate with number of glaucoma drops or surgical interventions although the study was not powered to detect associations [11]. Similar results were observed by Freedman et al. [41]. In a study published from China by Zhang et al., the postoperative QoL in children with congenital glaucoma correlated to surgical outcome and postoperative visual acuity [40]. However, all these were cross-sectional studies and were not particularly designed to study the influence of medications or surgery on QoL in children with glaucoma. The only longitudinal study published in this regard measures the QoL of caregivers before and after surgical intervention in congenital glaucoma [54]. They noticed that before surgery, all caregivers reported feelings of depression, anxiety, anger, irritability, lack of interest in leisure activities, decreased self-confidence, effect on appetite and sleep, and feelings of powerlessness related to the child's disease. However, there was a twofold improvement in QoL scores 6–8 weeks following their child's surgery. Interestingly, the authors did not find any correlation of caregiver's QoL scores to the degree of surgical success or failure.

Interventions for Improvement of Quality of Life

Although it seems intuitive to believe that the presence of disease itself has a negative effect on QoL and mood, there is a large variability in these parameters among people with the same condition and similar degree of impairment. Also, some studies have found that QoL and mood may be relatively preserved in other individuals with similar conditions and severe degree of impairment [112, 113]. These differences suggest that other psychological factors may dictate one's perception about one's QoL.

For management of children with glaucoma, enhanced outcomes and efforts to preserve maximum visual function, particularly best-corrected visual acuity, may help improve visual ability and QoL of both the affected children and their caregivers. Also, imparting education to the child and family about the disease could help alleviate some of the fears and clarify misconceptions that the patient-family unit may have in relation to the illness. There is also a need to adapt and utilize other strategies to help lower the stress associated with the illness. Research suggests that in addition to the psychological toll, adverse childhood experiences could result in neuroanatomical changes, increased levels of inflammation and dysfunction of the hypothalamus-pituitary axis [114]. One of the strategies shown to be effective in this regard is "mindfulness" [115]. Mindfulness is an evidence-based intervention that helps improve self-regulation and resilience in everyday life and in face of stress and trauma. This has been shown to improve QoL in multiple sclerosis and depression and anxiety in patients with cancer. [116, 117] "Mindfulness-based interventions" have also been found to be helpful in supporting parents of children with disabilities [118]. To reduce the stress of caring for a child with disability, several other strategies have also been reported to be effective. A form of therapy that has been shown to improve QoL in patients with chronic illnesses is "acceptance and commitment therapy" [119]. This is a modified and newer form of cognitive-behavior therapy that has been shown to reduce parental stress in children with acute traumatic brain injury, life-threatening illnesses, cerebral palsy, and other disabilities [119–122].

Evidence suggests that alternative strategies like yoga and meditation are effective in reducing stress in caregivers of individuals with Alzheimer's dementia, another condition that has been shown to be associated with significant caregiver stress [123–126]. Danucaloy et al. noted that an 8-week session on yoga and meditation produced a statistically significant reduction in stress, anxiety, and depression in such caregivers [123]. The other interventions that have been shown to significantly reduce caregiver stress in dementia are mindfulness-based cognitive therapy and caregiver education about self-care tools [125]. These tools help reduce personal stress, change negative self-talk, help them communicate their needs to family members and health-care and service providers, and make tough caregiving decisions.

The favorable results of such interventional therapies have also been supported by a number of physiological effects observed, namely, reduction in salivary cortisol, increase in telomerase activity, downregulation of pro-inflammatory NF-κB gene, and upregulation of antiviral interferon response factors [126].

Future Directions

There has been a fundamental shift in pediatric medicine toward a more collaborative partnership between patients, families, and their health-care providers, with patient- and family-centered care forming the backbone of high-quality pediatric care [127–129]. Collaborative decision-making, planning, delivery, and evaluation of health-care interventions can improve health, psychosocial, and educational outcomes in these individuals [127, 128]. This concept rests on thorough understanding of needs, beliefs, and expectations of the child-family unit through elaborate qualitative research.

There is a need to adapt this high-profile approach in the world of pediatric ophthalmology and childhood glaucoma. In order to understand the impact of this vision-threatening diagnosis and treatment on affected children and their caregivers, there is a need for larger trials investigating this issue. Clinicians and researchers need to produce robust disease-specific questionnaires that can be used in high-quality studies and daily practice. The development of these instruments should start with discussions with patients affected by the condition of interest so that the issues relevant to their lives can be captured accurately.

Efforts to understand and evaluate "quality of life" are incomplete if we do not devise appropriate interventions to help improve the same. Clinicians and paramedical staff need to educate the children and families and address knowledge gaps about the disease, management, and prognosis. There is a need for a multidisciplinary approach for management of chronic conditions like childhood glaucoma in pediatric ophthalmology. Strategies may involve development and streamlining of teams where health-care providers from various disciplines can identify stress related to illness, offer coping mechanisms, and direct affected individuals to various available psychological treatments and support services. In addition, QoL questionnaires can improve communication between clinicians and the families they care for and may also be a proxy measure of family well-being and have implications for community health.

Conclusion

There is evidence that childhood glaucoma has a significant negative effect on the QoL of affected children and their caregivers. However, there is an unmet need to identify and analyze this aspect in management of children with glaucoma. Ophthalmologists need to work in close association with mental health-care professionals and other supporting groups in order to provide a holistic treatment to affected children and their families.

References

1. Felce D, Perry J. Quality of life: its definition and measurement. Res Dev Disabil. 1995;16(1):51–74.
2. The World Health Organization Quality of Life assessment (WHOQOL): position paper from the World Health Organization. Soc Sci Med. 1995;41(10):1403–9.
3. United Nations. Office of the High Commissioner of Human Rights. Convention on the Rights of the Child. Adopted and opened for signature, ratification and accession by General Assembly resolution 44/25 of 20 Nov 1989. Entry into force 2 Sept 1990, in accordance with article 49.
4. Ben-Arieh A, Casas F, Frønes I, Korbin JE, editors. Handbook of child well-being. Theories, methods and policies in global perspective. Dordrecht: Springer Netherlands; 2014.
5. Wallander JL, Schmitt M, Koot HM. Quality of life measurement in children and adolescents: issues, instruments, and applications. J Clin Psychol. 2001;57(4):571–85.
6. Tadic V, Hogan A, Sobti N, Knowles RL, Rahi JS. Patient-reported outcome measures (PROMs) in paediatric ophthalmology: a systematic review. Br J Ophthalmol. 2013;97(11):1369–81.
7. Roberts MC, Steele RG. Handbook of pediatric psychology. 5th ed. New York: Guilford; 2017.
8. Eiser C, Jenney M. Measuring quality of life. Arch Dis Child. 2007;92(4):348–50. Review
9. Jozefiak T, Larsson B, Wichstrøm L, Mattejat F, Ravens-Sieberer U. Quality of life as reported by school children and their parents: a cross-sectional survey. Health Qual Life Outcomes. 2008;6:34.
10. Upton P, Lawford J, Eiser C. Parent-child agreement across child health-related quality of life instruments: a review of the literature. Qual Life Res. 2008;17(6):895–913.
11. Dahlmann-Noor A, Tailor V, Bunce C, Abou-Rayyah Y, Adams G, Brookes J, et al. Quality of life and functional vision in children with glaucoma. Ophthalmology. 2017;124(7):1048–55.
12. Mehta M, Bagga A, Pande P, Bajaj G, Srivastava RN. Behavior problems in nephrotic syndrome. Indian Pediatr. 1995;32(12):1281–6.
13. Rüth EM, Landolt MA, Neuhaus TJ, Kemper MJ. Health-related quality of life and psychosocial adjustment in steroid sensitive nephrotic syndrome. J Pediatr. 2004;145(6):778–83.
14. Dada T, Aggarwal A, Bali SJ, Wadhwani M, Tinwala S, Sagar R. Caregiver burden assessment in primary congenital glaucoma. Eur J Ophthalmol. 2013;23(3):324–8.
15. Zarit SH, Reever KE, Bach-Peterson J. Relatives of the impaired elderly: correlates of feelings of burden. Gerontologist. 1980;20(6):649–55.
16. Andolsek KM, Clapp-Channing NE, Gehlbach SH, Moore I, Proffitt VS, Sigmon A, et al. Caregivers and elderly relatives: the prevalence of caregiving in a family practice. Arch Intern Med. 1988;148(10):2177–80.
17. Parks SM, Novielli KD. A practical guide to caring for caregivers. Am Fam Physician. 2000;62(12):2613–22.
18. Stanley S, Balakrishnan S, Ilangovan S. Psychological distress, perceived burden and quality of life in caregivers of persons with schizophrenia. J Ment Health. 2017;26(2):134–41.
19. Tan JY, Molassiotis A, Lloyd-Williams M, Yorke J. Burden, emotional distress and quality of life among informal caregivers of lung cancer patients: an exploratory study. Eur J Cancer Care (Engl). 2018;27(1). https://doi.org/10.1111/ecc.12691.
20. Khare S, Rohatgi J, Bhatia MS, Dhaliwal U. Burden and depression in primary caregivers of persons with visual impairment. Indian J Ophthalmol. 2016;64(8):572–7.
21. Fridman M, Banaschewski T, Sikirica V, Quintero J, Erder MH, Chen KS. Factors associated with caregiver burden among pharmacotherapy-treated children/adolescents with ADHD in the Caregiver Perspective on Pediatric ADHD survey in Europe. Neuropsychiatr Dis Treat. 2017;13:373–86.
22. Arai Y, Noguchi C, Zarit SH. Potentially harmful behavior by caregivers may be predicted by a caregiver burden scale. Int J Geriatr Psychiatry. 2017;32(5):582–3.

23. Odberg T, Jakobsen JE, Hultgren SJ, Halseide R. The impact of glaucoma on the quality of life of patients in Norway. I. Results from a self-administered questionnaire. Acta Ophthalmol Scand. 2001;79(2):116–20.
24. Janz NK, Wren PA, Guire KE, Musch DC, Gillespie BW, Lichter PR, Collaborative Initial Glaucoma Treatment Study. Fear of blindness in the collaborative initial glaucoma treatment study: patterns and correlates over time. Ophthalmology. 2007;114(12):2213–20.
25. Agorastos A, Skevas C, Matthaei M, Otte C, Klemm M, Richard G, Huber CG. Depression, anxiety, and disturbed sleep in glaucoma. J Neuropsychiatry Clin Neurosci. 2013;25(3):205–13.
26. Popescu ML, Boisjoly H, Schmaltz H, Kergoat MJ, Rousseau J, Moghadaszadeh S, et al. Explaining the relationship between three eye diseases and depressive symptoms in older adults. Invest Ophthalmol Vis Sci. 2012;53(4):2308–13.
27. Wang SY, Singh K, Lin SC. Prevalence and predictors of depression among participants with glaucoma in a nationally representative population sample. Am J Ophthalmol. 2012;154(3):436–44.
28. Ramulu PY, West SK, Munoz B, Jampel HD, Friedman DS. Driving cessation and driving limitation in glaucoma: the Salisbury Eye Evaluation Project. Ophthalmology. 2009;116(10):1846–53.
29. Freeman EE, Munoz B, Rubin G, West SK. Visual field loss increases the risk of falls in older adults: the Salisbury eye evaluation. Invest Ophthalmol Vis Sci. 2007;48(10):4445–50.
30. Nutheti R, Shamanna BR, Nirmalan PK, Keeffe JE, Krishnaiah S, Rao GN, et al. Impact of impaired vision and eye disease on quality of life in Andhra Pradesh. Invest Ophthalmol Vis Sci. 2006;47(11):4742–8.
31. Parrish RK 2nd, Gedde SJ, Scott IU, Feuer WJ, Schiffman JC, Mangione CM, et al. Visual function and quality of life among patients with glaucoma. Arch Ophthalmol. 1997;115(11):1447–55.
32. Gordon MO, Kass MA. The ocular hypertension treatment study: design and baseline description of the participants. Arch Ophthalmol. 1999;117(5):573–83.
33. Mills T, Law SK, Walt J, Buchholz P, Hansen J. Quality of life in glaucoma and three other chronic diseases: a systematic literature review. Drugs Aging. 2009;26(11):933–50.
34. Hyman LG, Komaroff E, Heijl A, Bengtsson B, Leske MC, Early Manifest Glaucoma Trial Group. Treatment and vision-related quality of life in the early manifest glaucoma trial. Ophthalmology. 2005;112(9):1505–13.
35. Peters D, Heijl A, Brenner L, Bengtsson B. Visual impairment and vision-related quality of life in the Early Manifest Glaucoma Trial after 20 years of follow-up. Acta Ophthalmol. 2015;93(8):745–52.
36. van Gestel A, Webers CA, Beckers HJ, van Dongen MC, Severens JL, Hendrikse F, Schouten JS. The relationship between visual field loss in glaucoma and health-related quality-of-life. Eye (Lond). 2010;24(12):1759–69.
37. Black AA, Wood JM, Lovie-Kitchin JE. Inferior field loss increases rate of falls in older adults with glaucoma. Optom Vis Sci. 2011;88(11):1275–82.
38. Sawada H, Fukuchi T, Abe H. Evaluation of the relationship between quality of vision and the visual function index in Japanese glaucoma patients. Graefes Arch Clin Exp Ophthalmol. 2011;249(11):1721–7.
39. Musch DC, Lichter PR, Guire KE, Standardi CL. The collaborative initial glaucoma treatment study: study design, methods, and baseline characteristics of enrolled patients. Ophthalmology. 1999;106(4):653–62.
40. Zhang XL, Du SL, Ge J, Chen WR, Fan Q, Peng SX, et al. Quality of life in patients with primary congenital glaucoma following antiglaucoma surgical management. Zhonghua Yan Ke Za Zhi. 2009;45(6):514–21. (Article in Chinese)
41. Freedman BL, Jones SK, Lin A, Stinnett SS, Muir KW. Vision-related quality of life in children with glaucoma. J AAPOS. 2014;18(1):95–8.
42. Tailor VK, Dahlmann-Noor A, Adams G, Papadopoulos M. Survey of health- and vision-related quality of life and functional vision in children and young people with childhood glaucoma and cataract (abstract). J AAPOS. 2015;19(4):e64–5.
43. Chow MY, Morrow AM, Cooper Robbins SC, Leask J. Condition-specific quality of life questionnaires for caregivers of children with pediatric conditions: a systematic review. Qual Life Res. 2013;22(8):2183–200.
44. Basra MK, Finlay AY. The family impact of skin diseases: the greater patient concept. Br J Dermatol. 2007;156(5):929–37.
45. Knock J, Kline E, Schiffman J, Maynard A, Reeves G. Burdens and difficulties experienced by caregivers of children and adolescents with schizophrenia-spectrum disorders: a qualitative study. Early Interv Psychiatry. 2011;5(4):349–54.
46. Perkins S, Winn S, Murray J, Murphy R, Schmidt U. A qualitative study of the experience of caring for a person with bulimia nervosa. Part 1: the emotional impact of caring. Int J Eating Disord. 2004;36(3):256–68.
47. Punpanich W, Gorbach PM, Detels R. Impact of paediatric human immunodeficiency virus infection on children's and caregivers' daily functioning and well-being: a qualitative study. Child Care Health Dev. 2012;38(5):714–22.
48. Duguid A, Morrison S, Robertson A, Chalmers J, Youngson G, Ahmed SF, Scottish Genital Anomaly Network. The psychological impact of genital anomalies on the parents of affected children. Acta Paediatr. 2007;96(3):348–52.
49. Edmonds-Myles S, Tamborlane WV, Grey M. Perception of the impact of type 1 diabetes on low-income families. Diabetes Educ. 2010;36(2):318–25.

50. Forns D, Prat R, Tauler E. Evaluation of quality of life among the caregivers of asthmatic children: the new IFABI-R questionnaire. Allergol Immunopathol (Madr). 2011;39(1):32–8.
51. Sparacino PS, Tong EM, Messias DK, Foote D, Chesla CA, Gilliss CL. The dilemmas of parents of adolescents and young adults with congenital heart disease. Heart Lung. 1997;26(3):187–95.
52. Braich PS, Lal V, Hollands S, Almeida DR. Burden and depression in the caregivers of blind patients in India. Ophthalmology. 2012;119(2):221–6.
53. Toster H. Sources of stress in mothers of young children with visual impairments. J Vis Impair Blind. 2001;95(10):623–37.
54. Gothwal VK, Bharani S, Mandal AK. Impact of surgery on the quality of life of caregivers of children with congenital glaucoma. Ophthalmology. 2016;123(5):1161–2.
55. Power M, Harper A, Bullinger M. The World Health Organization WHOQOL-100: tests of the universality of Quality of Life in 15 different cultural groups worldwide. Health Psychol. 1999;18(5):495–505.
56. Skevington SM, Lotfy M, O'Connell KA. The World Health Organization's WHOQOL-BREF quality of life assessment: psychometric properties and results of the international field trial. A report from the WHOQOL Group. Qual Life Res. 2004;13(2):299–310.
57. Ware JE Jr, Sherbourne CD. The MOS 36-item short-form health survey (SF-36). I. Conceptual framework and item selection. Med Care. 1992;30(6):473–83.
58. Rabin R, de Charro F. EQ-5D: a measure of health status from the EuroQol Group. Ann Med. 2001;33(5):337–43.
59. Vandenbroeck S, De Geest S, Zeyen T, Stalmans I, Dobbels F. Patient-reported outcomes (PROs) in glaucoma: a systematic review. Eye (Lond). 2011;25(5):555–77.
60. Nelson P, Aspinall P, Papasouliotis O, Worton B, O'Brien C. Quality of life in glaucoma and its relationship with visual function. J Glaucoma. 2003;12(2):139–50.
61. Turano KA, Massof RW, Quigley HA. A self-assessment instrument designed for measuring independent mobility in RP patients: generalizability to glaucoma patients. Invest Ophthalmol Vis Sci. 2002;43(9):2874–81.
62. Walt JG, Rendas-Baum R, Kosinski M, Vaishali P. Psychometric evaluation of the glaucoma symptom identifier. J Glaucoma. 2011;20(3):148–59.
63. Burr JM, Kilonzo M, Vale L, Ryan M. Developing a preference-based glaucoma utility index using a discrete choice experiment. Optom Vis Sci. 2007;84(8):797–808.
64. Béchetoille A, Arnould B, Bron A, Baudouin C, Renard JP, Sellem E, et al. Measurement of health-related quality of life with glaucoma: validation of the Glau-QoL 36-item questionnaire. Acta Ophthalmol. 2008;86(1):71–80.
65. Janz NK, Wren PA, Lichter PR, Musch DC, Gillespie BW, Guire KE. Quality of life in newly diagnosed glaucoma patients: the Collaborative Initial Glaucoma Treatment Study. Ophthalmology. 2001;108(5):887–97.
66. Mangione CM, Berry S, Spritzer K, Janz NK, Klein R, Owsley C, et al. Identifying the content area for the 51-item National Eye Institute Visual Function Questionnaire: results from focus groups with visually impaired persons. Arch Ophthalmol. 1998;116(2):227–33.
67. Mangione CM, Lee PP, Gutierrez PR, Spritzer K, Berry S, Hays RD, National Eye Institute Visual Function Questionnaire Field Test Investigators. Development of the 25-item National Eye Institute Visual Function Questionnaire. Arch Ophthalmol. 2001;119(7):1050–8.
68. Pesudovs K, Gothwal VK, Wright T, Lamoureux EL. Remediating serious flaws in the National Eye Institute Visual Function Questionnaire. J Cataract Refract Surg. 2010;36(5):718–32.
69. Dreer LE, McGwin G Jr, Scilley K, Meek GC, Dyer A, Seker D, et al. Development of a nursing home vision targeted health-related quality of life questionnaire for older adults. Aging Ment Health. 2007;11(6):722–33.
70. Wolffsohn JS, Cochrane AL. Design of the low vision quality-of-life questionnaire (LVQOL) and measuring the outcome of low-vision rehabilitation. Am J Ophthalmol. 2000;130(6):793–802.
71. Lamoureux EL, Pallant JF, Pesudovs K, Hassell JB, Keeffe JE. The Impact of Vision Impairment Questionnaire: an evaluation of its measurement properties using Rasch analysis. Invest Ophthalmol Vis Sci. 2006;47(11):4732–41.
72. Atkinson MJ, Stewart WC, Fain JM, Stewart JA, Dhawan R, Mozaffari E, et al. A new measure of patient satisfaction with ocular hypotensive medications: the Treatment Satisfaction Survey for Intraocular Pressure (TSS-IOP). Health Qual Life Outcomes. 2003;1:67.
73. Barber BL, Strahlman ER, Laibovitz R, Guess HA, Reines SA. Validation of a questionnaire for comparing the tolerability of ophthalmic medications. Ophthalmology. 1997;104(2):334–42.
74. Lee BL, Gutierrez P, Gordon M, Wilson MR, Cioffi GA, Ritch R, et al. The Glaucoma Symptom Scale. A brief index of glaucoma-specific symptoms. Arch Ophthalmol. 1998;116(7):861–6.
75. Tadić V, Cumberland PM, Lewando-Hundt G, Rahi JS, Vision-Related Quality of Life Group. Do visually impaired children and their parents agree on the child's vision-related quality of life and functional vision? Br J Ophthalmol. 2017;101(3):244–50.
76. Cole SR, Beck RW, Moke PS, Celano MP, Drews CD, Repka MX, et al. The Amblyopia Treatment Index. J AAPOS. 2001;5(4):250–4.
77. Carlton J. Developing the draft descriptive system for the child amblyopia treatment questionnaire

(CAT-Qol): a mixed methods study. Health Qual Life Outcomes. 2013;11:174.
78. Hrisos S, Clarke MP, Wright CM. The emotional impact of amblyopia treatment in preschool children: randomized controlled trial. Ophthalmology. 2004;111(8):1550–6.
79. Angeles-Han ST, Yeh S, McCracken C, Jenkins K, Stryker D, Myoung E, et al. Using the effects of youngsters' eyesight on quality of life questionnaire to measure visual outcomes in children with uveitis. Arthritis Care Res (Hoboken). 2015;67(11):1513–20.
80. Rah MJ, Walline JJ, Jones-Jordan LA, Sinnott LT, Jackson JM, Manny RE, ACHIEVE Study Group, et al. Vision specific quality of life of pediatric contact lens wearers. Optom Vis Sci. 2010;87(8):560–6.
81. Hatt SR, Leske DA, Holmes JM. Comparison of quality-of-life instruments in childhood intermittent exotropia. J AAPOS. 2010;14(3):221–6.
82. Sacchetti M, Baiardini I, Lambiase A, Aronni S, Fassio O, Gramiccioni C, et al. Development and testing of the quality of life in children with vernal keratoconjunctivitis questionnaire. Am J Ophthalmol. 2007;144(4):557–63.
83. Felius J, Stager DR Sr, Berry PM, Fawcett SL, Stager DR Jr, Salomão SR, et al. Development of an instrument to assess vision-related quality of life in young children. Am J Ophthalmol. 2004;138(3):362–72.
84. Birch EE, Cheng CS, Felius J. Validity and reliability of the Children's Visual Function Questionnaire (CVFQ). J AAPOS. 2007;11(5):473–9.
85. Khadka J, Ryan B, Margrain TH, Court H, Woodhouse JM. Development of the 25-item Cardiff Visual Ability Questionnaire for Children (CVAQC). Br J Ophthalmol. 2010;94(6):730–5.
86. Cochrane GM, Marella M, Keeffe JE, Lamoureux EL. The Impact of Vision Impairment for Children (IVI-C): validation of a vision-specific pediatric quality-of-life questionnaire using Rasch analysis. Invest Ophthalmol Vis Sci. 2011;52(3):1632–40.
87. Rahi JS, Tadić V, Keeley S, Lewando-Hundt G, Vision-Related Quality of Life Group. Capturing children and young people's perspectives to identify the content for a novel vision-related quality of life instrument. Ophthalmology. 2011;118(5):819–24.
88. Gothwal VK, Sumalini R, Bharani S, Reddy SP, Bagga DK. The second version of the L. V. Prasad-functional vision questionnaire. Optom Vis Sci. 2012;89(11):1601–10.
89. Albrecht GL, Devlieger PJ. The disability paradox: high quality of life against all odds. Soc Sci Med. 1999;48(8):977–88.
90. Carretero S, Garcés J, Ródenas F. Evaluation of the home help service and its impact on the informal caregiver's burden of dependent elders. In: Garcés J, Carretero S, Ródenas F, editors. Readings of the social sustainability theory. Applications to the long-term care field. Valencia: Tirant lo Blanch; 2011. p. 119–44.
91. Shaw C, McNamara R, Abrams K, Cannings-John R, Hood K, Longo M, et al. Systematic review of respite care in the frail elderly. Health Technol Assess. 2009;13(20):1–224.
92. Werner S, Auslander GK, Shoval N, Gitlitz T, Landau R, Heinik J. Caregiving burden and out-of-home mobility of cognitively impaired care-recipients based on GPS tracking. Int Psychoger. 2012;24(11):1836–45.
93. Mosquera I, Vergara I, Larrañaga I, Machón M, del Río M, Calderón C. Measuring the impact of informal elderly caregiving: a systematic review of tools. Qual Life Res. 2016;25(5):1059–92.
94. Mohamed S, Rosenheck R, Lyketsos CG, Schneider LS. Caregiver burden in Alzheimer disease: cross-sectional and longitudinal patient correlates. Am J Geriatr Psychiatry. 2010;18(10):917–27.
95. Clark MC, Nicholas JM, Wassira LN, Gutierrez AP. Psychosocial and biological indicators of depression in the caregiving population. Biol Res Nurs. 2013;15(1):112–21.
96. Rudnick A. Burden of caregivers of mentally ill individuals in Israel: a family participatory study. Int J Psychosocial Rehabil. 2004;9(1):147–52.
97. Gitlin LN, Winter L, Dennis MP, Hodgson N, Hauck WW. Targeting and managing behavioral symptoms in individuals with dementia: a randomized trial of a nonpharmacological intervention. J Am Geriatr Soc. 2010;58(8):1465–74.
98. Löckenhoff CE, Duberstein PR, Friedman B, Costa PT Jr. Five-factor personality traits and subjective health among caregivers: the role of caregiver strain and self-efficacy. Psychol Aging. 2011;26(3):592–604.
99. Ducharme FC, Lévesque LL, Lachance LM, Kergoat MJ, Legault AJ, Beaudet LM, et al. "Learning to become a family caregiver." Efficacy of an intervention program for caregivers following diagnosis of dementia in a relative. Gerontologist. 2011;51(4):484–94.
100. Mackenzie CS, Wiprzycka UJ, Hasher L, Goldstein D. Associations between psychological distress, learning, and memory in spouse caregivers of older adults. J Gerontol. 2009;64(6):742–6.
101. Rezende TC, Coimbra AM, Costallat LT, Coimbra IB. Factors of high impacts on the life of caregivers of disabled elderly. Arch Gerontol Geriatr. 2010;51(1):76–80.
102. Schoenmakers B, Buntinx F, DeLepeleire J. Supporting the dementia family caregiver: the effect of home care intervention on general well-being. Aging Ment Health. 2010;14(1):44–56.
103. Löwe B, Unützer J, Callahan CM, Perkins AJ, Kroenke K. Monitoring depression treatment outcomes with the patient health questionnaire-9. Med Care. 2004;42(12):1194–201.
104. Kroenke K, Spitzer RL, Williams JB. The PHQ-9: validity of brief depression severity measure. J Geriatr Intern Med. 2001;16(9):603–13.
105. Casado B, Sacco P. Correlates of caregiver burden among family caregivers of older Korean Americans. J Gerontol B Psychol Sci Soc Sci. 2012;67(3):331–6.

106. Gonçalves LHT, Costa MAM, Martins MM, Nassar SM, Zunino R. The family dynamics of elder elderly in the context of Porto, Portugal. Rev Lat Am Enfermagem. 2011;19(3):458–66.
107. Juniper EF, Guyatt GH, Feeny DH, Ferrie PJ, Griffith LE, et al. Measuring quality of life in the parents of children with asthma. Qual Life Res. 1996;5(1):27–34.
108. Minaya P, Baumstarck K, Berbis J, Goncalves A, Barlesi F, Michel G, et al. The CareGiver Oncology Quality of Life questionnaire (CarGOQoL): development and validation of an instrument to measure the quality of life of the caregivers of patients with cancer. Eur J Cancer. 2012;48(6):904–11.
109. Gothwal VK, Bharani S, Mandal AK. Quality of life of caregivers of children with congenital glaucoma: development and validation of a novel questionnaire (CarCGQoL). Invest Ophthalmol Vis Sci. 2015;56(2):770–7.
110. Janz NK, Wren PA, Lichter PR, Musch DC, Gillespie BW, Guire KE, CIGTS Study Group, et al. The Collaborative Initial Glaucoma Treatment Study: interim quality of life findings after initial medical or surgical treatment of glaucoma. Ophthalmology. 2001;108(11):1954–65.
111. Arora V, Bali SJ, Gupta SK, Vashisht P, Agarwal T, Sreenivas V, Dada T. Impact of initial topical medical therapy on short-term quality of life in newly diagnosed patients with primary glaucoma. Indian J Ophthalmol. 2015;63(6):511–5.
112. Lulé D, Häcker S, Ludolph A, Birbaumer N, Kübler A. Depression and quality of life in patients with amyotrophic lateral sclerosis. Dtsch Arztebl Int. 2008;105(23):397–403.
113. Miglioretti M, Mazzini L, Oggioni GD, Testa L, Monaco F. Illness perceptions, mood and health-related quality of life in patients with amyotrophic lateral sclerosis. J Psychosom Res. 2008;65(6):603–9.
114. Danese A, McEwen BS. Adverse childhood experiences, allostasis, allostatic load, and age-related disease. Physiol Behav. 2012;106(1):29–39.
115. Ortiz R, Sibinga EM. The role of mindfulness in reducing the adverse effects of childhood stress and trauma. Children (Basel). 2017;4(3):pii: E16. https://doi.org/10.3390/children4030016.
116. Bogosian A, Hughes A, Norton S, Silber E, Moss-Morris R. Potential treatment mechanisms in a mindfulness-based intervention for people with progressive multiple sclerosis. Br J Health Psychol. 2016;21(4):859–80.
117. Jeitler M, Jaspers J, von Scheidt C, Koch B, Michalsen A, Steckhan N, et al. Mind-body medicine and lifestyle modification in supportive cancer care: a cohort study on a day care clinic program for cancer patients. Psychooncology. 2017;26(12):2127–34.
118. Rayan A, Ahmad M. Mindfulness and parenting distress among parents of children with disabilities: a literature review. Perspect Psychiatr Care. 2018;54(2):324–30. https://doi.org/10.1111/ppc.12217.
119. Graham CD, Gouick J, Krahé C, Gillanders D. A systematic review of the use of Acceptance and Commitment Therapy (ACT) in chronic disease and long-term conditions. Clin Psychol Rev. 2016;46:46–58.
120. Burke K, Muscara F, McCarthy M, Dimovski A, Hearps S, Anderson V, et al. Adapting acceptance and commitment therapy for parents of children with life-threatening illness: pilot study. Fam Syst Health. 2014;32(1):122–7.
121. Brown FL, Whittingham K, Boyd RN, McKinlay L, Sofronoff K. Improving child and parenting outcomes following paediatric acquired brain injury: a randomised controlled trial of Stepping Stones Triple P plus Acceptance and Commitment Therapy. J Child Psychol Psychiatry. 2014;55(10):1172–83.
122. Whittingham K, Sanders M, McKinlay L, Boyd RN. Interventions to reduce behavioral problems in children with cerebral palsy: an RCT. Pediatrics. 2014;133(5):e1249–57.
123. Danucalov MA, Kozasa EH, Ribas KT, Galduróz JC, Garcia MC, Verreschi IT, et al. A yoga and compassion meditation program reduces stress in familial caregivers of Alzheimer's disease patients. Evid Based Complement Alternat Med. 2013;2013:513149.
124. Lavretsky H, Epel ES, Siddarth P, Nazarian N, Cyr NS, Khalsa DS, et al. A pilot study of yogic meditation for family dementia caregivers with depressive symptoms: effects on mental health, cognition, and telomerase activity. Int J Geriatr Psychiatry. 2013;28(1):57–65.
125. Oken BS, Fonareva I, Haas M, Wahbeh H, Lane JB, Zajdel D, et al. Pilot controlled trial of mindfulness meditation and education for dementia caregivers. J Altern Complement Med. 2010;16(10):1031–8.
126. Black DS, Cole SW, Irwin MR, Breen E, St Cyr NM, Nazarian N, Khalsa DS, Lavretsky H. Yogic meditation reverses NF-κB and IRF-related transcriptome dynamics in leukocytes of family dementia caregivers in a randomized controlled trial. Psychoneuroendocrinology. 2013;38(3):348–55.
127. Kuo DZ, Houtrow AJ, Arango P, Kuhlthau KA, Simmons JM, Neff JM. Family-centered care: current applications and future directions in pediatric health care. Matern Child Health J. 2012;16(2):297–305.
128. Barry MJ, Edgman-Levitan S. Shared decision making--pinnacle of patient-centered care. N Eng J Med. 2012;366(9):780–1.
129. Hanson CS, Craig JC, Tong A. In their own words: the value of qualitative research to improve the care of children with chronic kidney disease. Pediatr Nephrol. 2017;32(9):1501–7.

Index

A. L. Grajewski et al. (eds.), *Surgical Management of Childhood Glaucoma*,
https://doi.org/10.1007/978-3-319-54003-0

C

D

MIX
Papier aus verantwortungsvollen Quellen
Paper from responsible sources
FSC® C105338

If you have any concerns about our products,
you can contact us on
ProductSafety@springernature.com

In case Publisher is established outside the EU,
the EU authorized representative is:
Springer Nature Customer Service Center GmbH
Europaplatz 3, 69115 Heidelberg, Germany

Printed by Libri Plureos GmbH
in Hamburg, Germany